Laboratory Medicine in India

Guest Editor

T.F. ASHAVAID, PhD, FACB, CSci

CLINICS IN LABORATORY MEDICINE

www.labmed.theclinics.com

Consulting Editor
ALAN WELLS, MD, DMSc

June 2012 • Volume 32 • Number 2

SAUNDERS an imprint of ELSEVIER, Inc.

W.B. SAUNDERS COMPANY
A Division of Elsevier Inc.

1600 John F. Kennedy Boulevard • Suite 1800 • Philadelphia, Pennsylvania 19103-2899

http://www.theclinics.com

CLINICS IN LABORATORY MEDICINE Volume 32, Number 2
June 2012 ISSN 0272-2712, ISBN-13: 978-1-4557-3884-7

Editor: Teia Stone

Reprints. For copies of 100 or more, of articles in this publication, please contact the Commercial Reprints Department, Elsevier Inc., 360 Park Avenue South, New York, New York 10010-1710. Tel. (212) 633-3813, Fax: (212) 462-1935, E-mail: reprints@elsevier.com.

Clinics in Laboratory Medicine (ISSN 0272-2712) is published quarterly by Elsevier Inc., 360 Park Avenue South, New York, NY 10010-1710. Months of issue are March, June, September, and December. Business and Editorial offices: 1600 John F. Kennedy Blvd., Suite 1800, Philadelphia, PA 19103-2899. Periodicals postage paid at NewYork, NY and additional mailing offices. Subscription prices are $240.00 per year (US individuals), $382.00 per year (US institutions), $128.00 (US students), $291.00 per year (Canadian individuals), $483.00 per year (foreign institutions), $176.00 (foreign students). Foreign air speed delivery is included in all *Clinics* subscription prices. All prices are subject to change without notice. POSTMASTER: Send address changes to *Clinics in Laboratory Medicine*, Elsevier Health Sciences Division, Subscription Customer Service, 3251 Riverport Lane, Maryland Heights, MO 63043. **Customer Service: 1-800-654-2452 (US). From outside of the US and Canada, call 1-314-447-8871. Fax: 1-314-447-8029. E-mail: journalscustomerservice-usa@elsevier.com (for print support) or journalsonlinesupport-usa@elsevier.com (for online support).**

Clinics in Laboratory Medicine is covered in *EMBASE/Exerpta Medica, MEDLINE/PubMed (Index Medicus), Cinahl, Current Contents/Clinical Medicine, BIOSIS* and *ISI/BIOMED.*

Printed and bound by CPI Group (UK) Ltd, Croydon, CR0 4YY

Transferred to Digital Print 2012

Contributors

CONSULTING EDITOR

ALAN WELLS, MD, DMSc
Department of Pathology, University of Pittsburgh, Pittsburgh, Pennsylvania

GUEST EDITOR

TESTER F. ASHAVAID, PhD, FACB, CSci
Consultant Biochemist, Head, Department of Laboratory Medicine; Joint
Director–Research, P. D. Hinduja National Hospital and Medical Research Centre, Veer
Savarkar Marg, Mahim, Mumbai, Maharashtra, India

AUTHORS

PRIYA ABRAHAM, MD, PhD
Professor of Microbiology, Department of Clinical Virology, Christian Medical College,
Vellore, Tamil Nadu, India

TESTER F. ASHAVAID, PhD, FACB, CSci
Consultant Biochemist, Head, Department of Laboratory Medicine; Joint
Director–Research, P. D. Hinduja National Hospital and Medical Research Centre, Veer
Savarkar Marg, Mahim, Mumbai, Maharashtra, India

NABAJYOTI CHOUDHURY, MBBS, PhD, MBA
Senior Consultant & Head, Transfusion Medicine, Tata Medical Centre, Kolkata, India

TULSI D. CHUGH, MD, FRCPath
Emeritus Professor, National Academy of Medical Sciences; Chairman, Department of
Microbiology, BLK Super Speciality Hospital, New Delhi, India

POONAM DAS, MD
Head, Laboratory and Transfusion Services, Max Healthcare, New Delhi, India

KEDAR K. DEODHAR, MD, FRCPath
Associate Professor and Pathologist, Department of Pathology, Tata Memorial Hospital,
Parel, Mumbai, Maharashtra, India

PRITI DESAI, MBBS, MD, DCP
Assistant Professor, Department of Transfusion Medicine, Tata Memorial Hospital, Parel,
Mumbai, Maharashtra, India

ALPA J. DHERAI, PhD
Consultant Biochemist, Department of Laboratory Medicine, P.D. Hinduja National
Hospital and Medical Research Center, Mahim, Mumbai, Maharashtra, India

RATNA DUA PURI, MD, DM
Senior Consultant, Clinical Genetics, Center of Medical Genetics, Sir Ganga Ram
Hospital, New Delhi, India

RAJNI GAIND, MD
Consultant and Associate Professor (Microbiology), Vardhman Mahavir Medical College; Associated, Safdarjung Hospital, New Delhi, India

AMAR DAS GUPTA, MD, PhD
Mentor, Hematology Services and President, International Super Religare Laboratories, Goregaon (West), Mumbai, Maharashtra, India

VIJAY GUPTA, PGDBM
Director, Marketing, P.D. Hinduja National Hospital and Medical Research Centre, Mahim, Mumbai, Maharashtra, India

ANIL HANDOO, MD
Senior Consultant Haematology and Director Laboratory Services, Quality Management Department, BLK Super Speciality Hospital, New Delhi, India

MONIKA JAWANJAL, MBBS
House Officer, Department of Cardiology, P.D. Hinduja National Hospital and Medical Research Centre, Mahim, Mumbai, Maharashtra, India

SHASHANK R. JOSHI, MBBS, MD, DM
Consultant Endocrinologist, Department of Endocrinology, Lilavati Hospital, Bhatia Hospital, Bandra (West); Department of Endocrinology, Grant Medical College and Sir J J Group of Hospitals; Immediate Past President, Research Society for Study Of Diabetes In India (RSSDI), Mumbai, Maharashtra, India

SUDHA KOHLI, PhD
Senior Consultant, Division of Molecular Genetics, Center of Medical Genetics, Sir Ganga Ram Hospital, Rajender Nagar, New Delhi, India

MEENA LALL, PhD
Senior Consultant, Division of Cytogenetics, Center of Medical Genetics, Sir Ganga Ram Hospital, New Delhi, India

PALAT K. MENON, MD, PhD
Senior Medical Director, Quest Diagnostics India Pvt. Ltd, Gurgaon, Haryana, India

SHOIBAL MUKHERJEE, MD, DM
Vice President and Head Asia Medical Sciences Group at Quintiles Research Private Limited, Gurgaon, Haryana, India

MICHAEL PEREIRA, MSc
National AIDS Research Institute, MIDC, Bhosari, Pune, India

CHANDRASHEKHAR K. PONDE, MD
Consultant Cardiologist, Department of Cardiology, P.D. Hinduja National Hospital and Medical Research Centre, Mahim, Mumbai, Maharashtra, India

CAMILLA RODRIGUES, MD
Department of Microbiology, P.D. Hinduja National Hospital and Medical Research Center, Mahim, Mumbai, Maharashtra, India

RENU SAXENA, PhD
Senior Consultant, Division of Molecular Genetics, Center of Medical Genetics, Sir Ganga Ram Hospital, Rajender Nagar, New Delhi, India

SWARUP SHAH, PhD
Senior Research Fellow, Research Laboratories, P.D. Hinduja National Hospital and Medical Research Centre, Mahim, Mumbai, Maharashtra, India

SHOBHONA SHARMA, PhD
Department of Biological Sciences, Tata Institute of Fundamental Research, Mumbai, Maharashtra, India

HARIPALSINGH M. SONAWAT, PhD
Department of Chemical Sciences, Tata Institute of Fundamental Research, Mumbai, Maharashtra, India

SWAROOP KRISHAN SOOD, MD, FISHBT
Senior Consultant Haematology and Chairman, Quality Management Department, BLK Super Speciality Hospital, New Delhi, India

SRIKANTH TRIPATHY, MBBS, MD
National AIDS Research Institute, MIDC, Bhosari, Pune, India

SRIRAM PRASAD TRIPATHY, MD
Honorary Consultant to the Indian Council of Medical Research 2, Radhika Vaibhav, Jagtapnagar, Wanawadi, Pune, India

VIRAL VADWAI, Doctorate Fellow (PhD), M Tech
Department of Microbiology, P.D. Hinduja National Hospital and Medical Research Center, Mahim, Mumbai, Maharashtra, India

ISHWAR C. VERMA, MBBS, FRCP, FAAP
Director, Center of Medical Genetics, Sir Ganga Ram Hospital, Rajender Nagar, New Delhi, India

Contents

> Viral hepatitis is a major public health problem in India, caused mainly by hepatitis A, B, C, D, and E viruses (HAV, HBV, HCV, HDV, HEV respectively). India is hyperendemic for the enterically transmitted HAV and HEV, though some epidemiologic transitions are beginning to occur. India has the second largest pool of HBV carriers, with a horizontal spread of HBV in early childhood playing an important role. HCV infection is acquired mainly through suboptimal blood banking services and poor injection practices. Though there is evidence of HDV coinfection and superinfection with HBV infection in India, HDV detection rates are low.

> HIV testing is key in influencing HIV management and control. After a peak incidence of HIV in 2000, there has been a steady decline in new infections. An extensive network of HIV testing centers has been established in different parts of India under the National AIDS Control Program in Phases I, II, III, and a Phase IV scheduled to start in 2013. The highly acclaimed program is ably supported by international agencies such as WHO, UNICEF, and UNAIDS and has been highly effective, as evidenced by a decline in incidence and prevalence of HIV and deaths due to AIDS.

> In India, cervical cancer is the most common fatal cancer in women. The primary underlying cause of cervical cancer is persistent infection with human papilloma virus (HPV). This article describes the etiology of HPV and screening efforts for cervical cancer: cytology, visual inspection with acetic acid, visual inspection with Lugol's iodine, and HPV screening. It also suggests future directions for cervical cancer screening.

Diagnostics in Life Style Acquired Diseases

> Asian Indians are uniquely predisposed to type 2 diabetes. India has the second largest diabetic population in the world with an average prevalence of 10% to 12%. This is because of the unique Asian Indian phenotype, which has higher body fat proportion with lower muscle mass (sarcopenia). There is a strong genomic and familial preponderance, although clear-cut genomic markers are not yet identified. Sedentary physical habit compounded with high-carbohydrate, high-fat diet is the prime driver of the

disease in the genetically vulnerable population. Often diagnosis is late and with associated complications. Prevention is the key, and early diagnosis and prompt therapy is mandatory.

Cardiovascular Disease in India   217

Tester F. Ashavaid, Chandrashekhar K. Ponde, Swarup Shah, and Monika Jawanjal

Cardiovascular disease (CVD) is a major financial and public health burden in India, with young Indians at higher risk. Various cardiac risk factors and biomarkers have been identified, which helps assess cardiac risk during different stages of CVD. Indians succumb to CVD much earlier than their Western counterparts and other Asian populations, underscoring the importance of genetic testing in Indians. Once individuals at higher risk are identified, preventive measures can be undertaken. This article focuses on CVD prevalence, incidence, pathogenesis, risk factors, cardiac risk assessment, role of cardiac biomarkers in acute coronary syndromes, and importance of genetic testing in Indians.

Diagnostics in Genetic Disorders

Down Syndrome in India—Diagnosis, Screening, and Prenatal Diagnosis   231

Ishwar C. Verma, Meena Lall, and Ratna Dua Puri

Down syndrome is the most common genetic cause of mental retardation. Its frequency at birth in a population varies with maternal age distribution at birth, gestational timing of diagnosis, and case loss because of prenatal diagnosis and termination of pregnancy. The clinical features are similar in all ethnic groups. Longevity varies depending on the presence of associated conditions, especially heart disease. The cytogenetic findings are similar around the world, the majority of which are free trisomy 21. The newer therapies, although currently executed in experimental animals, hold promise for use in humans.

Hemoglobinopathies in India—Clinical and Laboratory Aspects   249

Ishwar C. Verma, Renu Saxena, and Sudha Kohli

β-thalassemia is the most common single gene disorder in India. It is estimated that there are almost 39 million carriers of the disorder in India and that almost 12,000 infants with thalassemia major are born ever year. Micromapping studies are required to derive accurate figures for carriers and the affected. The interaction of the various globin genes has been studied to some extent, although studies of the nonglobin gene markers to predict prognosis are required. A number of centers provide prenatal diagnosis, but there is need to make the tests cheaper or subsidized for the poor.

Inborn errors of metabolism (IEM) often present with multisystemic or single organ manifestation primarily in childhood. Advances in laboratory techniques and knowledge of human genome have resulted in substantial changes in diagnosis and management of these disorders. Prompt diagnosis, appropriate counseling, prenatal testing, and carrier detection will help to dilute the mutant genetic pool. Newborn screening will further help to initiate early intervention to avoid irreversible neurologic damage in patients with IEM. Availability of diagnostic facilities in India is needed to elucidate the existence of IEM.

Regulation of Laboratories

There is a growing demand for quality in health care. Expeditious availability of reliable and accurate test results is vital to diagnosis of clinical disorders. A clinical laboratory performing these tests must implement a sound quality assurance program that ensures staff competence, safe environment, proper maintenance of calibrated equipment, use of standard procedures for patient preparation, sample collection, handling and analysis, communication with clinicians, maintenance of confidentiality, and timely dispatch of accurately transcribed test results. For results to be universally acceptable, the laboratory should be accredited by an authoritative accreditation body.

Blood bank regulation is intended to assure that the quality and safety of blood products meet appropriate standards. India has a regulatory system under the Drugs and Cosmetics Act that is being implemented by Drug Control authorities at central and state levels. It has a vigilant regulatory mechanism in place, and the Indian Blood Transfusion Service (BTS) is well regulated. Other competent authorities are in place to monitor technical standards by supplying blood bank consumables and nonconsumables; putting the emphasis on teaching, training, and research; and implementing a total quality management system in the Indian BTS to ensure a safe blood supply.

Unique Business Opportunities

Distant testing of patients' samples is necessitated by nonavailability of tests locally. In most cases it involves sending out of samples for complex and esoteric tests. This process entails understanding the variables and the nature and extent of changes. Temperature, time to testing, and transport-related conditions that exist in all clinical situations where testing facilities are not located by the side of patients are compounded when samples are transported across geographic regions. In this article the author examines these issues in the context of laboratory parameters of hematology tests and shares experiences at a leading reference laboratory in India.

Shoibal Mukherjee

Clinical trials are essential to the development of new disease therapies. With the world's highest disease burden, India must bear responsibility in the fight against disease. During the past decade the country has built clinical development capacity and capabilities. Contract research organizations (CROs) have led by providing training and employment. India's capabilities and capacity in the clinical development sciences reside largely within CROs. These organizations take health care interventions from laboratory to commercialization, and India holds great promise as a global hub for such capabilities. It remains to be seen whether this promise can be realized in the near future.

Vijay Gupta and Poonam Das

Medical tourism is travel to another country for health care that is not available or not affordable in one's own country. The term is debatable, and terms like *medical value travel* are alternately being used. The industry encompasses outbound, inbound, and intrabound (within one's own country) patients. Medical tourism is a fast-growing industry in many developing nations. In India, health care is one of the largest service sectors. The ratio of doctors to patients is high, although the quality of medical training varies, and there are internationally accredited multi- and superspecialty hospitals and some of the world's most talented doctors.

Palat K. Menon

This article provides an overview of international reference laboratories and their advent in India. International reference laboratory chains constitute Networks of Excellence in laboratory testing with best in trade quality management systems, good laboratory practices, laboratory information management systems, electronic document control, and a linked training management system. Its operations are Lean and

Six Sigma–driven. Reference laboratories invest in innovation, technology, large-scale operations, and cost-efficient testing. They provide high-quality as well as esoteric testing services and serve as models to evolve as centers of excellence in diagnostic testing. Policy and regulatory support can enhance the potential of these laboratories.

CLINICS IN LABORATORY MEDICINE

FORTHCOMING ISSUES

September 2012
Toxicology Testing
Michael G. Bissell, MD, PhD, MPH,
Guest Editor

December 2012
Conceptual Advances in Pathology
Zoltan Oltvai, MD, Guest Editor

RECENT ISSUES

March 2012
Nanobiotechnology
Kewal K. Jain, MD, FFPM, *Guest Editor*

December 2011
Cytogenetics
Caroline Astbury, PhD, FACMG,
Guest Editor

CLINICS IN LABORATORY MEDICINE

Preface

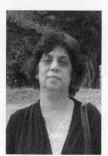

Tester F. Ashavaid, PhD, FACB, CSci
Guest Editor

It has been a great pleasure to serve as a guest editor for the Laboratory Medicine in India edition of the *Clinics in Laboratory Medicine* and I thank Dr Alan Wells for inviting me to do so and also for making this occasion an educational feast.

The series of articles for *Clinics in Laboratory Medicine* focuses on major issues faced by laboratories in India. This subject has grown by leaps and bounds across the world, and India, with approximately 50,000 laboratories, has also tried to keep pace with this advancement. India has an entire spectrum of labs starting from small labs housed in a single room to major international laboratories with their vast network of sample pickups and collection centers. Research is generally carried out in medical research institutes or hospital laboratories and standalone diagnostics labs also contribute to it.

I am extremely thankful for the cooperation I have received from various authors who are experts in their own field and who have kept to their deadlines.

In this issue, I have tried to group the articles under various subheadings, such as diagnostics in infectious diseases, diagnostics in lifestyle acquired diseases, and diagnostics in genetic diseases, and have also included the regulations, which are applicable to the labs in India, and upcoming unique business opportunities, which are currently available. While the main theme of the issue is on diagnostics, there is also a flavor of research as each author has also expounded on the research findings as well.

The articles provide insights into some of the vital medical issues faced by the country and the role of laboratory science in understanding them. The issue begins with an article on tuberculosis—laboratory diagnosis. Although tuberculosis is curable, it is unassailable, incurring human and economic losses. Dr Rodrigues and her coauthor have summarized the laboratory-based assays currently available for TB diagnosis and have given an overview of drug susceptibility testing for *Mycobacterium tuberculosis* by conventional and nonconventional phenotypic methods. They have elaborated on the genotypic methods, done a cost-effective analysis in terms of patient treatment outcome, and also drawn up a cost-effective algorithm using WHO-approved tests for TB diagnosis and drug resistance.

Clin Lab Med 32 (2012) xv–xviii
http://dx.doi.org/10.1016/j.cll.2012.05.001
0272-2712/12/$ – see front matter © 2012 Elsevier Inc. All rights reserved.

The next article continues with another scourge, ie, malaria, written by Dr Shobana Sharma and her colleague, who have given an extensive review of malaria that has hit various states of India time and again. They have also expounded on the resurgence of malaria and the measures and control strategies taken by the government to control the situation and explained various methodologies used by the labs for detection. Further to this, they have used NMR spectroscopy to study the in vivo metabolism as well as the overall glucose utilization rate of IRBCs.

Dr Chugh in his article on sexually transmitted infections (STI) has drawn the attention of how STI in India has increased 8-fold in 40 years. His article gives an overview of prevalence of STI in India in the general Indian population and also in various segments of society. The article touches on the WHO-developed assured criteria for evaluating rapid diagnostic tests, which are the need of the hour, and further emphasizes the mid-term review of national programs that are used for prevention and control of STIs.

The next two articles are on viral hepatitis and HIV testing in India by Dr Priya Abraham and Dr Srikanth Tripathy and his colleagues. Dr Abraham in her article on viral hepatitis quotes that India has the second largest pool of HBV carriers. HCV is mainly acquired by suboptimal blood banking services and through poor injection practices. Dr Abraham feels that the situation in India warrants a National Health Registry with the formulation and implementation of national prevention strategies. Dr Tripathy and his colleagues have tried to give a picture of the prevalence of HIV in India and have shown how after reaching a high peak of HIV incidence in the year 2000 there has been a steady decline in the incidence of new infections thanks to the extensive work and efforts put in by National AIDS Control Program as well as WHO, UNICEF, and UNAIDS, all of whom have contributed to the decline. They have also outlined the protocols followed for HIV testing in blood banks, in tuberculosis patients, and in antenatal clinics. Also, they have highlighted the NACO guidelines to be kept in mind for HIV testing and counseling as well as quality control procedures to be followed for HIV testing.

Cervical cancer, caused by persistent infection with the human papilloma virus (HPV), is one of the most common cancers in women in India. Cervical cancer screening by cytology has been a success story and has brought down the death rate for carcinoma cervix. However, India lacks a national screening program for cervical cancers. Dr Deodhar in his article entitled "Screening for Cervical Cancers/HPV" has looked at conventional cervical cytology techniques versus liquid-based cytology techniques as well as visual inspection tests and elaborated on their advantages and limitations. Although vaccines are available, their cost is a limiting factor for wider use in developing countries. He believes that, in India, visual inspection by acetic acid and by Lugol's iodine are acceptable alternatives for low-resource settings.

The second aspect of this issue deals with diagnostics in lifestyle acquired diseases, namely, type 2 diabetes in Asian Indians and cardiovascular diseases in India. Dr Shashank Joshi has made an often repeated point that India is a world leader in diabetes and that strong familial aggregation as well as lifestyle factors of imprudent diet and sedentary life style have contributed to "thin fat Indian" when compared to Caucasians and Africans. Also, Asian Indians have a higher fat composition. He has advocated aggressive screening and stringent treatment strategies to counteract this epidemic. He has also elaborated on the nutritional issues in Asian Indian type 2 diabetes and has expounded on how the diet of all income groups have moved away from whole-grain cereals to an increased intake of proteins and fats. It is the sedentary habits in Asian Indians that has led to the development of multifactorial diseases like type 2 diabetes and cardiovascular diseases. I along with my coauthors in the article entitled "Cardiovascular Diseases in India" especially coronary artery disease (CAD) have focused on various aspects of disease starting from prevalence, incidence, pathogenesis, risk factors, cardiac risk assessment, role of cardiac biomarkers in ACS, and the probable genetic links that may lead to CAD. Since CAD is a leading cause of mortality, this article stresses the need to identify genetic markers by developing assays for screening young asymptomatic Indians who seem to be more susceptible to CAD then their Caucasian, African, and other counterparts.

Under the section Diagnostics in Genetic Diseases are listed three articles. Dr Verma and his coauthors have contributed two articles, one on Down syndrome, which is the most common genetic disorder seen in India. He has explained the conditions associated with Down syndrome and its association with folate metabolism. His article touches on the various techniques used for the detection of Trisomy 21, genetic counseling, management, and treatment of patients with Down syndrome.

The second article, on Hemoglobinopathies–Clinical and Laboratory Aspects, elaborates on β-thalassemia, which is prevalent in India with a frequency of 1/1200. The prevalence of the β-thalassemia trait in different regions is different and varies from 1 to 17%. Also, this trait is more prevalent in certain communities and it is estimated that there are 36-39 million carriers of β-thalassemia in India.

The third article on inherited diseases is on inborn errors of metabolism (IEM) by Dr Dherai. These disorders, which are a group of greater than 500, are often neglected and not much was done in India, until recently. This is greatly due to the advanced technologies like GC/MS and LC/tandem mass, which have made forays into clinical laboratories. The various government bodies, ie, ICMR, DBT, and DST, are coordinating nationwide efforts to screen and bring about general awareness of these disorders along with facilities for newborn screening and IEM diagnostics so that it will help in the initiation of early intervention in newborns, thus avoiding irreversible neurological damage in patients.

The next aspect of this issue is on regulations pertaining to laboratories. In India, accreditation is not mandatory but National Accreditation Board of Testing and Calibration Laboratories (NABL), which works under the umbrella of ILAC (International Laboratory Accreditation) and its regional body APLAC (Asian Pacific Laboratory Accreditation Cooperation), has made untiring efforts in the awareness of lab accreditation for small, medium, and large laboratories and is becoming more and more popular.

NABL accredits laboratories against standard ISO 15189. Dr Sood, who has written this article, has put in pioneering efforts in the process and along with his colleague, Dr Handoo, has written a detailed and informative article on clinical lab accreditation in India.

The other aspect of laboratory regulations, ie, blood bank regulations, is written by Nabjyoti Choudhary. Blood banking in India is a legally empowered regulatory service and is regulated by the Drug and Cosmetics Act and its amendments. This act specifies the space, manpower, equipment, supplies, and reagents that need to be followed in Indian blood transfusion services. NACO (National AIDS Control Organization) is the facilitator to Indian blood transfusion services on behalf of the Ministry of Health and Family Welfare, Government of India. The goal of the National Blood Policy is to provide a safe and adequate quantity of blood and blood components to the general public.

The last aspect of this issue is on newer trends that are propelling Lab Medicine further in India. In the last 15 years, India has seen an emergence of standalone reference labs. Dr Amar DasGupta has elaborated on distant testing of patient samples, which is required due to nonavailability of tests locally. Sending tests from one area to the labs that are located in another geographic area entails understanding the variables that influence test results as it involves a time gap. He has reviewed preanalytical variables that alter cellular parameters in transit and on storage and how they affect interpretation of test results in Hematology, which in turn could influence medical management of the patients.

The issue also covers the insights of clinical trials and Contract Research Organization (CRO) in India, which is ably written by Dr Shoibal Mukherjee. CROs must assure quality and compliance to regulations, as well as tedious backroom operations to manage, analyze, and report data.

The article on medical tourism is written by Vijay Gupta and his coauthor, who have explained how India is uniquely placed in terms of skilled manpower, diverse medical conditions, and a large non-resident indian population, all of which contribute to make India a good destination for medical tourism, which will give a boost to the diagnostic industry in India.

The next article is on international reference labs written by Dr Palat Menon, who has elaborated on the advantages of reference labs in providing innovation, technology, large-scale operations, and cost-efficient testing. He has also indicated how these labs strive to drive their operations by Lean and Six Sigma principles, thereby enhancing diagnostic testing and providing globally harmonized testing for clinical trials.

This issue would not have seen the light of the day had it not been for the team effort put in by Sunita Makwana, who has worked alongside me. I also acknowledge help, sometimes almost instantly, provided by Dr Swarup Shah and Asha Rawal and Dr Apurva Sawant, to make this issue possible.

Tester F. Ashavaid, PhD, FACB, CSci
Department of Laboratory Medicine
P.D. Hinduja National Hospital and Medical Research Center
Veer Savarkar Marg
Mahim, Mumbai 400016

E-mail address:
dr_tashavaid@hindujahospital.com

Tuberculosis: Laboratory Diagnosis

Camilla Rodrigues, MD*, Viral Vadwai, Doctorate Fellow (PhD), M Tech

KEYWORDS

- *Mycobacterium tuberculosis* detection • Drug susceptibility testing
- Diagnostic algorithm • Molecular • Conventional

KEY POINTS

- Delay in laboratory diagnosis of tuberculosis (TB) is a major obstacle in TB control programs.
- There is an imperative need for scale-up of peripheral health care laboratories with conventional and molecular technologies for rapid and reliable diagnosis of TB.
- A cost-effective diagnostic algorithm for rapid diagnosis of TB should be implemented and followed, thereby reducing cost burden on patients.

Tuberculosis (TB), though curable, continues to be an unassailable infectious disease incurring both human and economic losses throughout the world. In 2010, an estimated 8.8 million incident TB cases occurred worldwide, with India alone and in combination with China accounting for 26% and 38% of all incident TB cases respectively.[1] This scenario is exacerbated further by an increasing prevalence of drug-resistant cases and smear-negative pulmonary and extrapulmonary TB cases, indicative of the need for highly sensitive and rapid diagnostic tools that would in turn facilitate early initiation of appropriate antitubercular treatment. The currently available laboratory-based assays for TB diagnosis are summarized in the section that follows.

A GLANCE AT THE PAST AND PROBLEMS OF THE PRESENT

Although TB has a long history, it was in 1991 when the World Health Assembly (WHA) declared it as a "global public health problem." For efficient TB control, the WHA set two important targets to be accomplished by 2005 for efficient TB control[2]:

1. To achieve a case detection rate (CDR) of 70% in new smear-positive cases
2. To achieve a treatment success rate of 85%.

The authors have nothing to disclose.
Department of Microbiology, P. D. Hinduja National Hospital and Medical Research Center, Lalita Girdhar Building, Veer Savarkar Marg, Mahim, Mumbai 400016, Maharashtra, India
* Corresponding author.
E-mail address: dr_crodrigues@hindujahospital.com

Clin Lab Med 32 (2012) 111–127
http://dx.doi.org/10.1016/j.cll.2012.03.002
0272-2712/12/$ – see front matter © 2012 Elsevier Inc. All rights reserved.

In an effort to achieve this target, in 1994, the World Health Organization (WHO), along with STOP TB Partnership (TBP), launched the now known as Directly Observed Therapy, Short-course (DOTS), ensuring proper case management to achieve favorable patient treatment outcomes. After failure to meet the set goals in 2005, the WHO and the TBP framed the Global Plan to STOP TB 2006–2015 with a target to reduce the number of TB deaths to half by 2015 in comparison to that in 1990.[3] It also advocated the need for additional funding for TB control; strengthening of diagnostic laboratories for ensuring availability of quality test results; and aiding research activities for developing rapid, highly sensitive, cost-effective TB diagnostic tools, novel anti-TB drugs, and vaccines. The same report also summarized the incompetence of the existing health care systems in diagnosis of TB cases, drug-resistant cases in particular. Envisaging the inability in the health care system, efforts have been put in to increase the proficiency of both private–public diagnostic laboratories to ensure rapid and accurate test results. The implementation has been planned in a phased manner and the scale-up has been appreciable, facilitating diagnosis of smear-positive TB. Efforts are being made to implement current diagnostic tools such as liquid TB culture and liquid phenotypic and molecular drug susceptibility assays especially for detection of smear-negative TB, drug-resistant (DR) TB, and TB in human immunodeficiency virus (HIV) patients. Current research focuses on development of point-of-care tests for its immediate feasibility and dissemination across health care systems.

DETECTION OF *M. TUBERCULOSIS*
Direct Tests

Microscopy
Acid-fast bacilli (AFB) smear microscopy plays an important role in the early diagnosis of mycobacterial infection because most mycobacteria grow slowly and culture results become available only after weeks of incubation. In addition, AFB smear microscopy is often the only available diagnostic method in developing countries. This method is rapid, simple, inexpensive, can be performed directly on clinical specimens, and does not require a high-tech laboratory. It can detect a minimum of 5000 to 10,000 bacilli per milliliter of sputum specimen. Various studies utilizing microscopy for diagnosis of pulmonary TB have reported variable sensitivities ranging from 20% to greater than 80%.[4] Thus, a method to improve the sensitivity of microscopy is the need of the hour.

Concentrating sputum specimens with or without chemical processing has been tested for increasing the sensitivity of smear microscopy. A systematic review summarized the findings of various published primary studies evaluating the various combinations of physical (centrifugation, sedimentation) and chemical methods (sodium hydroxide, *N*-acetyl-L-cysteine, bleach, ammonium sulfate, dithiothreitol) has reported chemical processing followed by centrifugation offers increased sensitivity without any compromise in specificity on comparison with direct microscopy (**Table 1**).[4] A study from India has reported 12- to 16- fold increase in sensitivity of smear microscopy when the specimen was processed by universal sample processing (USP) methodology.[5]

An alternative to increasing sensitivity is the use of fluorescent microscopy (FM). However, its feasibility in remote settings is limited because of its high cost. An alternative to FM is light-emitting diode (LED) microscopy, which is less expensive and capable of running on chargeable batteries, making it feasible in resource-limited settings. LED microscopy using auramine staining has been reported to have approximately 10% higher sensitivity compared to routine light microscopy, with no

Table 1

Studies comparing sensitivity and incremental yield for Ziehl–Neelsen direct smears and sputum smears chemically processed followed by centrifugation/sedimentation

Chemical Method	Physical Method	No. of Studies	Comparison Against Culture	Pooled Sensitivity[a]/Positivity[b] (%)		Difference in Sensitivity/ Positivity (%)	Collective Sensitivity/ Positivity (%)
				Direct Microscopy	Post-Processing		
NaOCl	Centrifugation[c]	6	Yes	44.5	57.1	+12.6	+18
NaOH	Centrifugation[c]	4	Yes	65.5	82.8	+17.3	
NALC-NaOH	Centrifugation[c]	2	Yes	81.5	90.5	+9	
USP	Centrifugation[d]	1	Yes	69	98	+2	
Chlorhexidine gluconate-NaOCl	Centrifugation[e]	1	Yes	74	89	+1	
NaOCl	Centrifugation[c]	11	No	15.7	25	+9.3	+7
NaOH	Centrifugation[c]	4	No	19	25	+6	
NaOH	Not performed	2	No	36.5	33	-3.5	
Not Performed	Centrifugation[c]	1	No	22	29	+7	
Chitin	Sedimentation 30-45 min	1	Yes	50	86	+36	9
NaOCl	Sedimentation 30-45 min	3	Yes	52	52.3	+0.3	
NaOCl	Sedimentation overnight	1	Yes	50	83	+33	23
(NH$_4$)$_2$SO$_4$-NaOH	Sedimentation overnight	2	Yes	57.5	86	+28.5	
Phenol (NH$_4$)$_2$SO$_4$	Sedimentation overnight	1	Yes	83	85	+2	
NaOCl	Sedimentation 30-45 min	3	No	26	29	+3	3
NaOCl	Sedimentation overnight	4	No	14.5	20.3	+5.8	5
(NH$_4$)$_2$SO$_4$-NaOH	Sedimentation overnight	1	No	9	26	+17	

[a] Sensitivity, calculated on comparing results of smear against culture.
[b] Positivity, estimated as the difference in the number of specimens reported as smear negative by direct microscopy but positive after processing.
[c] Centrifugation speed/force, 1500-3000 g/rpm; time, 15–20 minutes.
[d] Centrifugation force, 5000–6000 g; time, 10–15 minutes.
[e] Centrifugation speed, 2000 rpm; time, 5 minutes.

Table 2
Detailed analysis on the diagnostic performance of LED microscopy

Tests	Pooled Sensitivity (%)	Pooled Specificity (%)
Culture reference	83.6	98.2
Direct smears only	88.9	98.3
Concentrated smears only	72.7	97.9
400×/600× magnification	84.1	99.0
200× magnification	82.1	94.4
Microscopy reference	92.7	98.5
Direct smears only	93.6	98.5
Concentrated smears only	78.0	99.0
400×/600× magnification	95.0	98.0
200× magnification	90.0	99.0

significant compromise in specificity.[6] A recent systematic review has reported LED microscopy to have a sensitivity and specificity of +6 % and −1% respectively in comparison to Ziehl-Neelsen (ZN) microscopy.[7] **Table 2** provides a detailed analysis of the diagnostic performance of LED microscopy. The mean time saved to read slides compared to ZN slides was 46% (48% for smear-positive specimens, and 56% for smear negative specimens). In addition, the average cost per test is 10% to 12% less than for ZN microscopy. A recent study from Mumbai reported comparable diagnostic performance of LED microscopy in comparison with conventional smear microscopy (78% vs 83%, pulmonary specimens; 34% vs 37%, extrapulmonary specimens).[6] Fading characteristics were also studied, in which stained slides stored at various different environmental conditions (closed environment at room temperature, 22°C; exposed to light at room temperature, 22°C; refrigerator, 4°C; humidified incubator, 30°C) showed rapid fading with significant reduction in the proportion of positive slides; but storage of slides in a closed environment at room temperature remained positive the longest.[8]

A systematic review evaluating the diagnostic yield of each of the three sputum specimens inferred that microscopic analysis of the third specimen provided a low incremental diagnostic yield of 2% to 5%. Based on these findings, the WHO recommends the implementation of a "same-day-diagnosis" approach, emphasizing that all countries using the three-specimen case-finding strategy switch to the two-specimen case-finding strategy.[9,10]

Culture
Traditionally, culture is the gold standard and solid culture was the method used for confirmatory diagnosis of TB. Although having higher sensitivity compared to smear microscopy, it has a long turnaround time (TAT) of approximately 4 to 8 weeks. In addition, drug susceptibility testing (DST) takes 2 to 3 weeks, thus resulting in further delay in initiation of appropriate antitubercular treatment.

Broth-based liquid cultures have profound advantages over solid culture, capable of detecting as low a level as 10 to 10^3 viable bacilli per milliliter of the specimen, thereby increasing the case yield by 10%.[11] A systematic review has reported higher sensitivity of BACTEC MGIT 960 than solid culture (88% vs 76%); the pooled use of both these culture systems further increased the detection yield to 92%.[12] Also, BACTEC MGIT 960 was found to have a shorter TAT in comparison to solid cultures

(12.9 days vs 27 days),[12] in turn reducing the delay in obtaining drug susceptibility results to 10 days in comparison to 28 to 42 days for solid culture.[11] Similarly, a study from India has reported a higher recovery rate with a shorter TAT for BACTEC MGIT 960 in comparison to solid culture (9 days vs 38 days, smear-positive specimens; 16 days vs 48 days, smear-negative specimens).[13] Liquid culture was found to have a higher positivity rate against solid culture (7.5% vs 4.3%).[14] The WHO recommended the use of liquid medium for culture and DST, emphasizing the need for rapid diagnostic tools facilitating species identification.

These liquid culture systems, however, have limitations: (1) They are more prone to contamination by other nonmycobacterial organisms (8.6%)[12] or nontuberculous mycobacteria (NTM); even in experienced laboratories, approximately 5% to 7% of specimens do not yield results because of contamination. (2) Cross-contamination between samples during culture inoculation, that is, carryover of bacilli from positive to negative specimens, is possible (4%). A recent study reported that liquid culture systems are more accurate and cost-effective than solid cultures for diagnosis of TB in HIV-positive patients in a resource-limited setting.[15]

Thus, careful planning and systematic implementation of culture facilities should be considered with emphasis on biosafety equipments, training, supervision, and external quality assurance for efficient functioning of a laboratory.

As an alternative to these liquid cultures, use of novel in-house prepared bilayered media for rapid mycobacterial culture has been shown to achieve higher isolation rate in comparison to conventional solid media.[16] In addition, methods employing variable specimen processing techniques such as filtration of cerebrospinal fluid (CSF) samples[17] and USP protocol for sample processing[5] have reported increase in culture yield on solid and liquid media.

Species identification from positive cultures Assessment of the impact of liquid culture for its role in initiating early antitubercular treatment was blemished by the lack of rapid species identification test capable of distinguishing between *Mycobacterium tuberculosis* (MTB) complex and NTM. Conventional biochemical tests are slow, have a longer TAT, and require skilled labor, thereby delaying further DST and initiation of appropriate antitubercular treatment.

Rapid detection of MTB complex with minimal technical skill would be an ideal test for high-throughput laboratories. Immunochromatographic (ICT) assays are based on the principle of double-sandwich enzyme-linked immunosorbent assay (ELISA) detects MPT64 antigens specifically produced by MTB complex species without the need of additional special equipment. ICT assays have analytical sensitivity of 10^5 colony-forming units (cfu)/mL, providing a cost effective method, with results available with 15 minutes of processing. A recent systematic review evaluating the use of three commercially available ICT assays reported high sensitivity (range, 98.1%–98.6%) and high specificity (range, 99.2%–100%) for rapid identification of MTB complex from positive cultures (liquid or solid).[18]

Microscopic observation direct susceptibility and thin-layer agar

Microcolony culture techniques used for early MTB diagnosis are microscopic observation direct susceptibility (MODS), based on the microscopic observation of characteristic cord formation using an inverted microscope, while thin-layer agar (TLA) permits identification of isolates based on the characteristic morphology of mycobacteria in culture. Comparative performance of MODS and TLA for MTB diagnosis in comparison against culture are summarized in **Table 3**.[19]

Table 3
Performance characteristics of MODS and TLA

Characteristics	Diagnostic Assays	
	MODS[a]	TLA
Diagnostic performance		
Pooled sensitivity	92%	87%
Pooled specificity	96%	98%
For sputum specimens only		
Sensitivity	96%	NR[b]
Specificity	96%	NR[b]
Contamination rate	6.6%	12.3%
Operational characteristics		
TAT	9.2 d[c]	11.5 d[d]
Consumable cost per sample	$1.48	$2.42

[a] Three studies evaluating the use of MODS on extrapulmonary specimens such as CSF, gastric aspirate, nasopharyngeal aspirate, and stool samples reported lower sensitivity ranging from 51% to 85%.
[b] NR, not reported.
[c] MODS TAT, faster than solid culture and liquid culture by 16.1 days and 2.6 days, respectively.
[d] TLA TAT, faster than solid culture by 11.8 days but slower than liquid culture by 1.5 days.

Phage-based assays
The phage-based assay relies on the ability of MTB to support the growth of an infecting mycobacteriophage. Two main phage-based approaches used for MTB diagnosis are: (1) amplification of phages within viable MTB cells followed by detection of plaque formation due to progeny phages using helper cells and (2) detection of light produced by luciferase reporter phages by viable MTB cells. Phage-based tests are easy to perform, but require a high-tech infrastructure laboratory. The TAT of phage-based assays is 2 days compared to about 2 hours for smear microscopy or up to 2 months for culture. A systematic review based on the use of bacteriophage based assays for rapid detection of MTB reported high specificity (83%–100%) but inconsistent sensitivity (21%–88%).[20] For smear-positive specimens, the sensitivity and specificity ranged from 29% to 87% and 60% to 88% respectively while for smear-negative specimens, the sensitivity and specificity ranged from 13% to 78% and 89% to 99% respectively. Also in comparison against smear microscopy, difference in sensitivity (range, −58% to +30%) was highly variable with almost similar specificity (range, −0.07% to +0.26%). In a study done in Mumbai the FASTPlaque TB compared to liquid culture showed a sensitivity and specificity of 93.1% and 88.2% respectively.[21]

Mycobacterial antigen detection
Based on the principle of sandwich ELISA, these tests detect the presence of circulating mycobacterial antigens in clinical specimens such as CSF, sputum, serum, urine, and pleural fluid. For pulmonary TB, wide estimates of sensitivity (range, 2%–100%) and specificity (33%–100%) were reported.[22] When lipoarabinomannon (LAM)-based antigen kits were evaluated for diagnosis of TB in sputum specimens, the reported pooled sensitivity and pooled specificity was 87% and 70% respectively.

In case of extrapulmonary TB, finding of multiple antigens (such as LAM, ESAT-6, 65-kDa antigen, ES-20, ES-31, Ag85 complex) were collectively analyzed and evaluated on different specimen types such as serum, CSF, biopsy; pooled sensitivity and specificity was found to be 76% to 87% and 84% to 89% respectively.[22] A systematic review evaluating the use of LAM-based antigen assays for diagnosis of TB in urine specimens reported a sensitivity of 13% to 93% with a specificity of 87% to 99%.[23] Also the proportion of patients reported positive was higher for those with higher bacillary load in comparison with patients with lower bacillary load. It also reported 3% to 53% higher sensitivity in HIV-positive patients compared to HIV-negative patients. Another subgroup analysis showed no significant difference in the performance of LAM-based assays for diagnosis of TB using either fresh or frozen urine specimens (sensitivity, 59% vs 49%; specificity, 89% vs 97%). In India, several antigen-based tests have been developed and evaluated incorporating a single or cocktail of antigens specific for MTB complex. For example, certain studies have reported that the use of Ag 85 complex proteins[24] and hsp65 antigen[25] in antigen-based ELISA assays having higher sensitivity and specificity in pulmonary and extrapulmonary TB (TBM, pleural TB, ascitic TB, TB arthritis). Based on the variable diagnostic accuracy of each antigen for diagnosis of TB, attempts are being made to develop a large antigenic pool to enhance the sensitivity of the assay.

Nucleic acid amplification test assays

Nucleic acid amplification test (NAAT) assays such as polymerase chain reaction (PCR) have been heavily relied on for rapid diagnosis (<1 week) and accurate identification of MTB complex directly from clinical specimens. Although a plethora of both commercial and in-house tests exist, each targets a different method to amplify a particular sequence of mycobacterial genome, specific for MTB complex species. Commercial assays are expensive, require skilled labor and a high-infrastructure laboratory. Thus, use of commercial NAAT for rapid TB diagnosis as a replacement for conventional tests is not recommended. In-house tests are usually developed in resource-limited settings as an alternative to commercial assays. A systematic review of in-house studies has shown that the analytical sensitivity of PCR was not significantly affected by the kind of DNA extraction protocol (physical or chemical) employed but the use of IS*6110* as a PCR target and the use of nested amplification protocols significantly increased the diagnostic accuracy of PCR.[26] A number of Indian research laboratories have attempted to standardize an efficient, reliable PCR for diagnosis of both pulmonary and extrapulmonary TB, and have reported variable diagnostic accuracy for each different kind of gene being targeted.[27] Use of an in-house PCR (targeting gene encoding 38-kDa protein) has reported high accuracy for reliable diagnosis of extrapulmonary TB.[28–30] Also, amplification of shorter DNA fragments has been shown to achieve higher sensitivity in comparison to amplification of larger DNA fragments.[31] A recent study has reported the use of a single-tube multitarget, nested PCR assay for diagnosis of extrapulmonary TB with a sensitivity and specificity of 94.5% and 96.4% respectively, and the number of cases being reported positive increases with the increase in number of targeted genes.[32] Researchers in India have developed a multiplex PCR assay capable of simultaneously detecting MTB complex and NTM species from clinical specimens that has a higher reported diagnostic accuracy in comparison to both solid and liquid cultures.[33]

A major limitation in the use of these PCR assays is the risk of cross-contamination; hence to overcome these issues, many studies have coupled the use dUTP-uracil *N*-glycosylase (dUTP-UNG) with their amplification system for accurate reporting of test results. A systematic review reports the use of dUTP-UNG to be associated with increased specificity at the expense of lowering sensitivity.[34]

Indirect Tests

Serology

Serologic tests rely on antibody recognition of MTB antigens by the humoral immune response, as opposed to antigen recognition by the cellular immune response (eg, interferon-γ release assays). The major advantages of these tests are their speed (results may be available within hours) and technical simplicity compared to smear microscopy. Several commercial serologic tests differing in a number of features, including antigen composition, antigen source, chemical composition, extent and manner of purification of the antigen(s), and class of immunoglobulin detected (eg, IgG, IgM, or IgA) have been evaluated for rapid diagnosis of TB. However, a systematic review evaluating all commercially available serologic assays reported that none of the assays performed well enough (inconsistent sensitivity and specificity) to replace sputum smear microscopy, having little or no role in the diagnosis of pulmonary and extrapulmonary TB.[35] Based on this evidence, the WHO issued a negative recommendation based on the poor performance of all commercial serodiagnostics and the adverse impact of misdiagnosis and wasted resources on patients and health services when using these tests for the diagnosis of active TB.[36]

A recent study that performed a cost-effective analysis for the use of serologic tests in comparison with other available diagnostic assays in India inferred that serology was more costly and less effective than MGIT culture and hence does not recommend its use as an additional diagnostic test after smear microscopy for TB.[37]

Adenosine deaminase activity

Increase in adenosine deaminase activity (ADA) levels due to evaluated immune cellular response against MTB has been proposed as a rapid and inexpensive alternative for accurate diagnosis of TB in pleural, meningeal, and pericardial fluids, with high positive predictive value in TB-endemic countries. A systematic review evaluating the use of ADA for diagnosis of tuberculous pleurisy, tuberculous peritonitis, tuberculous meningitis, and tuberculous pericarditis have reported sensitivity and specificity of 92% and 89%, 100% and 96%, 79% and 91%, 88% and 83% respectively.[38-41]

DST FOR MTB

In 2008, there was an estimated 440,000 (range, 390,000–510,000) cases of multidrug-resistant (MDR) TB worldwide (India, 99,000), and 963 cases of extensively drug-resistant (XDR) TB were reported to WHO globally from 33 countries.[42]

Phenotypic Methods: Conventional Methods

The existing phenotypic methods used for TB diagnosis have been methodologically adapted to facilitate determination of drug resistance patterns of MTB strains.

Solid cultures (agar proportion method)

This method involves the inoculation of equal dilution of pure MTB culture strain (cell suspension) into a solid medium containing an appropriate concentration of antitubercular drug and other a drug-free medium, followed by incubation at 37°C with a mean TAT of 3 to 4 weeks. A bacterial growth greater than 1% on the drug-containing medium in comparison to the drug-free medium indicates the strain to be resistant to that particular drug. Although the use of Middlebrook 7H10 agar supplemented with OADC has been recommended in the Clinical and Laboratory Standards Institute guidelines, use of Lowenstein–Jensen medium has been the preferred choice in resource-limited countries.[43]

Liquid cultures (MGIT)

The principle of this assay is similar to that explained before for liquid culture using BACTEC MGIT 960. A homogeneous suspension of the viable bacilli is inoculated in both drug-containing and drug-free liquid medium, and the drug-susceptibility pattern of a particular MTB strain is automatically determined using the preset algorithm of the instrument. A recent study has successfully demonstrated the use of liquid MGIT culture for determination of drug susceptibility directly from clinical specimens. This reduced the reporting time by approximately 8 days in comparison to indirect DST. Also, concordance between direct and indirect DST for determination of isoniazid and rifampicin was found to be 95.1% and 96.1% respectively.[44]

Phenotypic Methods: Nonconventional Methods

These methods include MODS, TLA, phage-based methods, colorimetric redox indicator methods, and nitrate reductase assays (NRAs); they are optimized to facilitate rapid determination of drug-susceptibility pattern of MTB strains.

MODS and TLA

Based on the principle of the assay, the protocol was modified facilitating the determination of drug resistance to isoniazid and rifampicin. A recent systematic review has reported high sensitivity and specificity for determination of resistance to both first- and second-line drugs, in comparison against phenotypic DST (**Table 4**).[45]

Phage-based assays

Results of a recent systematic review have reported these assays not to be suitable as a replacement for conventional DST.[46] The pooled contamination rate/indeterminate results using these phage-based assays was found to be 5.8% (range, 0–36%). These rates were high for studies using direct patient specimens (mean, 21.2%) in comparison to studies using indirect specimen inoculation (mean, 2.1%). **Table 5** provides detailed results of phage-based assays evaluated for detection of rifampicin resistance.

Colorimetric redox indicator methods

These assays facilitate simultaneous detection of MTB and determination of drug resistance, observed by a change in the color (reduction reaction) of the culture medium containing antitubercular drugs due to in vitro MTB growth. Thus change in the color of the medium indicates the strain to be resistant to that particular drug. The different growth indicators evaluated are: tetrazolium salts: XTT [2,3-bis-(2-methoxy-4-nitro-5-sulfophenyl)-2*H*-tetrazolium-5-carboxanilide] and MTT [3(4,5-dimethylthiazol-2-yl)-2,5-diphenyltetrazoliumbromide] and the redox indicators Alamar blue and resazurin.

A recent systematic review has reported these assays to have high diagnostic accuracy for detection of resistance to rifampicin (sensitivity range, 89%–100%; specificity range, 97%–100%) and isoniazid (sensitivity range, 92%–100%; specificity range, 88%–100%), with an estimated TAT of 4 to 14 days.[47] Thus, these assays could be considered as a useful alternative for detection of multidrug resistance using clinical isolates, but also recommends its evaluation on direct clinical specimens to assess its true diagnostic potential.

Table 4
Diagnostic accuracy of MODS and TLA for determination of drug susceptibility pattern from clinical specimens

Specimen	Drug (concentration)	Sensitivity (%)	Specificity (%)	Contamination Rate (%)	TAT (days)
Microscopic observation: direct susceptibility					
Direct	Rifampicin (1 or 2 μg/mL)	96.8	99	7.4%	9.9
Indirect	Rifampicin (1 or 2 μg/mL)	100	100		
Direct	Isoniazid (0.1 μg/mL)	96.4	94.2		
Indirect	Isoniazid (0.1 μg/mL)	100	98		
Direct	Isoniazid (0.4 μg/mL)	88.6	98.5		
Indirect	Isoniazid (0.4 μg/mL)	93	100		
Indirect	Ofloxacin	100	100		
TLA					
Direct	Rifampicin (1 μg/mL)	100	100	1.4	11.1
Direct	Isoniazid (0.2 or 0.25 μg/mL)	100	100		
Direct	Ethambutol	100	99.5		
Direct	Streptomycin	100	100		
Direct	Pyrazinamide	100	100		
Indirect	Ofloxacin	100	100		
Indirect	Kanamycin	100	98.7		

Table 5
Performance of both commercial and in-house phage-based assays for determination of RIF resistance

Test	Pooled Sensitivity (%)	Pooled Specificity (%)
Commercial phage amplification assays	95.5	95
Indirect only	95.7	94.1
Direct only	93.6	96.3
Industry only	96.9	96.7
Non-industry only	92.6	85.1
In-house phage amplification assays	98.5	97.9
Luciferase reporter phage	99.3	98.6

NRA

The NRA is based on the conversion of nitrate to nitrite by nitroreductase enzymes of viable MTB cells, detected by a visual change in color of the culture medium (containing the Griess reagent) from pink to purple. A systematic review has reported direct NRA testing to be highly sensitive and specific. The sensitivity and specificity of NRA for detection of resistance to isoniazid and rifampicin and diagnosis of MDR TB has been reported to be 93% to 98% and 96% to 98%, with 92% specimens providing results within 14 days at a cost of US$3.58 per sample.[48]

Genotypic or Molecular Methods

Genetic studies have revealed the presence of certain mutations in specific regions of certain genes to be associated with conferring drug resistance. More than 95% of rifampicin-resistant isolates possess mutations in the Rifampicin Resistance Determining Region (RRDR: 81-bp region, codon 507–533) of the *rpoB* gene, while 70% to 80% of isoniazid-resistant isolates harbor mutations in the *katG* and *inhA* genes.

Subsequent genetic studies have also revealed the presence of certain mutations to be associated with conferring resistance to clinically important second-line antitubercular drugs. For example, mutations in the *gyrA* (codon 90–94) and *gyrB* (codon 510) region have been known to confer resistance in approximately 85% of the fluroquinolone-resistant isolates, while approximately 80% of aminoglycoside resistant isolates are known to possess mutations at codon 1401 and 1484 of the *rrs* gene. Using these molecular data, several commercial and in-house assays have been developed to facilitate rapid determination of XDR TB with a TAT of approximately 2 to 3 days.

Line probe assays

Inno-LiPA Rif TB test (Innogenetics NV, Ghent, Belgium) and Genotype MTB DRplus assay (Hain Lifescience, Nehren, Germany) are the two commercially available assays for rapid detection of MDR TB. Both assays include an MTB complex species-specific probe together with a number of wild-type probes encompassing the entire RRDR region of the *rpoB* and few mutant specific probes targeting the most highly prevalent mutations responsible for conferring drug resistance. The Genotype MTB DRplus assay also contains wild-type and mutant probes specific for *katG* and *inhA*-associated mutations known to confer isoniazid drug resistance.

A recent analysis reported LiPA assays to have high sensitivity (range, 82%–100%) and specificity (range, 92%–100%) for determination of rifampicin resistance, while subgroup analysis showed that use of clinical specimens reported a sensitivity of 80% to 100% with a uniform specificity, 100%.[49]

Similarly, a systematic review evaluated the use of Genotype MDRplus assays and reported higher diagnostic accuracy for determination of rifampicin resistance (pooled sensitivity, 98.1%; pooled specificity, 98.7%) than isoniazid resistance (pooled sensitivity, 84.3%; pooled specificity, 99.5%), for both clinical isolates and direct clinical specimens.[50]

In-house assays based on a similar principle have also been developed for use in resource-limited settings. Studies from Mumbai evaluating the use of these in-house assays have reported a sensitivity of greater than 98% for detection of resistance to rifampicin and isoniazid, and 95.3% for fluoroquinolones and 94.8% for aminoglycosides respectively.[51,52]

Real-time PCR assays

Xpert MTB/RIF (Cepheid Inc., Sunnyvale, CA, USA), the most recent commercial diagnostic tool, is based on the principle of hemi-nested real-time PCR using molecular beacons to facilitate simultaneous detection of MTB complex and determination of rifampicin resistance in less than 2 hours. This semi-automated system makes use of a single specimen processing step, followed by automated molecular protocols such as genomic DNA extraction, PCR amplification, and product detection within a closed cartridge, thus greatly reducing the chances of cross-contamination. For smear-negative sputum specimens, the diagnostic accuracy of Xpert MTB/RIF increases with multiple specimen processing.[53] Another study has reported high diagnostic accuracy (sensitivity, 81%; specificity, 99.6%) for diagnosis of extrapulmonary TB in comparison with a predefined composite reference standard.[54] Although limited data exist on its use for diagnosis in a high HIV prevalence setting,[55] for diagnosis of pediatric TB[56] and extrapulmonary TB, this assay appears to be a promising tool for diagnosis in such settings. Based on the evidence, the WHO has recommended and endorsed the use of Xpert MTB/RIF as an initial diagnostic tool in individuals suspected to have MDR TB or HIV-associated TB and to be used as an add-on test with smear microscopy in low MDR TB or HIV prevalence settings.[57]

Algorithms for Integrated Use of Conventional and Molecular Diagnostic Assays for Rapid TB Diagnosis and Determination of Drug Resistance

In spite of a pool of available diagnostic assays, there is still no single test completely reliable for the laboratory diagnosis of TB. Diagnostic algorithms in developed countries with a low incidence of TB focus on the screening process so as not to miss any patient with TB, while those in resource-limited settings with a higher incidence of HIV-associated and DR TB focus primarily on identifying patients at risk of MDR TB infection to facilitate initiation of appropriate antitubercular treatment and thereby interrupt further transmission. However, it is very important that all clinicians follow an algorithm so as to maintain a balance in the number of requests for a certain diagnostic procedures; otherwise, laboratory services will be overburdened with unnecessary testing and will also increase the cost burden on the patient. Thus, effective planning (**Fig. 1**) would facilitate successful integration of conventional and molecular methodologies for rapid diagnosis of MDR TB in a reference laboratory setting in a middle incidence country.[58]

TB DIAGNOSTICS: COST-EFFECTIVE ANALYSIS IN TERMS OF PATIENT TREATMENT OUTCOME, SCALEUP, AND NEED TO PROVIDE "UNIVERSAL ACCESS"

In recent years, the field of TB diagnostics research has reached a new echelon due to billion dollar funding provided by Global Fund, World Health Organization, World Bank, United States Agency for International Development, The Bill & Melinda Gates

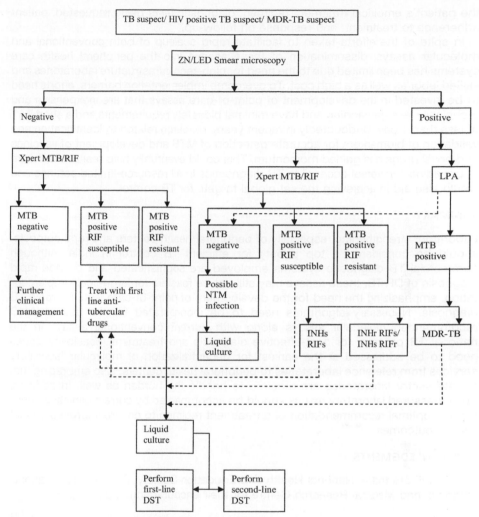

Fig. 1. A cost-effective algorithm using WHO-approved tests for rapid TB diagnosis and determination of drug resistance.

Foundation, International Union Against Tuberculosis and Lung Disease (The Union), World Vision, Foundation for Innovative New Diagnositcs, and Program for Appropriate Technology in Health along with many other governmental and nongovernmental agencies and institutions. This has facilitated a high-level scaleup of the primary diagnostic tools such as microscopy to all possible settings within the country. Efforts are also underway for scaleup, strengthening the existing laboratories for implementation of liquid culture, along with molecular assays for rapid determination of DR TB and early initiation of an appropriate treatment regimen.

Implementation of newer diagnostic tools also needs to be monitored through large-scale cost-effective analysis to measure the impact of these assays on patient treatment outcomes in terms of cost per disability-adjusted life years averted and cost for quality-adjusted life years gained. The cost-effective analysis relies primarily on the patient's empirical treatment regimen, diagnostic tests being requested, patient adherence to treatment, and response on follow-up.

In spite of the efforts taken to facilitate rapid scaleup of both conventional and molecular assays, dissemination of these assays into the peripheral health care systems has been limited due to the need for high-tech infrastructure laboratories and skilled labor as well as a high cost. To overcome implementation barriers, efforts need to be invested in the development of point-of-care assays that are inexpensive and technically less demanding and have minimal biosafety requirements and a short TAT of less than 1 day. Undoubtedly in recent years, research related to identification and validation of biomarkers for accurate detection of MTB and development of vaccines and novel drugs has gained momentum. This could eventually help realize the dream of providing "universal access" to TB diagnostics in all resource-limited settings and would also aid in achieving the set global targets for TB control.

SUMMARY

Laboratory strengthening, especially of peripheral health centers and rural outposts, should be considered a top priority for efficient TB control in India. Although commercial TB diagnostic systems employed are sophisticated and provide rapid diagnosis of DR TB, these assays may still not be feasible for large-scale implementation, emphasizing the need for the development of point-of-care tests for rapid TB diagnosis. Necessary algorithms need to be incorporated for the use of WHO recommended molecular assays along with current conventional assays in the national TB program for cost-effective diagnosis and treatment. Feasibility issues need to be addressed at the earliest for decentralization of molecular laboratory services from reference laboratories to peripheral health centers, also embracing that private sector laboratories are required to handle the burden as well. In addition, quality-assured laboratory results should be accompanied by correct clinical diagnosis and optimal recommendation of a treatment regimen to ensure improved patient clinical outcomes.

ACKNOWLEDGMENTS

The authors thank National Health and Education Society, P. D. Hinduja National Hospital, and Medical Research Centre for their encouragement and support.

REFERENCES

1. World Health Organization. Global tuberculosis control: WHO report. Geneva (Switzerland): World Health Organization; 2011. Available at: http://www.WHO/HTM/TB/2011.16. Accessed March 28, 2012.
2. World Health Organization. The STOP TB strategy: building on and enhancing DOTS to meet the TB-related Millennium Development Goals. Geneva (Switzerland): World Health Organization; 2006. Available at: http://www.WHO/HTM/TB/2006.368. Accessed March 28, 2012.
3. World Health Organization. The STOP TB Strategy: the global plan to stop TB 2011–2015. Geneva (Switzerland): World Health Organization; 2011.
4. Steingart KR, Ng V, Henry M, et al. Sputum processing methods to improve the sensitivity of smear microscopy for tuberculosis: a systematic review. Lancet Infect Dis 2006;6:664–74.
5. Chakravorty S, Tyagi JS. Novel multipurpose methodology for detection of mycobacteria in pulmonary and extrapulmonary specimens by smear microscopy, culture, and PCR. J Clin Microbiol 2005;43(6):2697–702.

6. Shenai S, Minion J, Vadwai V, et al. Evaluation of light emitting diode-based fluorescence microscopy for the detection of mycobacteria in a tuberculosis-endemic region. Int J Tuberc Lung Dis 2010;15(4):483–8.

7. Minion J, Brunet L, Pai M. Fluorescent light emitting diode (LED) microscopy for the detection of *Mycobacterium tuberculosis*: a systematic review. In: Approaches to improve sputum smear microscopy for tuberculosis diagnosis; WHO expert group meeting. Geneva (Switzerland); 2009.

8. Minion J, Shenai S, Vadwai V, et al. Fading of auramine-stained mycobacterial smears and implications for external quality assurance. J Clin Microbiol 2011;49(5):2024–6.

9. Mase SR, Ramsay A, Ng V, et al. Yield of serial sputum specimen examinations in the diagnosis of pulmonary tuberculosis: a systematic review. Int J Tuberc Lung Dis 2007;11(5):485–95.

10. World Health Organization. Same-day-diagnosis of tuberculosis by microscopy. Geneva (Switzerland); 2010.

11. World Health Organization. Use of liquid TB culture and drug susceptibility testing (DST) in low and medium income settings. Geneva (Switzerland): World Health Organization; 2007.

12. Cruciani M, Scarparo C, Malena M, et al. Systematic review of BACTEC MGIT 960 and BACTEC 460 TB, with or without solid media, for detection of mycobacteria. J Clin Microbiol 2004;42(5):2321–5.

13. Rodrigues C, Jani J, Shenai S, et al. Drug susceptibility testing of *Mycobacterium tuberculosis* against second-line drugs using the Bactec MGIT 960 System. Int J Tuberc Lung Dis 2008;12(12):1449–55.

14. Hillemann D, Richter E, Rusch-Gerdes S. Use of the BACTEC Mycobacteria Growth Indicator Tube 960 automated system for recovery of mycobacteria from 9,558 extrapulmonary specimens, including urine samples J Clin Microbiol 2006;44(11):4014–7.

15. Dowdy DW, Lourenco MC, Cavalcante SC, et al. Impact and cost-effectiveness of culture for diagnosis of tuberculosis in HIV-infected Brazilian adults. PLoS ONE 2008;3(12):e4057.

16. Bhattacharya S, Roy R, Chowdhury NR, et al. Comparison of a novel bilayered medium with the conventional media for cultivation of *Mycobacterium tuberculosis*. Indian J Med Res 2009;130:561,e6.

17. Kumar P, Srivatsava MV, Singh S, et al. Filtration of cerebrospinal fluid improves isolation of mycobacteria. J Clin Microbiol 2008;46:2824,e5.

18. Brent AJ, Mugo D, Musyimi R, et al. Performance of MGIT TBc identification test and systematic review of MPT64 assays for identification of *Mycobacterium tuberculosis* complex in liquid culture. J Clin Microbiol 2011;49(12):4343–6.

19. Leung E, Minion J, Benedetti A, et al. Microcolony culture techniques for tuberculosis diagnosis: a systematic review. Int J Tuberc Lung Dis 2012;16(1):16–23.

20. Minion J, Pai M. Bacteriophage assays for rifampicin resistance detection in *Mycobacterium tuberculosis*: updated systematic review. Int J Tuberc Lung Dis 2010;14(8):941–51.

21. Shenai S, Rodrigues C, Mehta AP. Evaluation of a new phage amplification technology for rapid diagnosis of tuberculosis. Ind J Med Microbiol 2002;20(4):194–9.

22. Flores LL, Steingart KR, Dendukuri N, et al. Systematic review of antigen detection tests for the diagnosis of tuberculosis. Clin Vaccine Immunol 2011;18(10):1616–27.

23. Minion J, Leung E, Talbot E, et al. Diagnosing tuberculosis with urine lipoarabinomannan: systematic review and systematic review. Eur Respir J 2011;38:1398–405.

24. Kashyap RS, Dobos KM, Belisle JT, et al. Demonstration of components of antigen 85 complex in cerebrospinal fluid of tuberculous meningitis patients. Clin Diagn Lab Immunol 2005;12:752,e8.
25. Rajan AN, Kashyap RS, Purohit HJ, et al. Serodiagnosis of tuberculosis based on the analysis of the 65 kD heat shock protein of *Mycobacterium tuberculosis*. Int J Tuberc Lung Dis 2007;11:792,e7.
26. Flores LL, Pai M, Colford JM, et al. In-house nucleic acid amplification tests for the detection of *Mycobacterium tuberculosis* in sputum specimens: systematic review and meta-regression. BMC Microbiol 2005;5:55.
27. Haldar S, Bose M, Chakrabarti P, et al. Improved laboratory diagnosis of tuberculosis: the Indian experience. Tuberculosis 2011;91(5):414–26.
28. Kulkarni SP, Jalil MA, Kadival GV. Evaluation of polymerase chain reaction for the diagnosis of tuberculous meningitis in children. J Med Microbiol 2005;54:369,e73.
29. Kulkarni SP, Vyas SP, Kadival GV. Use of polymerase chain reaction in the diagnosis of abdominal tuberculosis. J Gastroenterol Hepatol 2006;21:819,e23.
30. Jambhekar NA, Kulkarni SP, Madur BP, et al. Application of the polymerase chain reaction on formalin-fixed, paraffin-embedded tissue in the recognition of tuberculous osteomyelitis. J Bone Joint Surg [Br] 2006;88:1097,e101.
31. Chakravorty S, Pathak D, Dudeja M, et al. PCR amplification of shorter fragments from the *devR* (Rv3133c) gene significantly increases the sensitivity of tuberculosis diagnosis. FEMS Microbiol Lett 2006;257:306,e11.
32. Vadwai V, Shetty A, Rodrigues C. Using likelihood ratios to estimate diagnostic accuracy of a novel multiplex nested PCR in extra-pulmonary tuberculosis. Int J Tuberc Lung Dis 2012;16(2):240–7.
33. Gopinath K, Singh S. Multiplex PCR assay for simultaneous detection and differentiation of *Mycobacterium tuberculosis*, *Mycobacterium avium* complexes and other mycobacterial species directly from clinical specimens. J Appl Microbiol 2009;107:425,e35.
34. Sarmiento OL, Weigle KA, Alexander J, et al. Assessment by systematic review of PCR for diagnosis of smear-negative pulmonary tuberculosis. J Clin Microbiol 2003;41(7):3233–40.
35. Steingart KR, Flores LL, Dendukuri N, et al. Commercial serological tests for the diagnosis of active pulmonary and extrapulmonary tuberculosis: an updated systematic review. PLoS Med 2011;8(8):e1001062.
36. World Health Organization. Commercial serodiagnostic tests for diagnosis of tuberculosis: policy statement. Geneva (Switzerland): World Health Organization; 2011. Available at: http://www.WHO/HTM/TB/2011.5. Accessed March 28, 2012.
37. Dowdy DW, Steingart KR, Pai M. Serological testing versus other strategies for diagnosis of active tuberculosis in India: a cost-effectiveness analysis. PLoS Med 2011;8:e1001074.
38. Greco S, Girardi E, Masciangelo R, et al. Adenosine deaminase and interferon gamma measurements for the diagnosis of tuberculous pleurisy: a systematic review. Int J Tuberc Lung Dis 2003;7(8):777–86.
39. Tuon FF, Litvoc MN, Lopes MIBF. Adenosine deaminase and tuberculous pericarditis: a systematic review. Acta Tropica 2006;99:67–74.
40. Xu HB, Jiang RH, Li L, et al. Diagnostic value of adenosine deaminase in cerebrospinal fluid for tuberculous meningitis: a systematic review. Int J Tuberc Lung Dis 2010;14(11):1382–7.
41. Riquelme A, Calvo M, Salech F, et al. Value of adenosine deaminase (ADA) in ascitic fluid for the diagnosis of tuberculous peritonitis: a systematic review. J Clin Gastroenterol 2006;40:705–10.

42. World Health Organization. WHO report 2010: Global tuberculosis control. Geneva (Switzerland): World Health Organization; 2010. Available at: http://www.WHO/HTM/TB/2010.7. Accessed March 28, 2012.

43. Parsons LM, Somosko A, Gutierrez C, et al. Laboratory diagnosis of tuberculosis in resource-poor countries: challenges and opportunities. Clin Microbiol Rev 2011; 24(2):314–50.

44. Siddiqi S, Ahmed A, Asif S, et al. Direct drug susceptibility testing of *Mycobacterium tuberculosis* for rapid detection of multi-drug resistance using BACTECTM MGIT 960 System: a multicenter study. J Clin Microbiol 2012;50(2):435–40.

45. Minion J, Leung E, Menzies D, et al. Microscopic-observation drug susceptibility and thin layer agar assays for the detection of drug resistant tuberculosis: a systematic review and systematic review. Lancet 2010;10(10):688–98.

46. Minion J, Pai M. Bacteriophage assays for rifampicin resistance detection in Mycobacterium tuberculosis: updated systematic review. Int J Tuberc Lung Dis 2010;14(8): 941–51.

47. Martin A, Portaels F, Palomino JC. Colorimetric redox-indicator methods for the rapid detection of multidrug resistance in *Mycobacterium tuberculosis*: a systematic review and systematic review. J Antimicrob Chemother 2007;59:175–83.

48. Bwanga F, Haile M, Joloba ML, et al. Direct nitrate reductase assay versus microscopic observation drug susceptibility test for rapid detection of MDR-TB in Uganda. PLoS ONE 2011;6(5):e19565.

49. Morgan M, Kalantri S, Flores L, et al. A commercial line probe assay for the rapid detection of rifampicin resistance in *Mycobacterium tuberculosis*: a systematic review and systematic review. BMC Infect Dis 2005,5:62.

50. Ling DI, Zwerling AA, Pai M. GenoType MTBDR assays for the diagnosis of multidrug-resistant tuberculosis: a systematic review. Eur Respir J 2008;32:1165–74.

51. Shenai S, Rodrigues C, Mehta A. Rapid speciation of 15 clinically relevant mycobacteria with simultaneous detection of resistance to rifampin, isoniazid, and streptomycin in *Mycobacterium tuberculosis* complex. Int J Infect Dis 2009;13(1):46–58.

52. Ajbani K, Shetty A, Mehta A, et al. Rapid diagnosis of extensively drug resistant tuberculosis by use of a reverse line blot hybridization assay. J Clin Microbiol 2011;49(7):2546–51.

53. Boehme CC, Nabeta P, Hillemann D, et al. Rapid molecular detection of tuberculosis and rifampin resistance. N Engl J Med 2010;363(11):1005–15.

54. Vadwai V, Boehme C, Nabeta P, et al. Xpert MTB/RIF: a new pillar in diagnosis of extrapulmonary tuberculosis? J Clin Microbiol 2011;49(7):2540–5.

55. Theron G, Peter J, van Zyl-Smit R, et al. Evaluation of the XpertMTB/RIF assay for the diagnosis of pulmonary tuberculosis in a high HIV prevalence setting. Am J Respir Crit Care Med 2011;184:132–40.

56. Nicol MP, Workman L, Isaacs W, et al. Accuracy of the Xpert MTB/RIF test for the diagnosis of pulmonary tuberculosis in children admitted to hospital in Cape Town, South Africa: a descriptive study. Lancet Infect Dis 2011;11(11):819–24.

57. World Health Organization: Rapid implementation of the Xpert MTB/RIF diagnostic test: technical and operational 'how-to.' Practical considerations. Geneva (Switzerland): World Health Organization; 2011. Avaliable at: http://www.WHO/HTM/TB/2011.2. Accessed March 28, 2012.

58. Balabanova Y, Drobniewski F, Nikolayevskyy V, et al. An integrated approach to rapid diagnosis of tuberculosis and multidrug resistance using liquid culture and molecular methods in Russia. PLoS ONE 2009;4(9):e7129.

Host Responses in Malaria Disease Evaluated Through Nuclear Magnetic Resonance–Based Metabonomics

Haripalsingh M. Sonawat, PhD[a], Shobhona Sharma, PhD[b],*

KEYWORDS

- Plasmodium • Pathology • Cerebral malaria • Glucose flux • Metabonomics
- Nuclear magnetic resonance

KEY POINTS

- Malaria is a widespread disease caused by several species of *Plasmodium*. The parameters that render the hosts susceptible to severe disease complications are not completely understood.
- Nuclear magnetic resonance (NMR)–based studies offer a convenient platform to investigate the disease process in a noninvasive, nondestructive, and unbiased manner. NMR-based metabonomics allows a systems biological view of the global changes in host metabolism due to the parasite infection.
- Parasite-infected host red blood cells influence the neighboring uninfected host red blood cells metabolically.
- In the murine model of malaria, a sexually dimorphic host response is observed upon parasitic infection. Also the animals that are prone to cerebral malaria have different metabolic status vis-a-vis the ones that do not.
- Early prediction of susceptibility to cerebral malaria may be explored using such metabonomic methods.

Relationships between host and parasites are intimate, and cross-regulations at various levels are likely. Fascinating methods have been adopted by parasites to thrive and colonize living organisms. The parasites exhibit a fine-tuning of developmental modifications in response to the attack by the host immune

---

The authors have nothing to disclose.

Statement of Funding: The study was supported by in-house funds of Tata Institute of Fundamental Research, Department of Atomic Energy, Government of India.

[a] Department of Chemical Sciences, Tata Institute of Fundamental Research, Homi Bhabha Road, Mumbai 400005, Maharashtra, India; [b] Department of Biological Sciences, Tata Institute of Fundamental Research, Homi Bhabha Road, Mumbai 400005, Maharashtra, India

* Corresponding author.

E-mail address: sharma@tifr.res.in

system. On the other hand, the host fights the parasites through its armory of immune, behavioral, and metabolic responses.

Currently five species of *Plasmodium* are infectious for humans: *P falciparum, P vivax, P malariae, P ovale,* and the recent identification of *P knowlesi.*[1] Of these, *P falciparum* malaria causes maximum severity, and the severe disease pathology is usually defined according to World Health Organization (WHO) criteria.[2] However, only a small fraction of the *P falciparum*–infected population becomes susceptible to severe malaria disease, which can result in cerebral malaria (CM), severe anemia, multiorgan dysfunction, hypoglycemia, and acidosis. The mortality through malaria is largely caused by the severe disease, and it would be good to be able to develop methods to predict the susceptibility and progression to severe disease. Nuclear magnetic resonance (NMR) is a noninvasive method that can be used to monitor live erythrocytic stages in culture, as well as assess host body fluids for metabolic changes in the parasite and in the vertebrate host.

LIFE CYCLE OF MALARIA PARASITES

In the vertebrate host, malarial parasites exist broadly as free sporozoites, liver-stage parasites (collectively known as pre-erythrocytic stage), erythrocytic (including free merozoites), and gametocytic stages. Sporozoites, introduced by the female *Anopheles* mosquito in a vertebrate organism during a blood meal, find their way to the liver and infect hepatocytes. Inside the hepatocyte each sporozoite transforms itself and proliferates massively into the merozoites that will infect erythrocytes. Subsequent cyclic erythrocytic stages, consisting of rings, trophozoites, and schizonts, are responsible for the symptoms, complications, and fatality associated with malaria. The diagnosis of malaria and most of the therapeutic drug treatments are targeted to the erythrocytic stages. After a few cycles of asexual stages, some of the infected erythrocytes differentiate into gametocytes. These forms are ingested by the mosquito and progress through the reproductive phase of the parasites, eventually producing infective sporozoites that reside in the salivary glands.

MALARIA IN INDIA

Nearly all malaria in India is caused by *P falciparum* and *vivax* parasites, whereas several *Anopheles* species contribute as mosquito vectors. *Anopheles culicifacies* is widely distributed and is the principal vector of rural malaria, *An stephensi* is the primary urban vector, *An fluviatilis* is a vector in the hills and foothills, whereas three to four species contribute to the Northeastern regions of India. The National Institute of Malaria Research and National Vector Borne Disease Control Programme have prepared guidelines for the diagnosis and treatment of malaria in India.[3] The epidemiology of malaria is not uniform in India, because of its extreme ecological diversity. About 2 million confirmed malaria cases and about 1000 deaths are reported annually by the National Vector Borne Disease Control Program of India, although 15 million cases and 20,000 deaths are estimated by WHO South East Asia Regional Office. Whereas there is controversy about the number of persons infected and the exact mortality in India due to malaria,[4] specific pockets have been assessed, and clearer data are available for such pockets.[5,6]

In the 1950s a large reduction in malaria cases was effective in India because of the Global Malaria Eradication Programme of WHO, and it was estimated to be fewer than 50,000 cases per annum in 1961. However, in the 1970s the incidence increased to 1,322,398 by 1971 (annual parasite incidence [API]: 2.47; slide positivity rate [SPR]: 3.27%, and *P falciparum* [Pf]:11.2%) and then to 6,467,215 in 1976 (API:11.25;

SPR:11.6%, and Pf: 11.7%).[7] The emergence of resistance in mosquito vectors to commonly used insecticide DDT and in parasites to abundant use of the antimalarial chloroquine contributes significantly to this resurgence. It is remarkable that *P falciparum* has been showing steady increase in the post-resurgence phase in 1970s and accounts for nearly 45% of the total reported cases.[6] Currently, the states of Odisha, Jharkhand, West Bengal and the North Eastern States, Chhattisgarh and Madhya Pradesh contribute to the bulk of malaria. Urban areas contribute about 15% of the total malaria cases reported in India and are primarily associated with construction activities and migrant populations. Most of the malaria-attributable mortality is reported from Odisha and other forested areas occupied by ethnic tribes in the country.[5–7] Whereas most of the severity of malaria disease is ascribed to falciparum malaria cases, specific severe cases have also been reported for *P vivax* from Western regions of India. A recent study by the authors' group indicates the existence of an adult male bias in clinical malaria in hypoendemic regions of India. Women and prepubertal children in the study exhibited the lowest risk of clinical malaria; adult males demonstrated the highest risk.[8] This result may have implications in the development of malarial vaccines and the formulation of antimalarial health strategies.

Directorate of National Vector Borne Disease Control Programme (NVBDCP) has framed technical guidelines/policies and provides most of the resources for the program in India.[3] Suitable guidelines have been developed at the national level for monitoring of malaria; these have been issued to ensure that there is uniformity in collection, compilation, and onward submissions of data. Passive surveillance of malaria is carried out by primary health care clinics, Malaria Clinics, community health clinics, and other secondary and tertiary level health institutions that malaria patients visit for treatment. Active surveillance is carried out by health workers throughout the country. Apart from these, Accredited Social Health Activists (ASHAs)—village volunteers—are involved in the program to provide diagnostic and treatment services at the village level as a part of introduction of an intervention like Rapid Diagnostic Tests and use of artemisinin combination therapy for the treatment of Pf cases.[9]

The malaria control strategies in India include (a) early case detection and prompt treatment (EDPT), (b) vector control, (c) community participation and environmental management, and finally (d) monitoring and evaluation of the malaria control program. In EDPT, chloroquine continues to be the main antimalaria drug for uncomplicated malaria. Drug distribution centers and fever treatment depots have been established in rural areas for providing easy access to antimalarial drugs for the community. For severe malaria, currently monotherapy has been prohibited. In vector control, apart from the use of chemical insecticides, much more emphasis is placed on biological control measures such as use of larvivorous fish and biocides. Awareness of personal prophylactic measures that individuals/communities can take is spread. These include use of mosquito repellents, provision of the houses with wire mesh, use of bed nets treated with insecticide, and so forth. In community participation, sensitizing the community to detection of *Anopheles* breeding places and their elimination and involvement of non-governmental organization schemes in program strategies are associated. Toward monitoring and evaluation of the malaria control program, strategies are instituted including a monthly computerized management information system, field visits by State National Programme officers, and field visits by malaria research centers and other Indian Council of Medical Research institutes.[9]

NMR TOOLS AND METABONOMICS FOR INVESTIGATING DISEASE PROCESS

In vivo NMR is one of the frontier areas in the field of NMR spectroscopy and has several wide-ranging applications in both basic biological as well as biomedical studies. It has emerged as a separate field in itself and is used for routine clinical diagnosis. The technique is amenable for studying the control and regulation of metabolic pathways in humans and animals in a noninvasive and nondestructive manner. Development of magnetic resonance imaging and magnetic resonance spectroscopy has placed NMR as a versatile diagnostic tool in medicine. The study of intracellular or ex vivo or in vivo metabolism by NMR is especially important because it is nonselective and unbiased—a labeled substrate can be followed into several metabolic pathways in a single experiment. This ability provides a new platform for investigating disease progression and treatment at molecular level. However, because the disease process is usually complex involving multiple metabolic pathways in a multiorgan response of the host, the traditional single mode biochemical and clinical methods of investigation are clearly inadequate.[10] A systems biological strategy such as metabonomics could well be ideal for investigating such a phenomenon. Metabonomics is the quantitative measurement of the time-related multiparametric metabolic response of living systems to pathophysiologic stimuli.[11] The technique involves the generation of metabolic databases, based on the pattern of endogenous metabolites present in biofluids from control animals and humans, patients with disease(s).^{1}H NMR spectroscopy–based metabonomics requires little or no sample preparation, is rapid and nondestructive, and uses small sample sizes for detection of the metabolites.[11,12] The technique has been used to investigate/ diagnose diseases such as inborn errors of metabolism, diabetes, arthritis, Alzheimer disease, coronary heart disease, and diseases related to chronic renal failure. A biofluids fingerprint database of the progression of infection of the malarial parasite remains unexplored. It would be interesting to determine if malarial parasite–specific metabolite marker(s) are excreted in the patient urine or are present in blood plasma and if they are, then determine their temporal variation in terms of type and concentration with the progression of disease, specifically so in the initial stages of infection by the parasite.

NMR methods have been used earlier to assess metabolic processes in malaria.[13,14] The authors' laboratory has been investigating the malaria disease, and the host responses in both human and murine models have been studied.[15–20] In the mouse model perturbations were induced under controlled environment, whereas human samples such as urine and sera were assessed for understanding disease pathology and for a search of markers relating to severe pathologic conditions. The study has been conducted at several levels such as (a) assessment of glucose utilization and flux using labeled glucose in cultures of growing and developing parasites, (b) systems biology by ^{1}H NMR–based metabonomics in murine models, (c) lesions in specific metabolic pathways in various organs and compartments using labeled substrates, and (d) molecular metabolic epidemiology in human patients. In this article the authors review their recent work on the NMR investigations of the malaria disease process.

GLUCOSE METABOLISM AND PATHOLOGY

The clinical disease of malaria is concomitant with the occurrence of erythrocytic stages of *Plasmodium* in the blood. The pathology of the disease depends on parasite species (and perhaps strains), parasite numbers, host genetic makeup, and the nutritional and immune status of the host. In severe cases of malaria, hypoglycemia and lactic acidosis often occur, and one of the reasons for hyperlactatemia or acidosis is assumed to be the increased anaerobic glycolysis by the infected erythrocytes.[21,22] During its intraerythrocytic growth phase, the malarial parasite relies mainly on glycolysis for its energy requirements, and it has been documented that the parasite-infected red blood cells (IRBCs) use glucose at a rate much higher than that of the normal red blood cells (RBCs).[15,16,23] In a malaria patient the percentage of parasite-infected RBC rarely exceeds 3% to 4%, and is generally around 0.1% to 1% (4000–40,000/mL),[24] and thus the patient blood contains largely uninfected RBCs. Through Carbon-13 NMR (^{13}C-NMR) studies, the authors have demonstrated the remarkable ability of a small parasitized RBC cohort (IRBC) to downmodulate glucose utilization in normal uninfected red blood cells.[15]

The utilization of [2-^{13}C]glucose by *P falciparum*–infected red cells was measured using ^{13}C-NMR spectra under physiologic conditions. The quantitative estimates of metabolites and flux routed through various metabolic intermediates of a *P falciparum* culture consisting mainly of trophozoites have been assessed in the authors' laboratory. A typical NMR data profile is shown for the utilization of [2-^{13}C]glucose for both RBC and IRBC (3% parasitemia) (**Figs. 1**A, B), and the data are plotted to show the rates of utilization of glucose, and production of [2-^{13}C]lactate (see **Figs. 1**C, D). The glucose utilization of the IRBC was found to be significantly higher as compared with that of uninfected RBC. Concomitantly the rate of [2-^{13}C]lactate, which originates through glycolysis, was found to increase in the IRBC. The ^{13}C-NMR spectra showed no signatures of aerobic metabolism. NMR methods have been used elegantly[25] to implicate fumarate generated from the purine salvage pathway as being incorporated into nucleic acids and proteins. Fumarate is shown to get converted to malate and then subsequently to aspartate through a metabolic pathway that involves fumarate hydratase, malate quinone oxidoreductase, and aspartate aminotransferase. Various studies suggest functionality to a portion of the tricarboxylic acid cycle and also highlight possible metabolic cross-talks in *P falciparum*.[25,26]

The results from the authors' laboratory showed that the overall glucose utilization rate of IRBCs increases by about 100-fold, consistent with earlier observations in the field.[15,23] The actual mechanism(s) of this high increase in glucose utilization seem to be controlled by the properties of the parasite glycolytic enzymes, and their regulation. The authors' results also show significant downregulation in the rate of glucose utilization of the vast majority of uninfected red blood cells (URBCs) (>96%) in the presence of a small percentage (<4%) of *P falciparum* IRBCs. The inhibition of glucose utilization and 2,3-diphosphoglycerate (2,3-DPG) levels of the uninfected red cells could be reversed by increasing the glucose concentration in the medium.[15]

2,3-DPG is an allosteric regulator of hemoglobin oxygen affinity, and it is produced by diphosphoglycerate mutase, which is present in the erythrocyte but not in *Plasmodium*. A decrease in the 2,3-DPG level and 2,3-DPG/hemoglobin (Hb) ratio in *P knowlesi*– and *P yoelii*–infected animals has been observed earlier.[14,27,28] The decrease in the 2,3-DPG/Hb ratio was also postulated to be responsible for a shift in the oxyhemoglobin dissociation curve.[14] Increases in several glycolytic enzyme activities and concomitant reduction in pH (from 7.2 to 7.0) in freshly collected whole blood from *P berghei*–infected mice as compared with uninfected mice have been reported earlier, although no correlation was proposed.[28] The authors' experiments, with less than 4% parasitemia, simulated a real patient scenario, and it was observed that a decrease in initial pH, but not high lactate concentration, was an important factor in inhibiting the glucose utilization rate of normal RBCs.[15,16] In the authors' study the decline in 2,3-DPG was observed with less than 4% parasitized cells, and therefore the decrease cannot be explained through mechanisms exclusively

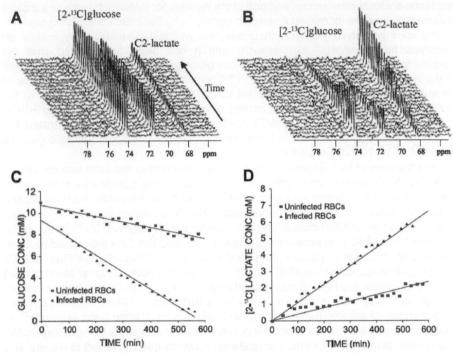

Fig. 1. Utilization of [2-13C]glucose by human RBCs infected with malarial parasite *P falciparum*. Stacked plot of the time-lapse ^{13}C-NMR spectra of RBC (*A*) and *P falciparum*–infected RBCs (IRBC) containing 3% parasitemia (*B*) after incubation with [2-^{13}C]glucose.^{13}C-NMR spectra were recorded and the data processed as mentioned in the methods section. Panels (*C*) and (*D*) show the concentration profiles of [2-^{13}C]glucose and C2-lactate of uninfected and infected red blood cells. The lines are linear fits for C2-glucose and C2-lactate obtained from the data shown in (*A*) and (*B*) respectively. (*From* Mehta M, Sonawat HM, Sharma S. Glycolysis in Plasmodium falciparum results in modulation of host enzyme activities. J Vect Borne Dis 2006;43:95–103; with permission.)

operating in the parasitized cells alone. The authors suggest that the changes in pH resulting from such activities in the infected cells may be largely responsible for lowered glycolysis in uninfected cells and hence lower levels of 2,3-DPG.

The glycolytic enzyme 6-phospho-1-fructokinase (PFK) is a key regulatory enzyme in glycolysis. The authors have characterized *P falciparum* PfPFK extensively.[29] Of the two putative PFK genes on chromosome 9 (PfPFK9) and 11 (PfPFK11), only the PfPFK9 gene possessed the catalytic features appropriate for PFK activity. The deduced PfPFK9 protein contains domains homologous to the plantlike pyrophosphate (PPi)-dependent PFK subunits, which are quite different from the human erythrocyte PFK protein. However, despite an overall structural similarity to plant PPi-PFKs, the recombinant PfPFK protein and the parasite extract exhibited only adenosine triphosphate (ATP)-dependent enzyme activity, and none with PPi. Unlike host PFK, the *Plasmodium* PFK was insensitive to fructose-2,6-bisphosphate (F-2,6-bP), phosphoenolpyruvate (PEP) and citrate. A comparison of the deduced PFK proteins from several protozoan PFK genome databases implicated a unique class of ATP-dependent PFK present among the apicomplexan protozoans.[29] The authors also demonstrated that the human red cell PFK is differentially inhibited by pH as compared with *P falciparum* PFK, thus providing a mechanism of differential rates of glucose utilization in the IRBCs and URBCs.[15,29] Extensive in vivo analysis of erythrocyte glycolysis has been carried out using NMR and, in addition to the glycolytic flux, the 2,3-DPG synthesizing enzyme is also significantly inhibited by low pH.[30] Indeed, it has been observed that all three regulatory enzymes of glycolysis, hexokinase, pyruvate kinase, and PFK, show differential pH sensitivities between human erythrocyte and *Plasmodium* enzymes. All the three *Plasmodium* enzymes are insensitive to acidic pH, whereas human RBC enzymes are affected considerably.[31]

MALARIA DISEASE PROGRESSION (MURINE MODEL) AND SEXUAL DIMORPHISM IN HOST RESPONSE

^{1}H NMR spectra of urine, sera and brain extracts of mice were analyzed over disease progression using principal component analysis (PCA) and orthogonal partial least square discriminant analysis (OPLS-DA). Analyses of overall changes in urinary profiles during disease progression demonstrate that females show a significant early postinfection shift in metabolism as compared with males (**Fig. 2**). In contrast, serum profiles of female mice remain unaltered in the early infection stages whereas those of the male mice changed (**Table 1**). Brain metabolite profiles do not show global changes in the early stages of infection in either sex.[17] By the late stages urine, serum, and brain profiles of both sexes are severely affected. Analyses of individual metabolites show significant increase in lactate, alanine and lysine, kynurenic acid, and quinolinic acid in sera of both males and females at this stage. Early changes in female urine are marked by an increase of ureidopropionate, lowering of carnitine, and transient enhancement of asparagine and dimethylglycine. When analyzed individually asparagine and dimethylglycine levels decrease and quinolinic acid increases early in sera of infected females. In brain extracts of females, an early rise in levels is also observed for lactate, alanine and glycerol, kynurenic acid, ureidopropionate, and 2-hydroxy-2-methylbutyrate. These results suggest that *P berghei* infection leads to impairment of glycolysis, lipid metabolism, metabolism of tryptophan, and degradation of uracil.[17]

^{1}H NMR–based metabonomics were further used to investigate the multimodal response of mice to malarial parasite infection by *P berghei* ANKA. Liver metabolism was followed by NMR spectroscopy through the course of the disease in both male and female mice.[18] On infection kynurenic acid, alanine, carnitine, and β-alanine showed significant alteration in the liver, suggesting altered kynurenic acid, glucose, fatty acid, and amino acid metabolism. Distinct sexual dimorphism was also observed in the global analysis of the liver metabolic profiles. Multiway principal component analysis (MPCA)–based correlation of liver and brain metabolic profile to the metabolite profile of serum also indicated distinct sexual dimorphism at early stage of the disease.[18] The females are able to regulate their liver metabolism so as to maintain homeostasis in the blood. In males, however, choline in liver showed anticorrelation to choline content of plasma indicating a higher phospholipid degradation process. The brain-plasma correlation profile showed an altered energy metabolism in both the sexes. Characterization of early changes along these pathways may be crucial for prognosis and better disease management in malaria patients. Additionally, the distinct sexual dimorphism exhibited in these responses has a bearing on the understanding of the pathophysiology of malaria.

CEREBRAL MALARIA AND PLEURAL EFFUSION

CM is a severe clinical manifestation of *P falciparum* infection. The cerebral manifestation is accompanied by various disorders and complications including fever, anaemia,

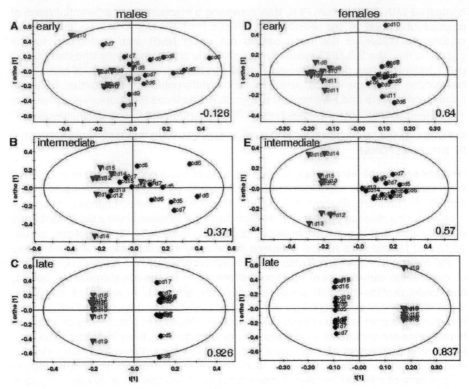

Fig. 2. Representative OPLS-DA scores of ^{1}H NMR spectra of mouse urine showing postinfection temporal changes. A-C male. D-F female. Data points of days −2 to 0 (preinfection) for three mice of a litter have been compared with A, D: days 1 to 4 (early stage infection); B, E: days 5 to 8 (intermediate stage infection) and C, F: days 9 to ~13 (late stage infection). Each point represents a sample corresponding to the day indicated. The first number in the label indicates the mouse. 1 = inf1, 2 = inf2, c = control. Black circle = uninfected, Red triangle = infected. The ellipse is a 95% Hotelling's T2 ellipse. For A and B, nonsignificant orthogonal components had to be calculated. R2X(cum), Q2(cum) = A. .569, −.126; B. .531, −.371; C. .925, .926; D. .752, .64; E. .558, .57; F. .911, .837. (*From* Basant A, Rege MM, Sharma S, et al. Alterations in urine, serum and brain metabolomic profiles exhibit sexual dimorphism during malaria disease progression. Malar J 2010;9:110.)

hemoglobinuria, retinal damage, acute lung injury/acute respiratory distress syndrome (ARDS), pulmonary edema and pleural effusion (PE).[32] ARDS is an important predictor of mortality in adults due to malaria and is associated with a greater than 70% fatality rate. Pulmonary edema and PE are thus important aspects to be investigated with this disease. Some of the clinical and pathologic aspects are known for these complications, like increased vascular permeability and vasodilatation that might lead to cardiac insufficiency. The increase in the vascular permeability and decrease in osmotic pressure of serum colloid play a crucial role in circulatory shock in CM. However, it is not understood why some people are susceptible and not others.

The murine model of the disease provides a convenient alternative for investigating changes in biofluids during the disease progression to CM. The model consists of *P berghei* (ANKA) as the causative agent used in combination with C57BL/6 mice, which shares many symptoms and features of human CM.[33] This mouse model has been

Table 1
Summary of postinfection temporal changes and gender differences in metabolic profiles of different samples

Sample	Male-Female Difference Q² (Cum)	Early Stage Q² (Cum)		Late Stage Q² (Cum)	
		Males	Females	Males	Females
Urine	0.81	−0.13	0.64	0.93	0.84
Serum	−0.16	0.53	−0.24	0.98	0.98
Brain	−0.28	0.08	−0.20	0.99	0.93
Liver	−0.78	−0.88	0.99	0.98	0.99

Values are in terms of Q^2(cum) from OPLS-DA analysis, representing extent of separation between infected and uninfected or male and female populations.
Data from Basant A. Host metabolic changes during malaria: 1H NMR investigations [MSc thesis]. Mumbai (Maharashtra): Tata Institute of Fundamental Research; 2010.

used in studies of malarial lung syndromes. The vascular permeability is known to be increased in brain, lungs, kidneys, and heart in murine model of CM. The fractions of infected mice that transit into CM exhibit variation. In the authors' experiments they monitored this combination of mice and parasite over the time of disease progression. During several such trials a consistent observation was that 40% to 60% of the animals exhibited symptoms of CM.[20] This result fortuitously allowed a direct comparison of the pleural fluids of mice with CM and those that remained with noncerebral malaria (NCM). The animals that transited into CM exhibited lower body temperature (**Fig. 3**B) and displayed neurologic symptoms such as ataxia, paralysis, convulsions, deviation of head, and so forth.

¹H NMR of the sera and the PE of CM–infected mice were analyzed using PCA, OPLS-DA, MPCA, and multivariate curve resolution (MCR). It has been observed that there was 100% occurrence of PE in the mice affected with CM, as opposed to those that are noncerebral and succumbing to hyperparasitemia (NCM/HP). An analysis of ¹H NMR and sodium dodecyl sulfate–polyacrylamide gel electrophoresis profile of PE and serum samples of each of the CM mice exhibited a similar profile in terms of constituents.[20] Multivariate analysis on these two classes of biofluids revealed that glucose, creatine, and glutamine contents were high in the PE and lipids content was high in the sera. MCR showed that changes in PE covaried with that of serum in CM mice. The increase of glucose in PE is negatively correlated to the glucose in serum in CM as obtained from the result of MPCA. This study for the first time led to the characterization of metabolites in PE formed during murine CM.[20] The study indicates that the origin of PE metabolites in murine CM may be the serum. The loss of the components like glucose, glutamine, and creatine into the PE may worsen the situation of patients, in conjunction with the enhanced glycolysis, glutaminolysis, and increased activity of creatine phosphokinase, which are already reported characteristic pathophysiologic features of malaria. Parameters that would be indicative of the prognosis of CM in specific animals are being explored. Early prediction of CM complications in humans would be of tremendous help in terms of patient management and care.

MALARIA IN HUMANS—VIVAX MALARIA

P vivax is responsible for 70% to 80% of malarial infection in the Indian subcontinent. This species of the parasite is generally believed to cause a relatively benign form of

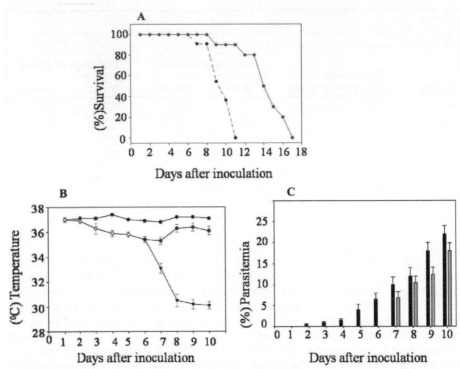

Fig. 3. Parameters of C57BL/6 mice monitored postinoculation with RBCs infected with *P berghei* ANKA (PbA). (*A*) % Survival of the NCM mice (*red circles*) and CM mice (*black circles*) postinoculation with the parasite. (*B*) The rectal temperature monitored in the uninfected controls (*filled black circles*) and the PbA–inoculated animals (*open circles*). The NCM mice are pink circles whereas the CM mice are black triangles. (*C*) The PbA–infected animals are represented by black bars until day 6. After day 6 the black bar refers to the CM and the grey bar to the NCM mice. (*From* Ghosh S, Sengupta A, Sharma S, et al. Multivariate modelling with ¹H NMR of pleural effusion in murine cerebral malaria. Malar J 2011;10:330.)

the disease. However, recent reports from different parts of the world indicate that vivax malaria can also have severe manifestations.[34] Host response to the parasite invasion is thought to be an important factor in determining the severity of manifestation. In order to better understand the disease pathology the authors attempted to determine the host metabolic response associated with *P vivax* infection. NMR spectroscopy of urine samples from *P vivax*–infected patients, healthy individuals, and nonmalarial fever patients were carried out followed by multivariate statistical analysis. As mentioned earlier, the statistical methods used were PCA and OPLS-DA. The urine metabolic profiles (**Fig. 4**) of *P vivax*–infected patients were distinct from those of healthy individuals as well as of nonmalarial fever patients.[19] A highly predictive model was constructed from urine profile of malarial and nonmalarial fever patients. Several metabolites varied significantly across these cohorts. Thus, the relative urinary levels of valerylglycine, pipecolic acid, and phenylpyruvic acid were higher and those of tyrosine, glucose, and N-acetylglutamate were lower in vivax patients in comparison with the healthy individuals. However, malaria patients showed high urinary glucose and ornithine, and lower levels of N-butyrate and acetate compared with nonmalaria febrile patients. Ornithine could, therefore, serve as a

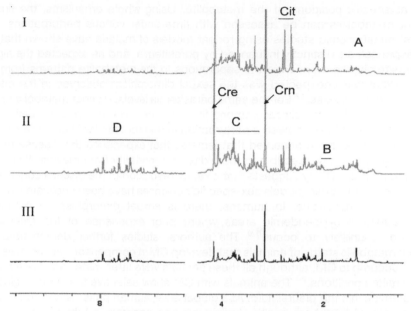

Fig. 4 Representative urine ^{1}H NMR spectral profile of I. Adult male patient with nonmalarial fever, II. Adult male healthy individual, and III. Adult male infected with *P vivax*. However, because of high variability in the urine profiles across individuals, a direct comparison of the spectral profile is not possible. Key: A: Branched chain amino acid and small chain fatty acids, B: acetate and N-acetyl groups of acetylated amino acids, C: glucose, carbohydrates and amino acid alpha protons, D: Aromatic amino acids and metabolites, Cit: citrate, Crn: creatine/phosphocreatine/creatinine and Cre: creatine. The Urea and water regions were excluded from the figure. (*From* Sengupta A, Ghosh S, Basant A, et al. Global host metabolic response to *Plasmodium vivax* infection: a ^{1}H NMR based urinary metabonomic study. Malar J 2011;10:384.)

potential biomarker of *vivax* malaria.[19] An increasing trend in pipecolic acid was also observed. This metabolite, a breakdown product of lysine, was suggested to be unique for the experiments with the murine model of the disease.[35] Overall, the authors' results suggest an impairment in the hepatic function and urea cycle. The results open up a possibility of noninvasive analysis and diagnosis of *P vivax* using urine metabolic profile. Distinct variations in certain metabolites were recorded, and among these, ornithine may have the potential of being used as a biomarker of vivax malaria.

SUMMARY

Currently large-scale metabonomic studies can be conducted using NMR and mass spectrometry. Whereas mass spectrometry has the advantage of being far more sensitive in terms of detection limits of metabolites, NMR studies have the advantage of being noninvasive and quantitative and can be used on whole organisms. The illustrations shown previously for the use of body fluids such as urine and plasma in NMR analysis allowed the authors to assess the global metabolic changes with malaria disease progression. They also allow specific questions on the fate of a particular metabolite through the follow-up of resultant metabolites starting with labels at specific positions of the metabolite. Using whole organisms, the flux of different metabolites can be assessed with time under various perturbations. The authors' metabonomic studies using rodent models of malaria have shown that the host responses are distinctly influenced by parasitemia, and as expected the higher the parasitemia, the more were the separations in the metabolite patterns from the normal. What was unexpected was the sexual dimorphism observed in the rate of sensitivity to the disease.[17] For the same parasitemia levels, distinct metabolic profile was detected early in the disease among female mice, even before overt pathologic symptoms set in. Males showed a perturbation in metabolites far later in the disease progression. It has been observed that females that experience the disease for the first time are far less susceptible to morbidity and mortality from malaria,[36] and this early metabolic sensitivity suggests that an early resolution of the disease could result from the same. In mouse models sex-specific hormones have been implicated in such differential susceptibilities. In humans, there is sexual dimorphism in pathology among adults in hypoendemic areas where prior experience of the disease in childhood is unlikely to occur.[5,9] The authors' studies further demonstrate the different metabolic status of animals that develop CM in comparison with animals that do not succumb to CM, although all these animals were litter-mates and were reared under similar conditions.[20] The animals with CM show selective transport of glucose and glutamine into the pleural fluid. At a global level, human patients with malaria are metabolically distinct from healthy individuals and nonmalaria febrile patients. The possibility of early detection of CM is being investigated. This research should lead to improvements in clinical management of such patients, and thus reduction in morbidity and mortality.

REFERENCES

1. Cox-Singh J, Singh B. Knowlesi malaria: newly emergent and of public health importance? Trends Parasitol 2008;24:406–10.
2. World Health Organization. Guidelines for the treatment of malaria. Geneva (Switzerland): World Health Organization; 2006.
3. Guidelines for diagnosis and treatment of malaria in India, 2011. Available at: http://www.mrcindia.org/Guidelines%20for%20Diagnosis2011.pdf. Accessed May 9, 2012.
4. Valecha N, Staedke S, Filler S, et al. Malaria-attributed death rates in India. Lancet 2011;377:992–3.
5. Kumar A, Valecha N, Jain T, et al. Burden of malaria in India: retrospective and prospective view. Am. J Trop Med Hyg 2007;77:69–78.
6. Singh N, Mishra AK, Shukla MM, et al. Forest malaria in Chhindwara, Madhya Pradesh, central India: a case study in a tribal community. Am J Trop Med Hyg 2003;68:602–7.
7. Sharma VP. Re-emergence of malaria in India. Indian J Med Res 1996;103:26–45.
8. Pathak S, Rege M, Gogtay NJ, et al. Age-dependent sex bias in clinical malarial disease in hypoendemic regions. PLoS One 2012;7(4):e35592.
9. Malaria Control Strategies, National Vector Borne Diseases Control Programme, Directorate General of Health Services, Ministry of Health & Family Welfare. Available at: http://nvbdcp.gov.in/malaria11.html. Accessed May 9, 2012.
10. Makinen VP, Soininen P, Forsblom C, et al. ^{1}H NMR metabonomics approach to the disease continuum of diabetic complications and premature death. Mol Syst Biol 2008;4:167.

11. Nicholson JK, Lindon JC, Holmes E, et al. 'Metabonomics': understanding the metabolic responses of living systems to pathophysiological stimuli *via* multivariate statistical analysis of biological NMR data. Xenobiotica 1999;29:1181–9.
12. Nicholson JK, Wilson ID. High resolution proton magnetic resonance spectroscopy of biological fluids. Prog Nucl Magn Reson Spectros 1989;21:449–501.
13. Deslauriers R, Ekiel I, Kroft T, et al. NMR studies of malaria. ^{31}P nuclear magnetic resonance of blood from mice infected with *Plasmodium berghei*. Biochim Biophys Acta 1982;721:449–57.
14. Krishna S, Shoubridge EA, White NJ, et al. *Plasmodium yoelii*: blood oxygen and brain function in the infected mouse. Exp Parasitol 1983;56:391–6.
15. Mehta M, Sonawat HM, Sharma S. Malaria parasite-infected erythrocytes inhibit glucose utilization in normal red cells. FEBS Lett 2005;579:6151–8.
16. Mehta M, Sonawat HM, Sharma S. Glycolysis in Plasmodium falciparum results in modulation of host enzyme activities. J Vect Borne Dis 2006;43:95–103.
17. Basant A, Rege MM, Sharma S, et al. Alterations in urine, serum and brain metabolomic profiles exhibit sexual dimorphism during malaria disease progression. Malar J 2010;9:110.
18. Sengupta A, Basant A, Ghosh S, et al. Liver metabolic alterations and changes in host intercompartmental metabolic correlation during progression of malaria. J Parasitol Res 2011;901854.
19. Sengupta A, Ghosh S, Basant A, et al. Global host metabolic response to *Plasmodium vivax* infection: a ^{1}H NMR based urinary metabonomic study. Malar J 2011;10: 384.
20. Ghosh S, Sengupta A, Sharma S, et al. Multivariate modelling with ^{1}H NMR of pleural effusion in murine cerebral malaria. Malar J 2011;10:330.
21. Agbenyega T, Angus BJ, Bedu-Addo G, et al. Glucose and lactate kinetics in children with severe malaria. J. Clin. Endocrinol Metab 2000;85:1569–76.
22. Lang-Unnasch N, Murphy AD. Metabolic changes of the malaria parasite during the transition from the human to the mosquito host. Annu Rev Microbiol 1998;52:561–90.
23. Roth EF Jr, Calvin MC, Max-Audit I, et al. The enzymes of the glycolytic pathway in erythrocytes infected with Plasmodium falciparum malaria parasites. Blood 1988;72: 1922–5.
24. Molineaux L, Muir DA, Spencer HC, et al. The epidemiology of malaria and its measurement. In: Wernsdorfer WH, McGregor I, editors. Malaria, vol. II. New York: Churchill Livingstone; 1988. p. 999–1089.
25. Bulusu V, Jayaraman V, Balaram H. Metabolic fate of fumarate, a side product of the purine salvage pathway in the intraerythrocytic stages of Plasmodium falciparum. J Biol Chem 2011;286:9236–45.
26. Olszewski KL, Mather MW, Morrisey JM, et al. Branched tricarboxylic acid metabolism in Plasmodium falciparum. Nature 2010;466:774–8.
27. Oelshlegel FJ Jr, Sander BJ, Brewer GJ. Pyruvate kinase in malaria host–parasite interaction. Nature 1975;255:345–7.
28. Kruckeberg WC, Sander BJ, Sullivan DC. Plasmodium berghei: glycolytic enzymes of the infected mouse erythrocytes. Exp Parasitol 1981;51:438–43.
29. Mony BM, Mehta M, Jarori GK, et al. Plant-like phosphofructokinase from Plasmodium falciparum belongs to a novel class of ATP-dependent enzymes. Int J Parasitol 2009;39;1441–53.
30. Mulquiney PJ, Bubb WA, Kuchel PW. Model of 2,3-bisphosphoglycerate metabolism in the human erythrocyte based on detailed enzyme kinetic equations: in vivo kinetic characterization of 2,3-bisphosphoglycerate synthase/phosphatase using ^{13}C and ^{31}P NMR. Biochem J 1999;342:567–80.

31. Mony BM. Understanding glucose metabolism in the malarial parasite and its effects on the host [PhD thesis]. Mumbai (Maharashtra): Tata Institute of Fundamental Research; 2010.
32. Trampuz A, Jereb M, Muzlovic I, et al. Clinical review: severe malaria. Crit Care 2003;7:315–23.
33. Hunt NH, Grau GE. Cytokines: accelerators and brakes in the pathogenesis of cerebral malaria. Trends Immunol 2003;24:491–9.
34. Kochar DK, Das A, Kochar SK, et al. Severe *Plasmodium vivax* malaria: a report on serial cases from Bikaner in Northwestern India. Am J Trop Med Hyg 2009;80:194–8.
35. Li JV, Wang Y, Saric J, et al. Global metabolic responses of NMRI mice to an experimental *Plasmodium berghei* infection. J Prteom Res 2008;7:3948–56.
36. Cernetich A, Garver LS, Jedlicka AE, et al. Involvement of gonadal steroids and gamma interferon in sex differences in response to blood-stage malaria infection. Infect Immun 2006;74:3190–203.

Sexually Transmitted Infections

Tulsi D. Chugh, MD, FRCPath[a,b],*, Rajni Gaind, MD[c]

KEYWORDS

- Sexually transmitted infections • Epidemiology • Behavioral risk factors
- Antimicrobial resistance • Point-of-care diagnosis • Prevention and control

KEY POINTS

- In developing countries, sexually transmitted infections (STIs) account for 10% to 20% of adult patients attending government health facilities.
- A young population, with 36% younger than 15 years, unbalanced male/female ratio (1000:933), increasing urbanization, illiteracy, poverty, sexual promiscuity, and lack of health education account for a high prevalence of STIs.
- Epidemiologic surveillance system and laboratory diagnostic facilities, especially point-of-care diagnosis, are inadequate in India.
- Antibiotic resistance in causative pathogens is an important hurdle in their control.
- Currently, syndromic management is the most common approach in India.

Sexually transmitted infections (STIs) are the most common group of notifiable infectious diseases in most countries, particularly in people aged 15 to 50 years and infants. In the United States, of the top 11 reportable diseases in 1996, 5 were transmitted sexually (gonorrhea, chlamydial infection, syphilis, hepatitis B, and acquired immunodeficiency syndrome [AIDS]). STI are also among the 5 leading causes of health problems in developing countries.[1] The World Health organization (WHO) estimated that in 1999, 340 million new cases of curable STI occurred globally, of which 150 million were reported from South and Southeast Asia, including 50 million from India.[2] These diseases are endemic in the tropics and may be responsible for up to 17% of productive years lost in certain regions.[3]

Medical descriptions of these diseases date back to the 15th century. The older terminology of *venereal diseases* (VDs) has been superseded in the past 50 years by *sexually transmitted diseases* (STDs), and more recently, by *sexually transmitted*

The authors have nothing to disclose.
[a] National Academy of Medical Sciences, Ansari Nagar, Mahatama Gandhi Marg, New Delhi 110029, India; [b] Department of Microbiology, BLK Super Specialty Hospital, Pusa Road, New Delhi 110005, India; [c] Department of Microbiology, Vardhman Mahavir Medical College, Safdarjung Hospital, Safdarjung Enclave, Mahatama Gandhi Marg, New Delhi 110029, India
* Department of Microbiology, Vardhman Mahavir Medical College, Safdarjung Hospital, Safdarjung Enclave, Mahatama Gandhi Marg, New Delhi 110029, India.
E-mail address: chughtd@gmail.com

infections (STIs).[4] The term STI is now preferred because it covers all diseases that can be transmitted by sexual intercourse. However, for all practical purposes, STI and STD are used synonymously.[5] The term *reproductive tract infections* (RTIs) refers to infections that affect the reproductive tract and include STI, endogenous infections, and iatrogenic infections. Endogenous infections are probably the most common RTI worldwide and result from an overgrowth of organisms normally present in vagina and include bacterial vaginosis and candidiasis. There is growing evidence that the presence of bacterial vaginosis, like a number of STIs, can increase the risk of sexual transmission of HIV. Preliminary data have also suggested that bacterial vaginosis may increase perinatal transmission of HIV.

STI are more dynamic than other diseases prevailing in the community[5] and differ from other diseases for the following reasons:

- Their incubation periods are highly variable.
- There is no effective vaccine because the pathogens associated with STIs are genetically diverse.
- They are spread primarily by a behavior that is inherently resistant to change and varies considerably within and between social and ethnic groups.

STI have tremendous impact on national health. They are responsible for a significant proportion of maternal morbidity, fetal death, ectopic pregnancy, infertility, infant illness and death, malignancies (cancer of cervix, vulva, penis, and anus associated with human papilloma virus type 16 and 18 or with human herpes simplex virus 2), and increased susceptibility to human immunodeficiency virus (HIV) infection.

The epidemiologic profile of STI varies depending on ethnographic, demographic, socioeconomic, behavioral, and health factors. The incidence and clinical presentation of these diseases are also influenced by factors such as lifestyle and susceptibility of the individual, pathogenicity and interaction among pathogens, prevailing therapy, and preventive and control interventions.

Some STIs are easily treatable; however, many others are not. HIV/AIDS is perhaps the most serious sexually transmitted infection as it eventually leads to death. Among bacterial STIs, cure after appropriate antibiotic therapy is no longer certain for some infections such as gonorrhea and chancroid because of the increasing resistance of the microbes to antibiotics.

STI–HIV RELATIONSHIP

It is now well established that the presence of other STIs greatly facilitates the transmission and acquisition of HIV (**Box 1**). An individual with HIV eventually suffers damage of immune system, making him or her more susceptible to other infections, including STIs. Furthermore, STIs are more difficult to treat in these patients; for example, lesions associated with syphilis can last longer and single-dose treatment of chancroid may be less successful. Recurrent episodes of herpes simplex virus infection and *Candida* are also more frequent. As a result, an HIV-infected person is more likely to transmit HIV in subsequent unprotected sexual contact. The National AIDS Control Organization (NACO) of India has identified surveillance and prompt treatment of STI an important thrust area for HIV prevention in the country.[6]

GLOBAL TRENDS

Although substantial progress has been made in preventing, diagnosing, and treating certain STI in recent years; the Centers for Disease Control and Prevention (CDC) estimates that 19 million new infections occur each year, almost half of them among

Box 1 STI/RTI–HIV relationship		
Type of RTI	Increased Risk of HIV Transmission	Mechanism of HIV Transmission
Ulcerative STI • Syphilis • Chancroid	3–9 times	Because HIV is transmitted and acquired through direct contact of body fluids, presence of open sores and blisters/ulcers allows for greater contact and access to the blood stream for the virus.
Herpes simplex virus	2 times	
Inflammation causing STI • Gonorrhea • Chlamydia • Trichomoniasis	3–5 times	The infections increase genital shedding of HIV infected cells. In addition, urethral and endocervical infections that cause inflammation allow for more efficient exchange of infectious particles.
Bacterial vaginosis	1.5–2 times	

young people (15–24 years). In developed countries, there has been a steady increase in the rates of STIs, especially viral STIs and chlamydial infections. These agents, which may be regarded as the second generation of STIs, are frequently more difficult to identify, treat, and control.[7]

Chlamydia infection remains the most commonly reported infectious disease in the United States. It is estimated that there are approximately 2.8 million new cases each year. The increase in reported cases may be partly due to increased surveillance and use of sensitive diagnostic tests. Gonorrhea is the second most reported infectious disease in the United States. Following a 74% decline in the rate of reported gonorrhea from 1975 through 1977, overall gonorrhea rates appear to have reached a plateau. The rate of primary and secondary syphilis—the most infectious stages of the disease—decreased throughout the 1990s, and in 2000 reached an all-time low.[7] However, over the past 5 years syphilis in the United States has been increasing. Between 2004 and 2005, the national syphilis rate increased 11.1%. The rate of syphilis among men is nearly six times the rate among women. Also, more than half of syphilis cases in recent years have occurred in men who have sex with men (MSM).[7]

SEXUALLY TRANSMITTED INFECTIONS IN INDIA

In developing countries, STIs account for 10% to 20% of adult patients attending government health facilities.[8] In Delhi, between 1954 and 1994 the number of STI cases increased eight times. However, these figures are an underestimate because these infections are often treated by traditional healers, quacks, pharmacists, or private practitioners who are more accessible and less judgmental in their attitudes. Also, an inadequate epidemiologic surveillance system,[9] laboratory diagnostic facilities, and financial resources make it difficult to obtain a reliable estimate of the problem.

Socioeconomic Vulnerabilities

National demographic characteristics in India reflect an environment vulnerable for their transmission of STIs, including the following[9]:

- A young population, with 36% younger than 15 years.
- An unbalanced male/female ratio (a ratio of 1000:933 in the 2001 census), leading to a greater proportion of men in cities.

- An increasing pace of urbanization.
- A geographic disparity in the levels of economic development has led to selective migration of men from rural areas to urban destinations.
- Illiteracy: Figures for the most recent (2005–2006) National Family Health Survey show that 26% girls and 11% boys 15 to 19 years of age are illiterate.
- Gender disparity in education, literacy, employment, and health that results in women being disproportionately affected by risk of STI transmission.
- Poverty: A 1990s World Bank study of 50 low-income countries noted that eight structural and behavioral level variables could explain up to two thirds of the variation in HIV prevalence between countries.[10] India is a low-income country and has inequalities in income distribution.
- Other factors associated with increased disease burden are loss of traditional values of sexual behavior, increased sexual promiscuity, and failure to seek early medical treatment, thereby increasing the reservoir of infection.

Behavioral Risk Factors

The Human Rights Watch (HRW) reports that Indian female commercial sex workers (CSWs) are treated with contempt, Men who have sex with men (MSM) are severely marginalized and injecting drug use (IDU) is illegal. Because of complex social and political dynamics, reaching CSWs, MSM, and IDUs with STI/HIV prevention services remains a major challenge.

EPIDEMIOLOGY OF STIS/RTIS AND HIV IN INDIA

The exact burden of STIs in India remains relatively unknown. Community-based surveys are rarely undertaken due to epidemiologic diversity, high cost, and inadequate capacity.[11]

Burden of STI/RTI in the General Population

The prevalence of STI/RTI among the general population based on data of a Mid-Term Review (MTR) of the National AIDS Control Program III (NACP) of the studies conducted after 2000 is summarized in **Table 1**.[11] The studies highlight the following:

- **Rates of STI in general population were almost similar in urban and rural areas.** A large facility-based study from Delhi in 2002–2004 of symptomatic and asymptomatic women attending rural and urban peripheral health centers to determine the laboratory prevalence of STI and RTI was conducted.[12] A total of 4090 women in four study groups showed no significant difference in infection rates in women from urban (33.4%) and rural (30.9%) areas. Overall, in both urban and rural areas, *Candida* infection was predominant, followed by HSV-2 IgM, bacterial vaginosis (BV), and trichomoniasis.
- **A high proportion of STI/RTI identified by screening tests among the female general population were asymptomatic.** In a study from Chennai (2001),[13] only 33.3% and 22.5% of gonococcal and trichomonal infections respectively were symptomatic, whereas all chlamydial infections were asymptomatic. Similarly in a community-based STI prevalence study in Delhi (2002),[14] 31.2% of asymptomatic women had bacterial vaginosis.
- **Syphilis seropositivity.** All population-based surveys except the one from Delhi[11] showed that the prevalence of reactive syphilis serology (**Venereal Disease Research Laboratory Test/Rapid Plasma Reagin** Test confirmed by Treponema Pallidum Hemaglutination Assay/**Particle Agglutination Assay**) in

Table 1 Prevalence of STI/RTI in general population (%)	Females	Males
Clinical Examination: STI Syndrome		
Genital discharge	8–51	0.2–6.6
Genital ulcer	0–7.8	0.7–2
Lower abdominal pain/PID	0.6–37	—
Scrotal swelling	—	0–1.5
Inguinal swelling	—	0.3–1.7
Laboratory Investigations		
Syphilis	0–4.7	1–10.1
Gonorrhea	0–1.9	0–3.9
Chlamydia infection	0–1.3	0–1.1
Trichomoniasis	1.2–8	1.5–3.6
Candidiasis	7.2–23.9	—
Bacterial vaginosis	17.8–63.7	—
HSV-2 serology (IgG)	8.6–17.9	7–10.6
HIV	0–0.95	0–1.4

Data from National AIDS Control Programme III: report on mid-term review of sexually transmitted infection services. Available at: http://nacoonline.org/upload/STI%20RTI%20services/STI%20RTI%20 MONOGRAPH%20_NACP-III-.pdf. Accessed May 14, 2012. Findings from 25 studies for female and 15 for male general population are included.

the male general population was 2% or less, whereas in females it was 1.2% or less. Seroprevalence of syphilis among antenatal care (ANC) attendees in Delhi during 2003–2007 ranged from 0.1% to 11.3% and showed a consistently declining pattern.[15] Analysis of Computerized Management Information System data at the national level showed a declining trend in syphilis positivity in the ANC women from 1.7% in 2005–2006 to 0.8% in 2008–2009.[16]

- **Prevalence of *Neisseria gonorrhea* (NG) and *Chlamydia trachomatis* (CT).** In the female general population, prevalence of NG was 1.9% or less, and CT was 1.3% or less. In the male general population, although the prevalence of CT was low (<1.1%), the prevalence of NG infection was higher as compared to that in females (≤3.9%).
- **There is a considerable burden of RTI among the female general population.** Across studies, in women, the prevalence of candidiasis ranged from 7.2% to 23.9% and bacterial vaginosis, 17.8% to 63.7%.[11,17] Community-based prevalence studies in Delhi have shown variable RTI prevalence rates: candidiasis (16.9%–23.9%) and bacterial vaginosis (32.8%–63.7%).[11]A community-based cross-sectional study among 263 married women in Rajasthan (2002) detected a prevalence of candidiasis and bacterial vaginosis in 14% and 26% respectively. The study also showed that the prevalence of RTI was highest (76%) in women aged 30 to 34 years and lowest (33%) in those 15 to 19 years of age.
- **HSV-2 seropositivity (IgG)** was somewhat higher in women (8.6%–17.9%) compared to men (7%–10.6%) in the general population. A community-based cross-sectional survey in the tribal population of Central India (2004–2005)[10] showed a prevalence of HSV-2 IgG 20.8% in STI patients (males, 12%; females,

Table 2 Prevalence of STI/RTI in FSWs (%)	
Clinical Examination: STI Syndrome	%
Genital discharge	3.7–77.1
Genital ulcer	0–7.3
Lower abdominal pain/PID	0–33.9
Laboratory Investigations	**Females**
Syphilis	1.7–39.7
Gonorrhea	0–16.9
Chlamydia infection	0.9–22.6
Trichomoniasis	2–54
Candidiasis	8.9–25
Bacterial vaginosis	11.3–52.6
HSV-2 serology (IgG)	34.6–100
HIV	2.2–54

Data from National AIDS Control Programme III: report on mid-term review of sexually transmitted infection services. Available at: http://nacoonline.org/upload/STI%20RTI%20services/STI%20RTI%20MONOGRAPH%20_NACP-III-.pdf. Accessed May 14, 2012. Summary data derived from a total of 21 studies on FSW.

25.8%), compared to 7.3% in males and 17.9% in females . A recent study by the Indian Council of Medical Research (ICMR) (2006–2009) assessed the seroprevalence of HSV-2 in pregnant women in the northeastern states (Regional Medical Research Centre, Indian Council of Medical Research. Seroprevalence of HSV-2 in pregnant women in northeastern states, Unpublished data, 2012).

- The overall prevalence in 1640 pregnant women was 8.7%. The highest seropositivity was observed in the 18- to 24-year age group (49.3%), followed by the 25- to 29-year age group (29.6%).[18]

Burden of STI in Female CSWs

As per NACO estimates, 0.6% to 0.7% of the adult female urban population is engaged in transactional sex.[19] There are approximately 1.25 million female CSWs in India,[20] and the prevalence of STI/RTI is summarized in **Table 2**.[11] The prevalence varies in different parts of the country. In a study from Pune (1993–2002),[21] the prevalence of HIV infection remained stable (46% in 1993 and 50% in 2002; $P = .80$). The presence of genital ulcer disease decreased over time ($P<.001$) and the prevalence of syphilis increased during this period ($P = .001$).However, genital discharge diseases remained stable over a period of 10 years. In Gujarat, two rounds of population-based surveys during 1999–2003 showed a highly significant decline in the levels of trichomoniasis, gonorrhea, Chlamydia, and syphilis.[22] Integrated Behavioural and Biological Assessment (IBBA) studies conducted in Karnataka 2004 and 2009[23] showed that there was a reduction in the prevalence of HIV (19.6% vs 16.4%, $P = .04$); high-titer syphilis (5.9% vs 3.4%, $P = .001$); and chlamydia and/or gonorrhea (8.9% vs 7.0%, $P = .02$). The Frontiers Prevention Project (FPP) in Andhra Pradesh, based on two cross-sectional surveys conducted 4 years apart in female CSWs, showed reduction in various STI.[24]

Table 3 Prevalence of STI/RTI in MSM/transgender (%)	
	%
Clinical Examination: STI Syndrome	
Genital discharge	0–8.5
Genital ulcer	0–7.3
Scrotal swelling	0.7
Inguinal swelling	0–0.6
Warts/*Condyloma acuminata*	0.3–5.9
Laboratory Investigations	
Syphilis	MSM: 3–17 TG: 16.5–57
Gonorrhea	Oropharyngeal: 0.9–4.7 Rectal: 1.9–11.1 Urethral: 1.6–6.3
Chlamydia infection	0.6–4.0
Trichomoniasis	0.3–1.3
HSV-2 serology (IgG)	16–61.5
HIV	MSM: 2.2–54 TG: 12–68

Data from National AIDS Control Programme III: report on mid-term review of sexually transmitted infection services. Available at: http://nacoonline.org/upload/STI%20RTI%20services/STI%20RTI%20 MONOGRAPH%20_NACP-III-.pdf. Accessed May 14, 2012. Summary data derived from a total of 13 studies on MSM.

Burden of STI in MSM and Transgender

There is an estimated 2.35 million MSM (including 0.24 million male/transgender sex workers) in India. The data of 13 studies on MSM from India are shown in **Table 3**.[11] Syphilis and HIV seroprevalence is higher in transgender as compared to MSM. While prevalence of chlamydial infection is low in the MSM population, a significant percent of MSM suffered from oropharyngeal and rectal gonorrhea (4.7% and 7.4% respectively). HSV-2 seropositivity (IgG) is also high among these groups. In a study among STI clinic attendees in Pune (1993–2002) in MSM, 18.9% were HIV positive, 21.5% had genital ulcer disease, 5.8% had syphilis, and 4.3% had gonorrhea. Over the decade, neither HIV nor NG prevalence changed among MSM, but syphilis and genital ulcer disease decreased significantly.[25] Two rounds of population-based studies in Gujarat, conducted during 2004 and 2006,[11] showed that except for trichomoniasis, there was a significant decline in all STIs.

CURRENT STATUS OF THE HIV EPIDEMIC IN INDIA

The HIV/AIDS was first recognized in India in 1986. In 2008, an estimated 2.27 million people between the ages of 15 and 49 years were living with HIV (PLHIV).[26] In India, infection may be due to HIV-1 or the less pathogenic HIV-2. Of persons infected with HIV in India, fewer than 5% have been reported due to HIV-2 and dual infection due to HIV-1 and -2 is seen in 3.3% to 20.1%, being more common in IDU in eastern states of India. HIV-1 subtype C is predominant, while HIV-1 A/C recombinants have been described in Maharashtra. In the northeastern states, other subtypes, that is, subtypes B', E, C, and B'/C recombinants are reported.[27] The epidemic in India shows an overall declining trend. HIV prevalence among adult population declined from 0.34% in 2007 to 0.29% in 2008. There is also a declining number of PLHIV in the country, from 2.73 million in 2002 to 2.27 million in 2008. Women account for 39% while children account for 3.8% of PLHA.

Analyses of information from approximately 300,000 HIV-positive persons show unprotected heterosexual sex as the principal mode of HIV. In 2009–2010, this mode of transmission accounted for 87% of all reported HIV cases. In 5.4%, the route of transmission was from mother to child, whereas 1.5% of all HIV cases reported homosexual sex and 1.6% were IDUs. Thus, the primary drivers of the HIV epidemic in India are unprotected paid/commercial sex, unprotected anal sex between men, and IDUs. It is estimated that there are 1.26 million female CSWs, 351,000 high-risk MSM, and 186,000 IDUs in India. Given that condom use is not optimal or consistent in many places, men who buy sex or clients of sex workers are the single most powerful driving force in India's HIV epidemic. As more than 90% of women acquire HIV infection from their husbands or their intimate sexual partners, they are at increased risk for HIV not due to their own sexual behavior, but because they are partners of men who are within a high-risk group (HRG).

HIV in India shows geographic variance. Six states (Andhra Pradesh, Karnataka, Maharashtra, Manipur, Nagaland, and Manipur) with high HIV prevalence account for an approximate 66% of the HIV burden. India has 195 priority districts identified according to the prevailing HIV prevalence rates for focused programmatic interventions. [28] Of these, 156 districts are category A with a 1% or lower prevalence among ANC attendees. Another 39 districts are category B with lower than 1% but 5% or greater prevalence among HRGs. Among sex workers, there is a decline of HIV in south Indian states, indicating a possible impact of interventions, while rising trends are evident in the northeast, suggesting a dual nature of the epidemic. Fifty-five districts have shown greater than 5% HIV prevalence among female CSWs in 2008–2009.

The latest round of surveillance provides evidence that although there is an overall decline in adult HIV prevalence—particularly in the high-prevalence states—there is an increase in many of the low-prevalence states. A steady decline in HIV prevalence among female CSWs has been noted, HIV prevalence among MSM is stable, and a varied trend in prevalence has emerged among IDUs.

ANTIBIOTIC RESISTANCE

Antibiotic resistance in etiologic pathogens associated with STIs could pose an important obstacle in their control. There have been reports of drug resistance, particularly in *Neisseria gonorrheae*, herpes simplex virus, and HIV. The emerging drug resistance warrants constant monitoring, a need to look at new drugs, and a change of operative plans to control the spread of STDs.

Neisseria gonorrheae

Over the last decade, *N. gonorrheae* isolates have developed a high level of resistance against several antimicrobial agents such as sulfonamides, penicillin, tetracycline, and quinolones, posing an increasing problem in its management.

In India, the majority of the studies on antibiotic resistance of *N. gonorrhea* have been conducted in North India and tertiary referral centers. The data generated may not be indicative of antibiotic susceptibility pattern at the community level. A Gonococcal Antimicrobial Susceptibility Program (GASP) under the WHO Southeast Asia Region became functional in 1997. Antimicrobial resistance patterns of *N. gonorrheae* were studied in seven different focal-point laboratories using the National

Committee for Clinical Laboratory Standards (NCCLS/CLSI) method or calibrated dichotomous sensitivity (CDS) technique, using high- and low-potency discs, respectively. Penicillinase-producing *N. gonorrheae* (PPNG) were reported from all seven laboratories and varied between 20% and 79%. PPNG were reported from Delhi (10%), Nagpur (13.5%), and the WHO Regional Reference Laboratory (RRL), New Delhi (26.8%). Resistance to ciprofloxacin was reported from all the laboratories and varied considerably (11%–100%).[29]

The regular monitoring of antimicrobial susceptibility has been conducted at the Regional STD Center (RRL) since 1995.[30] Data of the first 14 years (1995–2008) have documented the pattern of antimicrobial resistance in highlighting the alarming increase in ciprofloxacin and penicillin resistance. Ciprofloxacin resistance increased from 3.4% in 1996 to 83.3% in 2008. PPNG strains varied from 3.4% to 35.1%. A rising trend was observed in the isolation of tetracycline-resistant *N. gonorrheae* (TRNG), from 1.7% in 1996 to 19.3% in 2008. Ceftriaxone less susceptible strains were detected for the first time in 2001. Only nine isolates were found to be less sensitive to ceftriaxone during 2002 to 2006. These isolated were always resistant to quinolones and penicillin. All isolates were found to be sensitive to spectinomycin except one in 2002. The frequency of multiresistant isolates was 23.3%. However, there were considerable differences in the rates of quinolone resistance in different studies in India.[30]

Decreased susceptibility to third-generation cephalosporins, cefixime, and ceftriaxone, is being observed in an increasing proportion of gonococcal isolates submitted to Gonococcal Resistance to Antimicrobials Surveillance Programme—England and Wales (GRASP).[31] In 2009, 0.3% of GRASP isolates exhibited decreased susceptibility to ceftriaxone (minimum inhibitory concentration [MIC] $\geq$.125 mg/mL), and 1.2% to cefixime (MIC $\geq$.25 mg/mL) and this figure was 10.6% for cefixime at the slightly lower cutoff of MIC $\geq$.125 mg/mL. Gonococcal isolates reported as "less sensitive" to ceftriaxone were described in India as early as 1999. However, in all 10 patients from RRL, having strains less susceptible to ceftriaxone, responded to treatment with ceftriaxone or cefixime. Treatment failures are documented with oral third-generation cephalosporins such as cefixime, cefdinir, and ceftibuten from some countries but not as yet with ceftriaxone.[31]

The first-line treatment currently recommended for *N. gonorrheae* is a single 400-mg oral dose of cefixime or a 250-mg intramuscular dose of ceftriaxone. The use of quinolone antibiotics for the treatment of gonorrhea has been discontinued in India because of reported high levels of resistance.[11] Pharmacodynamic modeling suggests that therapeutic failures will occur with current treatment regimens (400 mg cexifime, 250 mg ceftriaxone), because peak serum concentrations are not maintained for a sufficient time period to eradicate gonococci with MICs of 0.125 mg/L or greater. The British Association for Sexual Health and HIV has issued new draft guidelines, which recommends ceftriaxone 500 mg IM (up from 250 mg) as the first-line treatment; cefixime 400 mg oral as second-line treatment, only in cases in which injections are refused or contraindicated; and co-treatment with 1 g of azithromycin in all cases regardless of chlamydial infection status. Test of cure is recommended in all cases.[31]

Spectinomycin, an alternative drug of choice for cases resistant or hypersensitive to cephalosporins, is not easily available in India, and this may explain the retention of efficacy of this antibiotic in *N. gonorrheae*. Resistance to spectinomycin usually occurs via single-step chromosomal mutation, resulting in high-level resistance. Resistance in other bacterial, parasitic, and viral agents associated with STIs have

Box 2
Reports of resistance to other bacterial and parasitic and viral agents associated with STI reported in literature with limited or no reports from India

Pathogen	Resistance Reports
H. ducreyi	Sulphonamides, penicillins, tetracycline
Herpes simplex virus	Acylovir
Treponema pallidum	Clinical resistance to penicillin in neurosyphilis
Human papilloma virus-6	Interferon-α
Chlamydia trachomatis	Tetracycline, azithromycin, and ofloxacin
Trichomonas vaginalis	Metronidazole
HIV	Zidovudine, nucleoside analogue reverse transcriptase, protease inhibitors

From Sharma M, Sethi S. Drug resistance in sexually transmitted diseases. In: Sharma VK, editor. Textbook of sexually transmitted diseases and HIV/AIDS. New Delhi (India): Viva Books; 2009. p. 610–18.

been reported in the literature (**Box 2**).[32] However, there are no significant reports from India.

DIAGNOSIS AND POINT-OF-CARE TESTING

The syndromic approach works well with men but in women it has proved less effective. Studies in several developing countries have shown that syndromic management of women with the common complaint of vaginal discharge is neither sensitive nor specific in identifying women who have an STI.[33]

It is not sensitive because most women with STIa have no symptoms. It is not specific because most women who complain of vaginal discharge are not suffering from an STI but from bacterial vaginosis or candidiasis. Low specificity, resulting in overtreatment on a massive scale, is a particular drawback in populations with a low prevalence of STIs but a high prevalence of symptomatic vaginal discharge, as is often found in Asia. Attempts to improve the performance of the syndromic management flowchart for vaginal discharge by use of simple laboratory tests, such as microscopy and the leucocyte esterase dipstick, which detects pus cells in urine, have not been very successful.[33]

Point-of-Care Testing

A wide range of tests for the diagnosis of STI are now on the market. Nucleic acid amplification tests are commercially available for the diagnosis of Chlamydia trachomatis and Neisseria gonorrheae infection. These tests are highly sensitive and specific, and have become the "gold standard." These tests are expensive and technically demanding.

As part of WHO 2001 Sexually Transmitted Diseases Diagnostics Initiative, the organization explored the need for simple, affordable, point-of-care (POC) STI testing for curable bacterial STIs, including syphilis, gonorrhea, and chlamydial infection.[34] The focus of the initiative was the need in the developing world for diagnosis and treatment of these common STI in a single health care visit through the use of rapid testing. Diagnosis and treatment in a single visit is an important step in areas where limited health care facilities and transportation can make return visits for test results difficult and treatment improbable. Diagnosis of patients based on POC testing leads to treatment of more infected patients, ultimately decreasing transmission.[35] However, a rapid test that has a low sensitivity, more infected patients will be falsely reassured by a negative test result, which could increase the number of people exposed. False-negative test results can be problematic particularly in women, in whom untreated bacterial endocervical infections can progress to become pelvic inflammatory disease, which has serious long-term fertility sequelae. Another consequence of false-negative tests that lead to untreated STI is the increased risk patients have for acquiring HIV infection when bacterial STIs are present. Alternatively, if clinics use a rapid test that has a low specificity, it will result in a high number of false-positive results. False-positive tests for bacterial STI result in the administration of antibiotics to noninfected patients, potentially increasing the rates of antibiotic resistance. False-positive STI tests also can be psychologically detrimental to patients through the stigma of STI or from undermining an intimate relationship when confronting a partner.

Accordingly, WHO developed the ASSURED criteria for evaluating new rapid diagnostic tests. The following are the seven ASSURED criteria[35]:

A Affordable
S Sensitive (probability of infected patients testing positive for the disease)
S Specific (probability of noninfected patients testing negative for the disease)
U User friendly (easily performed in a few steps with minimal training)
R Rapid and robust (results available in <30 minutes)
E Equipment free
D Deliverable to those who need them

In assessing the sensitivity and specificity of a new rapid test, it should be compared against the gold standard for that particular infection.

The rapid tests are currently available for five common STI: syphilis, gonorrhea, chlamydial infection, HIV, and genital herpes. Most rapid tests are based on the principle of immunochromatography, in which antigen–antibody reactions are trapped on the strips and appear as colored lines or spots on membrane strips. For genital chlamydial and gonococcal infections the diagnostic target is antigen, and for syphilis and viral STIs the target is antibody. Most rapid tests are designed for room temperature storage, can be performed in less than 30 minutes with minimal training, and require little or no equipment. Availability of these rapid tests at different health care centers can facilitate STI management in India where, as per NACO reports wet mount examination, Gram stain, VDRL/RPR, HIV, and hepatitis B tests were available in 60% to 100% of district hospitals but were largely not available at community health centers.[33]

The majority of patients who have syphilis, are asymptomatic, and serologic testing is required to make a diagnosis. Rapid syphilis testing has been developed and is being implemented in developing countries. Currently there are two varieties of rapid syphilis tests, both of which are treponema-specific tests that use *Treponema pallidum* antigens to provide a visual test result:

1. The immunochromatographic tests (ICTs) work by using a test strip that is impregnated with treponemal antigens that react with antibodies to syphilis in whole blood or serum to produce a readable change on the test strip.
2. Particle agglutination tests use gelatin particles coated with treponemal antigens that clump together on a test tray when combined with whole blood or serum containing antibodies to syphilis.

The rapid tests cannot distinguish active infection from previously treated infection.[33] Thus, in areas with a high prevalence of syphilis, the test returns more positive results because there are more people who have prior treated infections and test positive. In settings with patients at high risk for syphilis and poor follow-up care, rapid testing with same-day treatment may offset the risk for overtreatment from tests positive from prior infections. However, due to associated serious sequelae of congenital syphilis, CDC recommends rapid screening and treatment for positive tests at the first prenatal visit in populations "in which use of prenatal care is not optimal."[35] Similarly rapid tests are available for other STIs and **Table 4** lists the tests available and their estimated performance characteristics.

PREVENTION AND CONTROL OF STIS

The National STD Control Program was initiated in 1946 (before the establishment of independent India) and was in operation until 1991. The program focused on the health-seeking behavior of individuals with STDs and on combating social stigma associated with these infections. With the emergence of HIV epidemic, the Government of India initiated a program of prevention and raising awareness of HIV/AIDS under the Medium Term Plan (1990–1992), the first plan (NACP-I, 1992–1999), and the second plan (NACP-II, 1999–2006) followed by ongoing NACP-III. Currently the NACP-III programmatic response to address prevention, management, and control of STI largely falls under the National Reproductive and Child Health (RCH 2) program, which was launched in 2005. The program draws its mandate from the National Population Policy (2000), which makes a strong reference "to include STD/RTI and HIV/AIDS prevention, screening and management in maternal and child health services." As a part of NACP-III, a Mid-Term Review (MTR) of the program was performed in 2009. The findings are important to formulate targeted interventions and strengthening and implementating the STD control program in India.

1. There were some missed opportunities for syphilis screening at the STI and ANC clinics. Only 30% of new STI clinic attendees were screened for syphilis. Syphilis screening of pregnant women was reported for 30% to 50% of those attending ANC services. Only 10% of the new STI clinic attendees were referred for HIV testing.
2. Though screening had been performed only for a small proportion of those attending STI and ANC clinics, there was a definite decline in syphilis seropositivity.
3. The genital ulcer disease/urethral discharge (GUD/UD) ratio revealed that there was a geographical diversity in the distribution of STI. A higher overall GUD/UD ratio indicates that reservoirs of infections still persist.
4. Syndromic diagnosis showed higher nonherpetic to herpetic GUD, indicating that there is still a preponderance of treatable bacterial STI in various states.

The major objectives of the current STD Control Program are to reduce STD cases and control HIV transmission and to prevent short- and long-term morbidity and mortality due to STDs. To strengthen implementation of the National STD control and preventive program the following steps have been recommended[10]:

- Build capacity of targeted interventions for STI service delivery to HRGs in terms of training, drug procurement, infrastructure, outreach, provider attitudes, and accessibility.
- Ensure optimal synergy with NRHM through regular convergence meetings at the national and state levels for STI program planning and service quality.
- Review and strengthen systems for supportive supervision and monitoring at STI service delivery sites, including availability of appropriate drugs, and ensure appropriate documentation.

Table 4
Rapid tests for diagnosis of STIs

Condition	Type	Target	Specimens	Sensitivity	Specificity	Comments
Chlamydia trachomatis infection	Immunochromatographic strips	Antigen	Urethral, cervical swabs	50%–75%	98%–99%	Performance compared with NAAT and/or culture
Neisseria gonorrheae infection	Gram stain	Morphology	Urethral, cervical swabs	>90% M (male) 45%–65% (female)	>95% (male) 90%–95% (female)	Performance compared with culture
	Immunochromatographic strips	Antigen	Urethral, cervical swabs	50%–70%	98%–99%	Performance compared with culture
Trichomonas vaginalis infection	Wet mount	Motile trichomonad	Vaginal secretions	50%–70%	99%–100%	Performance compared with culture
Bacterial vaginosis	Gram stain Wet mount	Clue cells Clue cells	Vaginal swab Vaginal secretions	Not known 38%–70%	Not known 90%–95%	Performance compared with Nugent score
	Card test	Proline amino-peptidase	Vaginal swab	93%	93%	
Syphilis	Non–*Treponema*-specific tests	Antibody	Serum	90%–98%	90%–95%	Requires centrifuge and rotator
	Treponema-specific tests	Antibody	Serum, plasma, or whole blood	90%–99%	99%–100%	Current and past infection indistinguishable
	Dark-field microscopy	Motile spirochaete	Lesion material	<50%	95%–100%	Requires special microscope, not useful in latent syphilis
Herpes simplex virus type 2	Immunochromatographic strips	Antibody	Serum	96%	98%	Performance compared with culture and sensitivity and immunoblot for specificity

- Strengthen implementation of 100% syphilis screening and treatment of all ANC women and HRG populations. Besides laboratory strengthening for implementation of 100% syphilis screening, HIV screening and syphilis screening should be integrated in STI clinics. To ensure quality of syphilis screening, at least one microbiology department per state should be upgraded to provide laboratory support to STI clinics.
- Consider using WHO approved POC testing technologies for syphilis to improve coverage of syphilis screening among ANC women and HRGs.
- Increase involvement of nongovernmental organization (NGO) and link worker roles in STI programming for improving health care–seeking behavior, and in identification and referrals to the program.
- Improve uptake of STI services. Health care–seeking behavior can be improved by raising awareness of STI and promoting early treatment at medical facilities. In addition, routine counseling should include a focus on STIs.
- Strengthen capacities in the regional STI research and training reference centers to undertake operational research by providing the necessary training, infrastructure, and equipment.

REFERENCES

1. Centers for Disease Control and Prevention (CDC). Summary of notifiable diseases in the United States, 1996. MMWR Morb Mortal Wkly Rep 1997;45:1–87.
2. World Health Organization (WHO). World Health Report. Geneva (Switzerland): WHO, 2001.
3. Laga M, Nzila N, Goeman J. The interrelationship of sexually transmitted diseases and HIV infection: implications for the control of both epidemics in Africa. AIDS 1991; 5(Suppl. 1):S55–S63.
4. Judson F. Introduction. In: Kumar B, Gupta S, editors. Sexually transmitted infections. 1st edition. New Delhi (India): Elsevier; 2005. p. 1–4.
5. Sharma VK, Khandpur S. Changing patterns of sexually transmitted infections in India. Natl Med J India 2004;17:310–9.
6. National AIDS Control Organization, India. Programme priorities and thrust areas: 2007. Available at: http://www.nacoonline.org. Accessed January 15, 2012.
7. Centers for Disease Control and Prevention (CDC). Trends in reportable sexually transmitted diseases in United States, 2005. Available at: http://www.cdc.gov/std/stats/trends2005.htm. Accessed January 15, 2012.
8. Arya OP, Lawson JB. Sexually transmitted diseases in tropics: epidemiological, diagnostic, therapeutic and control aspects. Trop Doct 1977;7:51–6.
9. Hawkes S, Santhya KG. Diverse realities: understanding sexually transmitted infections and HIV in India. Working paper series. New Delhi (India): Population Council; 2001.
10. Anvikar AR, Rao VG. Seroprevalence of sexually transmitted viruses in the tribal population of Central India. Int J Infect Dis 2009;13(1):37–9.
11. National AIDS Control Programme III. Report on mid-term review of sexually transmitted infection services. Available at: http://nacoonline.org/upload/STI%20RTI%20services/STI%20RTI%20MONOGRAPH%20_NACP-III-.pdf. Accessed January 15, 2012.
12. Ray K, Bala M, Bhattacharya M, et al. Prevalence of RTI/STI agents and HIV infection in symptomatic and asymptomatic women attending peripheral health set-ups in Delhi, India. Epidemiol Infect 2008;136:1432–40.

13. Panchanadeswaran S, Johnson SC, Mayer KH, et al. Gender differences in the prevalence of sexually transmitted infections and genital symptoms in an urban setting in southern India. Sex Transm Infect 2006;82(6):491–5.

14. Bhalla R, Sodhani P. Prevalence of bacterial vaginosis among women in Delhi, India. Indian J Med Res 2007;125(2):167–72.

15. HIV Sentinel Surveillance and HIV Estimation in India 2007. A technical brief. Available at: http://www.nacoonline.org. Accessed January 15, 2012.

16. National AIDS Control Organization (NACO). CMIS bulletin. Available at: http://www.nacoonline.org/upload/Publication/M&E%20Surveillance,%20Research/Quarterly%20CMIS%20Bulletin%20April-Sept%2008%20Bookmark.pdf. Accessed January 15, 2012.

17. Madhivananan P, Batman MT, Pasulti L, et al. Prevalence of *Trichomonas vaginalis* infection among young reproductive age females in India: implications of therapy and prevention. Sexual Health 2009;6:339–44.

18. Chandrasekaran P, Dallabetta G, Loo V, et al. Containing HIV/AIDS in India: the unfinished agenda. Lancet Infect Dis 2006;6:508–21.

19. National Behavioral Surveillance Survey (BSS). 2006. Available at: http://www.nacoonline.org. Accessed January 15, 2012.

20. National AIDS Control Programme Phase III. 2006–2011. Report of the Expert Group on Size Estimation of Population with High Risk Behavior November 30, 2006. National AIDS Control Organization Ministry of Health and Family Welfare, Government of India, New Delhi, India.

21. Brahme R, Mehta S, Sahay S, et al. Correlates and trend of HIV prevalence among female sex workers attending sexually transmitted disease clinics in Pune, India (1993–2002). J Acquir Immune Defic Syndr 2006;41(1):107–13.

22. Talsania NJ, Rathod D, Shah R, et al. STI/HIV prevalence in Sakhi Swasthya Abhiyan, Jyotisangh, Ahmedabad: a clinico-epidemiological study. Indian J Sex Transm Dis 2007;28:15–8.

23. Hernandez AL, Lindan CP, Mathur M, et al. Sexual behavior among men who have sex with women, men, and Hijras in Mumbai, India—multiple sexual risks. AIDS Behav 2006;10(4 Suppl):S5–16.

24. Gutierrez J, McPherson S, Fakoya A, et al. Community-based prevention leads to an increase in condom use and a reduction in sexually transmitted infections (STIs) among men who have sex with men (MSM) and female sex workers (FSW): the Frontiers Prevention Project (FPP) evaluation results. BMC Public Health 2010;10:497.

25. Gupta A, Mehta S, Godbole SV, et al. Same-sex behavior and high rates of HIV among men attending sexually transmitted infection clinics in Pune, India (1993–2002). J Acquir Immune Defic Syndr 2006;43(4):483–90.

26. UNGASS Country Progress Report 2010, India. Available at: http://www.unaids.org/en/dataanalysis/monitoringcountryprogress/2010progressreportssubmittedbycountries/india_2010_country_progress_report_en.pdf. Accessed January 15, 2012.

27. Ying-Ru J Lo, Shetty P, Reddy DSC, et al. Controlling the HIV/AIDS epidemic in India. Available at: http://whoindia.org/LinkFiles/Commision_on_Macroeconomic_and_Health.

28. HIV Sentinel Surveillance and HIV Estimation in India 2007. A technical brief. Available at: http://www.nacoonline. Accessed January 15, 2012.

29. Ray K, Bala M, Kumari S, et al. Antimicrobial resistance of *Neisseria gonorrheae* in selected World Health Organization Southeast Asia Region countries: an overview. Sex Transm Dis 2005;32(3):178–84.

30. Bala M. Antimicrobial resistance in *Neisseria gonorrheae* in South-East Asia. Regional Health Forum 2011;15(1):63–73.

31. Lowndes C. STI global update. Newsletter of the International Union against Sexually Transmitted Infections. Available at: http://www.iust.org. Accessed January 15, 2012.

32. Sharma M, Sethi S. Drug resistance in sexually transmitted diseases. In: Sharma VK, editor. Textbook of sexually transmitted diseases and HIV/AIDS. New Delhi (India): Viva Books; 2009. p. 610–8.

33. Mabey D, Peeling WR. Rapid diagnostic tests for sexually transmitted infections. IPPF Med Bull 2002;36(3):1–3.

34. Peeling RW, Holmes KK, Mabey D, et al. Rapid tests for sexually transmitted infection (STIs): the way forward. Sex Transm Infect 2006;82(Suppl V):1–6.

35. Greer L, Wendel GD Jr. Rapid diagnostic methods in sexually transmitted infections. Infect Dis Clin N Am 2008;22:601–17.

Viral Hepatitis in India

Priya Abraham, MD, PhD

KEYWORDS

- Viral hepatitis • India • Water-borne epidemics • Injection practices
- Blood donor

KEY POINTS

- Hepatitis in India is caused mainly by hepatitis A virus (HAV), hepatitis B virus (HBV), hepatitis C virus (HCV), and hepatitis E virus (HEV).
- HAV infection occurs frequently in children, though in parts of India there is an evolving epidemiology.
- HEV is the most common cause of acute sporadic hepatitis in India and has been associated with several large-scale epidemics in the past.
- India belongs to the intermediate endemicity zone for HBV carriers. HBV is the major cause of chronic liver disease and liver cancer. Horizontal transmission of HBV plays an important role. Genotypes D, A, and C have been reported in India.
- HCV is transmitted mainly through suboptimal blood banking and injection practices in India. Genotype 3 is the most predominant, followed by genotype 1.

Viral hepatitis is a major public health problem in India, caused mainly by hepatitis viruses A through E.[1] Though both of the enterically transmissible viruses, hepatitis A virus (HAV) and hepatitis E virus (HEV), are hyperendemic in India, it is HEV that has been the leading cause of past epidemics and sporadic acute and fulminant hepatitis among adults.[2–10] Frequent exposure to HAV in childhood leads to 90% to 100% seropositivity by adolescence.[11–13] However, in recent years, changing trends in exposure to HAV are being increasingly reported.[14]

After HEV, HBV is the second most common causative agent of acute, subacute, and fulminant hepatitis in India.[15] HBV is the major cause of chronic liver disease (CLD) among Indian patients.[16] The overall hepatitis B surface antigen (HBsAg) prevalence rate for India constitutes an intermediate HBV endemicity.[17] Hepatitis C virus (HCV) rarely causes acute icteric hepatitis but is the leading cause of post-transfusion hepatitis in the country. Hepatitis D virus (HDV) coinfection and superinfection appear to be infrequent among various populations studied in the country.[18]

The full burden of illness due to fulminant hepatitis, chronic infection, cirrhosis, liver failure, and hepatocellular carcinoma (HCC) in India is not fully known. Based on data

The author has nothing to disclose.
Department of Clinical Virology, Christian Medical College, Vellore 632 004, Tamil Nadu, India
E-mail address: priyaabraham@cmcvellore.ac.in

Clin Lab Med 32 (2012) 159–174
http://dx.doi.org/10.1016/j.cll.2012.03.003   labmed.theclinics.com
0272-2712/12/$ – see front matter © 2012 Elsevier Inc. All rights reserved.

Box 1
Summary of HAV in India

- Causes a mild self-limiting hepatitis.
- Is an enterically transmitted virus.
- Chronic infection does not occur.
- India is hyperendemic for HAV.
- Frequent exosure in childhood makes 90%–100% immune by adolescence.
- A changing epidemiology is seen in some segments of the population.
- Mortality due to HAV infection is low.
- Safe, effective vaccine available; universal use in India still debated.

---

from hospitals in India, about 250,000 people die annually of viral hepatitis or its sequelae.[18] To realize the true burden and take appropriate public health measures, there is a need to establish a hepatitis registry nationally.

HEPATITIS A VIRUS

HAV belongs to a novel genus, *Hepatovirus*, and virus family *Picornaviridae*. In developing countries such as India, HAV infection in early childhood is mostly asymptomatic or mildly symptomatic (**Box 1**).[13] However, in children with dual infection with HAV and HEV, which is not uncommon, acute liver failure can result.[19] A recent overview of the seropositivity profile among children and adults suggests an epidemiologic shift in certain geographic areas and populations in the country.[14] Recent epidemics and seroepidemiologic studies show a consistent decline in childhood seroprevalence, with an increasing number of susceptible older children and young adults to HAV.[14] Outbreaks of HAV infections are thus likely to occur in cleaner environments with better standards of living. However, heterogeneous pockets of exposed and susceptible persons probably coexist within a region that makes the decision about universal HAV vaccination a complex one.

The HAV seroprevalence among high-risk groups such as those with preexisting chronic liver disease is not significantly different from that among those without chronic liver disease, suggesting that routine vaccination in these groups is not warranted.[13,20] Mathur and Arora[14] have suggested that the cost of vaccination and screening a given population as well as the HAV seroprevalence of the population be taken into account before HAV vaccination programs are planned.

Screening for acute HAV-related hepatitis is achieved by various immunoglobulin M (IgM) anti-HAV enzyme-linked immunosorbent assays (ELISAs) (**Table 1**). Seroprevalence in a community is measured by employing anti-HAV or total antibody detection ELISA. HAV RNA testing is rarely used in a diagnostic setting but can be very useful in an outbreak setting to identify the source of infection and take appropriate measures.

HEPATITIS B VIRUS

On the global scale, India is in the intermediate endemicity range for HBV infection; the HBV carrier rate is between 2% and 7%.[16,17] HBV carriers are those who are positive for hepatitis B surface antigen (HBsAg) for 6 months or longer (see **Table 1**). HBsAg is also the most widely used marker used in India to screen for HBV infection. Considering an earlier estimated average carrier rate of 5%,[17] the projected burden of carriers in this country is more than 50 million. India thereby harbors the second

Table 1
Nomenclature for common hepatitis viruses and summary of viral hepatitis markers

Disease	Causative Agent	Diagnostic Marker	Interpretation
Hepatitis A	HAV	HAV RNA	Detectable in stool/serum, even before symptoms. Useful to investigate outbreaks.
		IgM anti-HAV	IgM antibodies to HAV. Indicates current or recent infection. Positive for 4–6 mo after infection.
		Anti-HAV	Total (mainly IgG) antibodies to HAV. Persists for many years. Used to study seroprevalence.
Hepatitis B	HBV	HBV DNA	Most sensitive marker of HBV replication. HBV DNA titers used to monitor individuals on antiviral therapy.
		HBsAg	Hepatitis B surface antigen—detectable in large quantity in serum. Most common marker used to screen carriers.
		HBeAg	Hepatitis B e antigen—high titers associated with high levels of replication and increased infectivity of serum.
		HBcAg	Hepatitis B core antigen—seen only within hepatocytes.
		IgM anti-HBc	IgM antibodies to the hepatitis B core antigen. Indicates current or recent infection. Positive for 4–6 mo after infection.
		Anti-HBe	Antibody to the HBeAg. Usually suggest lower titer of HBV in liver.
		Anti-HBc	Total (mainly IgG) antibodies to hepatitis B core antigen. Indicates exposure (current or past) to HBV.
		Anti-HBs	Antibody to hepatitis B surface antigen. Indicates immunity from past infection or HBV vaccination.
Hepatitis C	HCV	HCV RNA	Earliest marker of acute HCV infection. In chronic infection, continue to be detectable. HCV RNA titers used to monitor individuals on antiviral therapy.
		Anti-HCV	Antibody to HCV. Indicates exposure (current or past) to HCV. Most common marker used to screen carriers.
Hepatitis D	HDV	HDV RNA	Most sensitive marker of current HDV infection—detected using RT-PCR.
		HDV antigen	Hepatitis D virus or delta antigen. Antigenemia is seen in acute infection and persists in chronic HDV infection.
		IgM anti-HDV	IgM antibodies to the hepatitis D virus. Seen in acute HDV infection.
		Anti-HDV	Total (mainly IgG) antibodies to HDV. Indicates past or current infection.
Hepatitis E	HEV	HEV RNA	Detectable in stool/serum, even before symptoms. Viremia may last for a week to a month.
		IgM anti-HEV	IgM antibodies to HEV. Indicates current or recent infection. Positive for 3–6 mo after illness.
		Anti-HEV	Total (mainly IgG) antibodies to HEV. Indicates past or current infection. Titers may decline with time.

Table 2

A. Studies of HBsAg prevalence in the general population in India

Region	References	Technique	No. of Subjects	% HBsAg Positive
North India	Uppal et al[95]	ELISA	260	10.4
East India	Chowdhury et al[96]	ELISA	7653	2.97
West India	Bhagyalakshmi et al[97]	ELISA	702	1.42
South India	Singh et al[98]	ELISA	737	3.3
South India	Singh et al[98]	ELISA	816	4.2
South India	Kurien et al[99]	ELISA	1981	5.75

B. Studies of HBsAg prevalence in blood donors

Region	References	Technique	No. of Subjects	% HBsAg Positive
North India	Nanu et al[100,b]	Enzyme immunoassay	132,093	2.5
North India	Pahuja et al[101,b]	ELISA	28,956	2.23
North India	Meena et al[102,b]	ELISA	94,716	1.43
East India	Das et al[103,a]	ELISA	3745	2.25
West India	Elavia et al[104]	ELISA	3455	2.0
West India	Satoskar and Ray[105,b]	ELISA	3104	4.7
West India	Nijhawan et al[106,a]	ELISA	69,330	2.1–3.1
South India	Singhvi et al[107,b]	ELISA	8569	0.7–3.8
South India	Singh et al[108,b]	ELISA	30,428	0.62

[a] Volunteer blood donors.
[b] Volunteer and replacement blood donors.

largest pool of HBV carriers in the world. Chronic HBV infection can lead to the development of liver cirrhosis and HCC, thus constituting a major public health problem for this country.

HBV prevalence has been studied in the normal population, blood donor population, pregnant women, and also high-risk individuals. Earlier studies had utilized less sensitive techniques such as gel diffusion, immunoelectrophoresis, and counterimmunoelectrophoresis. In the 1990s screening assays evolved to reverse passive hemagglutination (RPHA) and finally radioimmunoassay (RIA) or ELISA. HBsAg prevalence rates in the normal population and among blood donors using ELISA for screening ranges between 1.42% and 10.3% and 0.62% to 4.7% respectively **(Tables 2**A, B). Among pregnant women, the seropositivity varies between 0.9% and 11.2%.[17,21,22] Hepatitis B e antigen (HBeAg) status, which is mostly reflective of high replicative activity of the virus in the liver, was less than 30% in most earlier studies on pregnant women, though a recent study revealed a HBeAg seropositivity of 56.8%.[21] Variations in seropositivity could be contributed by the heterogeneity of populations studied including known and unknown risk factors, differing study size, and the various HBsAg ELISA systems used across the country. Most studies among nonprofessional blood donors comprise a mix of replacement donors and volunteer donors. The antibody to hepatitis B core antigen (anti-HBc) seropositivity (a marker of exposure to the virus) among blood donors varies between 8.4% and 18.9%.[23,24] This level of anti-HBc positivity precludes its use as a screening marker in Indian blood banks. Further, most studies are point prevalence studies and do not fit into the strict definition of a HBV carrier-HBsAg positivity lasting for 6 months or longer. It may be summarized,

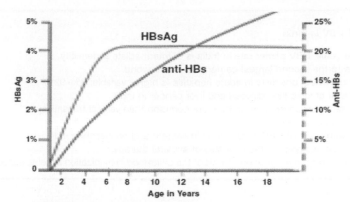

Fig. 1. Age-stratified prevalence of HBsAg and the antibody to hepatitis B surface antigen (anti-HBs). (*Reprinted from* Acharya SK, Madan K, Dattagupta S, et al. Viral hepatitis in India. Natl Med J India 2006;19(4):203–17; with permission.)

however, that across most studies among the general population, blood donors, and pregnant women, the HBsAg positivity ranges between 2% and 4%.

Earlier studies on age-stratified HBsAg seropositivity reveal that by the age of 5 years, HBsAg seropositivity is 2% to 3% (**Fig. 1**).[25] Low levels of HBeAg positivity among antenatal mothers suggest that perinatal transmission of the virus is perhaps less important than horizontal transmission in early childhood.[26,27]

Indian patients with thalassemia and hemophilia have HBsAg seropositivity rates of 6.6% to 10.34% and 6% respectively.[28,29] Among prerenal transplant patients, HBsAg seropositivity is between 4% and 5.7%, with seropositivity increasing to 7.5% after renal transplantation.[30] Among those attending sexually transmitted infection clinics, 3.6% are HBsAg positive, with up to 43.2% showing evidence of exposure to the virus (presence of antiHBc).[31] Among prison inmates with high-risk sexual practices, HBsAg seropositivity is higher.[32] HBsAg positivity among professional blood donors was found to be 11.7%,[33] with earlier studies showing higher positivity rates.

Alarming rates of HBV exposure have been reported in male human immunodeficiency virus (HIV)–positive intravenous drug users (100%) and their noninjecting spouses (92%) in Manipur, northeast India.[34] The Nicobarese, Shompen, and Jarawa tribes of the Andaman and Nicobar islands have been recently found to have HBsAg positivity rates ranging from 23.3% to 65%.[35,36]

In adults, frequent percutaneous injuries, frequently administered parenteral medications adopting poor injection practices, and poor knowledge about sterilization practices in the primary care centers contribute to the spread of this and other parenterally transmissible agents.[37,38]

The HBV genome is prone to random errors and mutations that occur after long periods of persistence within the host and immune pressure. This has led to the emergence of distinct genotypes and subgenotypes in a given population. Specific phases of chronic HBV infection causes certain mutations to merge (basic core promoter [BCP] and precore [PreC] mutations) while vaccine and antiviral therapy select out other (surface) variants of the virus. Studies from northern, western, and southern India reveal a predominance of genotype D in these regions followed by genotype A.[39–41] Eastern India has a unique distribution of genotypes D, A, and in addition genotype C.[40,42] There has been a single report of genotype G from north

---

Box 2
Summary of HBV in India

- On a global scale, HBV carrier rate in India is of intermediate endemicity.
- Contributes to the second largest carrier pool in the world.
- Frequency of HBsAg positivity in acute hepatitis is highly variable: 6%–92%.
- Major cause of chronic liver disease and liver cancer in India.
- Horizontal transmission appears to be more common than vertical transmission.
- Genotypes A and D are most common.
- Unique epidemiology of HBV strains seen in eastern and northeastern India.
- Oral nucleoside analogs are the mainstay of antiviral therapy.
- HBV vaccine has been introduced as part of the childhood immunization in some states of India.

India.[43] A novel HBV recombinant (genotype I) similar to strains from Vietnam and Laos has been identified in a primitive tribe in Arunachal Pradesh, in eastern India.[44] A diversity of HBV subgenotypes have been reported from eastern India, that is, As/A1, Cs/C1, D1, D2, D3, and D5.[45,46] Varying clinical outcome and frequencies of PreC mutation (1896) and BCP mutations (A/C1753 and T1762/A1764) have been detected among these subgenotypes.[46] A steady increase in trade, trafficking, and use of illicit drugs has impacted on the unique epidemiology of HBV in this northeastern region of India.

Frequency of HBsAg-positive acute hepatitis varies widely from 9% to 62%.[17] Variability of HBsAg detection could be due to the populations studied and the assays employed. Likewise, the proportion of HBsAg positivity among patients with fulminant hepatic failure ranges from 12.7% to 31%.[17] HBsAg positivity among chronic liver disease patients and those with cirrhosis ranges from 33% to 75% and 56% to 70% respectively.[17]

Indian patients with chronic HBV infection have been treated with interferon-α2b, interferon-α2a, pegylated interferon, and oral nucleoside analogs such as lamivudine, adefovir, entacavir, and tenofovir. The calculated cost and side effects are the major constraints to the wider use of interferon in this country.[47] Hence, oral nucleoside analogs are the mainstay of antiviral therapy for HBV (**Box 2**).

The HBV vaccine has been introduced in the immunization programs of more than 153 countries. Inclusion of the vaccine in the universal immunization schedule is likely to be the most cost-effective approach to reduce HBV carrier rates and the disease burden for India, especially with the available licensed, indigenous vaccines. Health is a state issue and some states of India have already incorporated the HBV vaccine in their immunization schedules.[48]

HEPATITIS C VIRUS

Hepatitis C virus is also a parenterally transmissible hepatitis causative agent, belonging to the virus family *Flaviviridae* and genus *Hepacivirus*. This virus causes disease that is typified by a silent, insidious onset in most individuals with high rates of persistence, with a high potential of developing worsening chronic liver disease with a disease spectrum of chronic hepatitis, cirrhosis, and occasionally HCC.

As reviewed by Acharya and colleagues,[18] HCV contributes to 15% to 20% of the chronic liver disease and HCC in India. HCV is believed to be spread in this country mainly through suboptimal blood banking and injection safety practices.[38,49] HCV antibody (HCV-Ab) is the widely used marker to screen for HCV (see **Table 1**).

HCV-Ab prevalence in the largest community based study in India was 0.87%, with HCV-Ab positivity increasing with age.[50] Using India's latest population census, a current estimate of HCV-Ab–positive individuals would be more than 10 million HCV seropositive individuals.

HCV-Ab is screened for in India using simple rapid immunofiltration (flow through) and immunochromatographic (lateral flow) membrane tests and third-generation ELISAs. Again, variability in data results from the composition of population tested, study size, assays used, as well as the level of adherence of good laboratory practices.

As reviewed by Mukhopadhya,[49] most studies involving volunteer and/or replacement donors have noted a seropositivity rate below 2%. Two studies comprising professional donors in western India have yielded an alarming prevalence of 55.3% and 87.3%.[51,52] These earlier findings reiterate the need for increased stringency in blood banks throughout the country. Nationwide, mandatory screening for HCV-Ab in blood banks was introduced as late as 2002.

Among thalassemia patients, the prevalence of HCV-Ab was between 16.7% and 21%.[53,54] In the latter study, HCV-Ab positivity correlated with advancing age, suggesting that HCV infection may have been acquired when mandatory screening in blood banks was not yet in place. Among the multiply transfused hemophilia patients, HCV-Ab seropositivity was found to be 23.9%.[29]

Hemodialysis patients are also at increased risk of acquiring HCV because of cross-contamination from the dialysis circuits and after multiple transfusions to treat anemia. HCV-Ab positivity among these patients was reported to be 9.93%.[55] Among renal transplant patients HCV-Ab detection rates are higher. However, in both hemodialysis patients and renal transplant patients, the antibody response is poor due to immunosuppression. Hence HCV-Ab detection in such patients may underestimate the burden of HCV infection. Of the 38 postrenal transplant patients who were HCV RNA positive, only 60% were HCV-Ab positive.[56] These findings emphasize the need to use direct markers of HCV replication such as HCV RNA detection.

Prison inmates from north India with risk factors such as intravenous drug use and high-risk sexual behavior have a HCV-Ab of 5%.[32] Intravenous drug use is a significant and alarming problem in northeast India, where 92% of the intravenous drug users studied, who were also HIV positive, showed HCV-Ab seropositivity.[34] Variability in the HCV-Ab positivity among HIV-infected individuals has been recorded in India.[49] A high seropositivity has been seen among patients with kala-azar (visceral leishmaniasis), especially in those who have had multiple injections of anti-leishmanial drugs. HCV-Ab was positive in these 32.9% of patients versus 4% of geographically matched controls among individuals who came mainly from the northern state of Bihar.[57]

A high degree of genetic variability is a hallmark feature of the HCV genome. HCV is classified into six major genotypes and more than 90 different subtypes.[58] The genotype of HCV and pretreatment virus load are major predictors of sustained virus response to antiviral therapy. The standard of care therapy for chronically infected HCV patients has been pegylated interferon and ribavirin for either 48 weeks (genotypes 1, 4, 6) or 24 weeks (for genotypes 2 and 3).[59] India has a predominance of genotype 3 in northern, eastern, and western India as compared to genotype 1, which is seen mainly in southern India.[18] In addition, the presence of genotypes 4 and 6 has been reported from within the country.[60,61]

The major constraint to providing standard of care therapy to HCV-infected individuals in India is cost. Unlike HBV, there is no vaccine for HCV. Therefore prevention of HCV infection rests on stringent blood banking and injection practices. Recently larger blood banks and blood collection centers have introduced nucleic

> **Box 3**
> **Summary of HCV in India**
>
> - Prevalence of anti-HCV antibody (HCV-Ab) in the general population is <1%.
> - HCV is spread mainly through poor blood bank screening and injection practices.
> - Predominant HCV genotype in India is genotype 3, followed by genotype 1.
> - Genotype 4 and 6 infections are less frequent.
> - Pegylated interferon and ribavirin are the standard of care for antiviral therapy in India.

acid amplification tests in their screening. Based on findings of a recent multicenter study, the Procleix Ultrio assay (Chiron Corp., Emeryville, CA, USA) can be predicted to interdict 3272 infected donations (2454 HBV-infected, 409 HCV-infected, and 818 HIV-infected donations) per 5 million units screened annually nationwide.[62]

Globally, HBV and HCV are the major etiologic causes for HCC.[63] Though the incidence of HCC in India appears to be lower than in other Asian countries and African countries, 80% of HCC in India is a result of virus-related liver disease.[64] HBV and HCV are associated with 36% to 47% and 30% of HCC in India[64] (**Box 3**).

HEPATITIS D VIRUS

HDV is a 36-nm virus particle that has a single-stranded circular RNA comprising 1700 nucleotides. Hepatitis D occurs only in individuals infected with HBV because HDV is a defective RNA viroid that requires HBsAg for its transmission.[65]

HDV infection is common in central Africa, the Amazon basin, and in the Mediterranean region, including Italy and the Eastern Europe. Globally there are about 15 to 20 million infected individuals.[66] HDV is transmitted parenterally among HBV-infected individuals as a coinfection (simultaneous infection of HBV and HDV) or as a superinfection (HDV infection superimposed on a preexisting chronic HBV infection).[67] During HDV infection, HDV RNA, HDV (δ) antigen, IgM anti-HDV, and IgG anti-HDV can be detected in serum (see **Table 1**). These markers are accompanied by the markers of acute or chronic HBV infection in HDV coinfection and HDV superinfection respectively.[68]

Acute HDV and HBV coinfection leads to complete virus clearance in 90% of cases but it can cause severe acute hepatitis with a propensity to lead to fulminant hepatitis.[65] In contrast to individuals with coinfection, individuals with chronic HBV infection with HDV superinfection rarely clear their HDV infection. As reviewed by Wedemeyer and Manns,[65] chronic HDV infection leads to much more severe liver disease as compared to HBV monoinfection. It is associated with an accelerated course of fibrosis progression, higher risk of hepatocellular carcinoma, and early decompensation of liver function in patients with cirrhosis. HDV infection is best confirmed by the detection HDV RNA using reverse-transcriptase polymerase chain reaction (RT-PCR).

At least eight different genotypes of HDV have been described and each genotype is associated with a characteristic geographic region and differing clinical course.[65] Genotype 1 is the most common genotype and has been detected throughout the world.

Serologic evidence of HDV infection (IgM and IgG) among HBV-related acute hepatitis, fulminant hepatitis, chronic hepatitis, cirrhosis, and hepatocellular carcinoma patients was found to be 3.1, 20, 8.1, 15.2, and 33.3 respectively.[69] Overall only 4 patients of the 123 subjects in this study had IgM anti-HDV.[69] Though there is

> **Box 4**
> **Summary of HDV in India**
>
> - Serologic evidence of HDV infection in cases of acute hepatitis, fulminant hepatitis, chronic hepatitis, cirrhosis, and liver cancer in India.
> - Seroprevalence rates are on the decline.

evidence of HDV coinfection and superinfection in India as reviewed by Acharya and colleagues,[18] more recent studies seem to suggest that the HDV epidemiology in India may be transitioning to lower rate of prevalence.[69–71] It is hoped that with greater HBV vaccination coverage in the country, HDV will play a smaller role in liver disease in the country (**Box 4**).

HEPATITIS E VIRUS

HEV is today classified as a hepevirus, in the family *Hepeviridae*. It is a spherical nonenveloped virus of about 27 to 34 nm. It has a single-stranded positive sense of approximately 7.5 kb with three partially overlapping open reading frames (ORFs) designated as ORF1, ORF2, and ORF3. ORF1 codes for a large nonstructural protein with several functional motives and domains. ORF2 encodes the capsid protein of HEV of 660 amino acids. ORF3 encodes a small protein of 123 amino acids that may act as an adaptor to link the intracellular transduction pathways, thus promoting HEV replication and assembly.[72]

HEV is transmitted mainly through fecally contaminated water and food. Over the past five and a half decades, several epidemics of HEV infection have occurred in India.[2–8] HEV infection is also an important cause of acute and subacute liver failure in the country.[9,10,73] Pregnant women with jaundice and acute viral hepatitis of HEV etiology showed higher mortality rates and poorer obstetric and fetal outcomes as compared to those with other types of hepatitis.[74,75] The precise mechanisms leading to this difference are not known but a shift in Th1/Th2 balance toward Th2 has been seen in pregnant women with HEV as compared to nonpregnant women with HEV, pregnant women without HEV, and nonpregnant women.[76] Another recently demonstrated mechanism is the selective suppression of nuclear factor kappa B NF p65 in pregnant versus nonpregnant women with fulminant hepatitis, which has been proposed to cause liver degeneration, severe immunodeficiency, and multiorgan failure.[77]

Less common modes of transmission are the vertical route[78] and via blood transfusions.[79] Person-to-person contact transmission is low.[80]

Increased morbidity and mortality are also documented in chronic liver disease patients with superinfection with HEV.[81,82] In organ transplant patients there is evidence of chronic HEV infection.[83] In a study among children, HEV was associated with at least one other hepatitis causing virus in 88% of cases with acute viral hepatitis.[84]

Genotypes 1, 2, 3, and 4 have been described that distribute to separate geographic regions.[72] The avian HEV strain was proposed to belong to the new genotype 5.[85] The circulation of genotype 1 and at least two subgenotypes within this genotype has been reported.[86] Related HEV strains have been also identified in pigs, deer, and wild boar.[72] It is postulated that any high anti-HEV prevalence in nonendemic parts of the world may be due to zoonotic transmission of nonhuman hosts.[72] The swine HEV strains in India differ genetically from the human strains, suggesting that pigs do not play a role in the spread of HEV in this endemic region.[87]

Box 5
Summary of HEV in India

- HEV is today classified as a hepevirus belonging to the family Hepeviridae.
- India is hyperendemic for HEV infection.
- Responsible for most of the hepatitis epidemics in India.
- Transmitted mainly through fecally contaminated water.
- Severe disease in pregnant women and in persons with preexisting chronic liver disease.
- HEV genotype 1 is seen in India.
- IgM anti-HEV used to diagnose acute HEV infection.
- Prevention currently rests on ensuring clean and safe water supply, improved sanitation, and public education.

In acute HEV infection, both IgM and IgG anti-HEV are detectable. IgG alone is detectable from past infection. Thus in an endemic region such as the Indian subcontinent, IgM anti-HEV is useful to detect acute infection while IgG anti-HEV testing is of value for seroprevalence studies (see **Table 1**). Commercial assays are available to detect these antibodies. The most definitive evidence of current HEV infection is the presence of HEV RNA in serum and stool. Viremia as detected by RT-PCR appears before liver enzyme elevation and may last for 1 week to 1 month.[88]

Efforts toward a vaccine have been hampered by the lack of a robust system to propagate HEV in vitro. The four genotypes known to circulate among humans share a common serotype. A subunit vaccine based on a truncated ORF2 protein produced in insect cells using recombinant baculovirus has been tested in humans and has shown 95% efficacy.[89] Until such time that the vaccine is licensed and is marketed at an affordable price, the mainstay of prevention of HEV infection will be ensuring clean water supplies, improving sanitation, and providing continuous public education (**Box 5**).

NEWER CANDIDATE HEPATITIS VIRUSES

GB virus C/hepatitis G virus (GBV-C/HGV) and Torque teno (TT) viruses were initially identified as candidate hepatitis viruses. Studies in India have shown a prevalence of 4% in the general population and up to 47% in healthy commercial blood donors.[90] GBV-C/HGV viremia was seen in 39.7% of thalassemic children, 52.9% of renal transplant patients, 14.3% of acute viral hepatitis patients, and 26.6% of acute liver failure patients.[91–93] TT viruses were detected in 32.9% of renal transplant patients and 21.5% to 73.6% of patients with various forms of liver disease.[92,94] These infections were mostly in association with the hepatitis viruses A to E and did not appear to contribute to pathogenesis in the liver.

SUMMARY

Viral hepatitis in India is a major public health challenge. India is hyperendemic for the two enterically transmitted hepatitis viruses, HAV and HEV. HAV-related infection occurs largely in children, and seroprevalence studies show that by adolescence, 90% to 100% have protective antibody. However, that pattern is slowly changing in segments of the population with better hygiene and living standards. Many large epidemics have been reported from India, and HEV continue to be the major cause of acute sporadic hepatitis among adults. India belongs to the intermediate endemicity zone for HBV and harbors the second largest pool of HBV carriers. It is the major cause of chronic liver disease and HCC in the country. Genotypes A, D, and C have been reported in the country. HCV prevalence (as measured by HCV-Ab) in the general population is less than 1%. However, based on India's population, the burden of HCV carriers is significant. HCV contributes to 10% to 15% of chronic liver disease and HCC in India. HCV genotype 3 is the most frequent, followed by genotype 1. HDV infection, though present, is relatively infrequent.

HAV and HBV vaccines are licensed and marketed in the country. India is yet to include the HBV vaccine in its national immunization program, though some Indian states have taken this initiative.

This high disease burden of liver disease caused by hepatitis viruses warrants the setting up of a national hepatitis registry and the formulation and implementation of national prevention and control strategies.

REFERENCES

1. Viswanathan R. Epidemiology. Indian J Med Res 1957;45(Suppl):1–29.
2. Dhamdhere MR, Nadkarni MG. Infectious hepatitis at Aurangabad: report of an outbreak. Indian J Med Sci 1962;16:1006–15.
3. Bhattacharji LM, Saha AL, Sampathkumaran MA, et al. Investigation of an outbreak of infectious hepatitis in a small town in West Bengal during July–October, 1960. Indian J Med Res 1963;51:550–62.
4. Pattanayak S, Singha P, Pal SC, et al. An outbreak of infectious hepatitis in Siliguri, 1966. Indian J Med Res 1968;56(11):1605–16.
5. Khuroo MS. Study of an epidemic of non-A, non-B hepatitis: possibility of another human hepatitis virus distinct from post-transfusion non-A, non-B type. Am J Med 1980;68(6):818–24.
6. Naik SR, Aggarwal R, Salunke PN, et al. A large waterborne viral hepatitis E epidemic in Kanpur, India. Bull World Health Organ 1992;70(5):597–604.
7. Ray R, Aggarwal R, Salunke PN, et al. Hepatitis E virus genome in stools of hepatitis patients during large epidemic in north India. Lancet 1991;338(8770):783–4.
8. Bansal J, He J, Yarbough PO, et al. Hepatitis E virus infection in eastern India. Am J Trop Med Hyg 1998;59(2):258–60.
9. Nanda SK, Yalcinkaya K, Panigrahi AK, et al. Etiological role of hepatitis E virus in sporadic fulminant hepatitis. J Med Virol 1994;42(2):133–7.
10. Madan K, Gopalkrishna V, Kar P, et al. Detection of hepatitis C and E virus genomes in sera of patients with acute viral hepatitis and fulminant hepatitis by their simultaneous amplification in PCR. J Gastroenterol Hepatol 1998;13(2):125–30.
11. Arankalle VA, Tsarev SA, Chadha MS, et al. Age-specific prevalence of antibodies to hepatitis A and E viruses in Pune, India, 1982 and 1992. J Infect Dis 1995; 171(2):447–50.
12. Mohanavalli B, Dhevahi E, Menon T, et al. Prevalence of antibodies to hepatitis A and hepatitis E virus in urban school children in Chennai. Indian Pediatr 2003;40(4):328–31.
13. Acharya SK, Batra Y, Bhatkal B, et al. Seroepidemiology of hepatitis A virus infection among school children in Delhi and north Indian patients with chronic liver disease: implications for HAV vaccination. J Gastroenterol Hepatol 2003;18(7):822–7.
14. Mathur P, Arora NK. Epidemiological transition of hepatitis A in India: issues for vaccination in developing countries. Indian J Med Res 2008;128(6):699–704.
15. Tandon BN, Gandhi BM, Joshi YK. Etiological spectrum of viral hepatitis and prevalence of markers of hepatitis A and B virus infection in north India. Bull World Health Organ 1984;62(1):67–73.
16. Tandon BN, Acharya SK, Tandon A. Epidemiology of hepatitis B virus infection in India. Gut 1996;38(Suppl 2):S56–9.

17. World Health Organization. Prevention of hepatitis B in India. New Delhi: World Health Organization Regional Office for South-East Asia; 2002.
18. Acharya SK, Madan K, Dattagupta S, et al. Viral hepatitis in India. Natl Med J India 2006;19(4):203–17.
19. Arora NK, Nanda SK, Gulati S, et al. Acute viral hepatitis types E, A, and B singly and in combination in acute liver failure in children in north India. J Med Virol 1996;48(3): 215–21.
20. Anand AC, Nagpal AK, Seth AK, et al. Should one vaccinate patients with chronic liver disease for hepatitis A virus in India? J Assoc Physicians India 2004;52:785–7.
21. Dwivedi M, Misra SP, Misra V, et al. Seroprevalence of hepatitis B infection during pregnancy and risk of perinatal transmission. Indian J Gastroenterol 2011;30(2):66–71.
22. Prakash C, Sharma RS, Bhatia R, et al. Prevalence of North India of hepatitis B carrier state amongst pregnant women. Southeast Asian J Trop Med Public Health 1998; 29(1):80–4.
23. Dhawan H-K, Marwaha N, Sharma R-R, et al. Anti-HBc screening in Indian blood donors: still an unresolved issue. World J Gastroenterol 2008;14(34):5327–30.
24. Asim M, Ali R, Khan LA, et al. Significance of anti-HBc screening of blood donors & its association with occult hepatitis B virus infection: implications for blood transfusion. Indian J Med Res 2010;132:312–7.
25. Tandon BN, Irshad M, Raju M, et al. Prevalence of HBsAg & anti-HBs in children & strategy suggested for immunisation in India. Indian J Med Res 1991;93:337–9.
26. Nayak NC, Panda SK, Zuckerman AJ, et al. Dynamics and impact of perinatal transmission of hepatitis B virus in North India. J Med Virol 1987;21(2):137–45.
27. Banerjee A, Chakravarty R, Mondal PN, et al. Hepatitis B virus genotype D infection among antenatal patients attending a maternity hospital in Calcutta, India: assessment of infectivity status. Southeast Asian J Trop Med Public Health 2005;36(1): 203–6.
28. Khakhkhar V, Joshi PJ. HBsAg seropositivity among multi-transfused thalassemic children. Indian J Pathol Microbiol 2006;49(4):516–8.
29. Ghosh K, Joshi SH, Shetty S, et al. Transfusion transmitted diseases in haemophilics from western India. Indian J Med Res 2000;112:61–4.
30. Murthy KK, John GT, Abraham P, et al. Profile of hepatitis B and hepatitis C virus infections in dialysis and renal transplant patients 1997–2001; CMCH Vellore. Indian J Nephrol 2003;13:24–8.
31. Risbud A, Mehendale S, Basu S, et al. Prevalence and incidence of hepatitis B virus infection in STD clinic attendees in Pune, India. Sex Transm Infect 2002;78(3):169–73.
32. Singh S, Prasad R, Mohanty A. High prevalence of sexually transmitted and blood-borne infections amongst the inmates of a district jail in Northern India. Int J STD AIDS 1999;10(7):475–8.
33. Irshad M, Singh YN, Acharya SK. HBV—status in professional blood donors in north India. Trop Gastroenterol 1992;13(3):112–4.
34. Saha MK, Chakrabarti S, Panda S, et al. Prevalence of HCV & HBV infection amongst HIV seropositive intravenous drug users & their non-injecting wives in Manipur, India. Indian J Med Res 2000;111:37–9.
35. Murhekar MV, Murhekar KM, Das D, et al. Prevalence of hepatitis B infection among the primitive tribes of Andaman & Nicobar Islands. Indian J Med Res 2000;111:199–203.
36. Murhekar MV, Murhekar KM, Sehgal SC. Alarming prevalence of hepatitis-B infection among the Jarawas—a primitive Negrito tribe of Andaman and Nicobar Islands, India. J Viral Hepat 2003;10(3):232–3.
37. Hutin YJF. Acting upon evidence: progress towards the elimination of unsafe injection practices in India. Indian Pediatr 2005;42(2):111–5.

38. Kermode M, Muani V. Injection practices in the formal & informal healthcare sectors in rural north India. Indian J Med Res 2006;124(5):513–20.
39. Gandhe SS, Chadha MS, Arankalle VA. Hepatitis B virus genotypes and serotypes in western India: lack of clinical significance. J Med Virol 2003;69(3):324–30.
40. Vivekanandan P, Abraham P, Sridharan G, et al. Distribution of hepatitis B virus genotypes in blood donors and chronically infected patients in a tertiary care hospital in southern India. Clin Infect Dis 2004;38(9):e81–6.
41. Chattopadhyay S, Das BC, Kar P. Hepatitis B virus genotypes in chronic liver disease patients from New Delhi, India. World J Gastroenterol 2006;12(41):6702–6.
42. Banerjee A, Datta S, Chandra PK, et al. Distribution of hepatitis B virus genotypes: phylogenetic analysis and virological characteristics of genotype C circulating among HBV carriers in Kolkata, Eastern India. World J Gastroenterol 2006;12(37):5964–71.
43. Kumar GT, Kazim SN, Kumar M, et al. Hepatitis B virus genotypes and hepatitis B surface antigen mutations in family contacts of hepatitis B virus infected patients with occult hepatitis B virus infection. J Gastroenterol Hepatol 2009;24(4):588–98.
44. Arankalle VA, Gandhe SS, Borkakoty BJ, et al. A novel HBV recombinant (genotype I) similar to Vietnam/Laos in a primitive tribe in eastern India. J Viral Hepat 2010;17(7):501–10.
45. Banerjee A, Kurbanov F, Datta S, et al. Phylogenetic relatedness and genetic diversity of hepatitis B virus isolates in Eastern India. J Med Virol 2006;78(9):1164–74.
46. Chandra PK, Biswas A, Datta S, et al. Subgenotypes of hepatitis B virus genotype D (D1, D2, D3 and D5) in India: differential pattern of mutations, liver injury and occult HBV infection. J Viral Hepat 2009;16(10):749–56.
47. Aggarwal R, Ghoshal UC, Naik SR. Treatment of chronic hepatitis B with interferon-alpha: cost-effectiveness in developing countries. Natl Med J India 2002;15(6):320–7.
48. Puri S, Bhatia V, Singh A, et al. Uptake of newer vaccines in Chandigarh. Indian J Pediatr 2007;74(1):47–50.
49. Mukhopadhyaya A. Hepatitis C in India. J Biosci 2008;33(4):465–73.
50. Chowdhury A, Santra A, Chaudhuri S, et al. Hepatitis C virus infection in the general population: a community-based study in West Bengal, India. Hepatology 2003;37(4):802–9.
51. Nandi J, Bhawalkar V, Mody H, et al. Detection of HIV-1, HBV and HCV antibodies in blood donors from Surat, western India. Vox Sang 1994;67(4):406–7.
52. Jha J, Banerjee K, Arankalle VA. A high prevalence of antibodies to hepatitis C virus among commercial plasma donors from Western India. J Viral Hepat 1995;2(5):257–60.
53. Agarwal MB, Malkan GH, Bhave AA, et al. Antibody to hepatitis-C virus in multi-transfused thalassaemics—Indian experience. J Assoc Physicians India 1993;41(4):195–7.
54. Jaiswal SPB, Chitnis DS, Jain AK, et al. Prevalence of hepatitis viruses among multi-transfused homogenous thalassaemia patients. Hepatol Res 2001;19(3):247–53.
55. Reddy AK, Murthy KVD, Lakshmi V. Prevalence of HCV infection in patients on haemodialysis: survey by antibody and core antigen detection. Indian J Med Microbiol 2005;23(2):106–10.
56. Radhakrishnan S, Abraham P, Raghuraman S, et al. Role of molecular techniques in the detection of HBV DNA & HCV RNA among renal transplant recipients in India. Indian J Med Res 2000;111:204–11.
57. Singh S, Dwivedi SN, Sood R, et al. Hepatitis B, C and human immunodeficiency virus infections in multiply-injected kala-azar patients in Delhi. Scand J Infect Dis 2000;32(1):3–6.
58. Hoofnagle JH. Course and outcome of hepatitis C. Hepatology 2002;36(5 Suppl 1):S21–9.

59. Ghany MG, Strader DB, Thomas DL, et al. Diagnosis, management, and treatment of hepatitis C: an update. Hepatology 2009;49(4):1335–74.
60. Raghuraman S, Abraham P, Sridharan G, et al. HCV genotype 4 — an emerging threat as a cause of chronic liver disease in Indian (south) patients. J Clin Virol 2004;31(4): 253–8.
61. Raghuraman S, Abraham P, Sridharan G, et al. Hepatitis C virus genotype 6 infection in India. Indian J Gastroenterol 2005;24(2):72–3.
62. Makroo RN, Choudhury N, Jagannathan L, et al. Multicenter evaluation of individual donor nucleic acid testing (NAT) for simultaneous detection of human immunodeficiency virus-1 & hepatitis B & C viruses in Indian blood donors. Indian J Med Res 2008;127(2):140–7.
63. Ince N, Wands JR. The increasing incidence of hepatocellular carcinoma. N Engl J Med 1999;340(10):798–9.
64. Dhir V, Mohandas KM. Epidemiology of digestive tract cancers in India. III. Liver. Indian J Gastroenterol 1998;17(3):100–3.
65. Wedemeyer H, Manns MP. Epidemiology, pathogenesis and management of hepatitis D: update and challenges ahead. Nat Rev Gastroenterol Hepatol 2010;7(1):31–40.
66. Hadziyannis SJ. Review: hepatitis delta. J Gastroenterol Hepatol 1997;12(4):289–98.
67. Casey JL. Hepatitis delta virus: molecular biology, pathogenesis and immunology. Antivir Ther (Lond) 1998;3(Suppl 3):37–42.
68. Taylor JM. Hepatitis delta virus. Intervirology 1999;42(2–3):173–8.
69. Chakraborty P, Kailash U, Jain A, et al. Seroprevalence of hepatitis D virus in patients with hepatitis B virus-related liver diseases. Indian J Med Res 2005;122(3):254–7.
70. Irshad M, Sharma Y, Dhar I, et al. Transfusion-transmitted virus in association with hepatitis A-E viral infections in various forms of liver diseases in India. World J Gastroenterol 2006;12(15):2432–6.
71. Saravanan S, Velu V, Kumarasamy N, et al. Seroprevalence of hepatitis delta virus infection among subjects with underlying hepatic diseases in Chennai, southern India. Trans R Soc Trop Med Hyg 2008;102(8):793–6.
72. Chandra V, Taneja S, Kalia M, et al. Molecular biology and pathogenesis of hepatitis E virus. J Biosci 2008;33(4):451–64.
73. Ramachandran J, Ramakrishna B, Eapen CE, et al. Subacute hepatic failure due to hepatitis E. J Gastroenterol Hepatol 2008;23(6):879–82.
74. Khuroo MS, Teli MR, Skidmore S, et al. Incidence and severity of viral hepatitis in pregnancy. Am J Med 1981;70(2):252–5.
75. Patra S, Kumar A, Trivedi SS, et al. Maternal and fetal outcomes in pregnant women with acute hepatitis E virus infection. Ann Intern Med 2007;147(1):28–33.
76. Pal R, Aggarwal R, Naik SR, et al. Immunological alterations in pregnant women with acute hepatitis E. J Gastroenterol Hepatol 2005;20(7):1094–101.
77. Prusty BK, Hedau S, Singh A, et al. Selective suppression of NF-kBp65 in hepatitis virus-infected pregnant women manifesting severe liver damage and high mortality. Mol Med 2007;13(9-10):518–26.
78. Khuroo MS, Kamili S, Jameel S. Vertical transmission of hepatitis E virus. Lancet. 1995;345(8956):1025–6.
79. Khuroo MS, Kamili S, Yattoo GN. Hepatitis E virus infection may be transmitted through blood transfusions in an endemic area. J Gastroenterol Hepatol 2004;19(7): 778–84.
80. Somani SK, Aggarwal R, Naik SR, et al. A serological study of intrafamilial spread from patients with sporadic hepatitis E virus infection. J Viral Hepat 2003;10(6):446–9.
81. Hamid SS, Atiq M, Shehzad F, et al. Hepatitis E virus superinfection in patients with chronic liver disease. Hepatology 2002;36(2):474–8.

82. Ramachandran J, Eapen CE, Kang G, et al. Hepatitis E superinfection produces severe decompensation in patients with chronic liver disease. J Gastroenterol Hepatol 2004;19(2):134–8.

83. Kamar N, Selves J, Mansuy J-M, et al. Hepatitis E virus and chronic hepatitis in organ-transplant recipients. N Engl J Med 2008;358(8):811–7.

84. Kumar A, Yachha SK, Poddar U, et al. Does co-infection with multiple viruses adversely influence the course and outcome of sporadic acute viral hepatitis in children? J Gastroenterol Hepatol 2006;21(10):1533–7.

85. Huang FF, Sun ZF, Emerson SU, et al. Determination and analysis of the complete genomic sequence of avian hepatitis E virus (avian HEV) and attempts to infect rhesus monkeys with avian HEV. J Gen Virol 2004;85(Pt 6):1609–18.

86. Arankalle VA, Paranjape S, Emerson SU, et al. Phylogenetic analysis of hepatitis E virus isolates from India (1976–1993). J Gen Virol 1999;80 (Pt 7):1691–700.

87. Shukla P, Chauhan UK, Naik S, et al. Hepatitis E virus infection among animals in northern India: an unlikely source of human disease. J Viral Hepat 2007;14(5):310–7.

88. Chauhan A, Jameel S, Dilawari JB, et al. Hepatitis E virus transmission to a volunteer. Lancet 1993;341(8838):149–50.

89. Shrestha MP, Scott RM, Joshi DM, et al. Safety and efficacy of a recombinant hepatitis E vaccine. N Engl J Med 2007;356(9):895–903.

90. Kar P, Bedi P, Berry N, et al. Hepatitis G virus (HGV) infection in voluntary and commercial blood donors in India. Diagn Microbiol Infect Dis 2000;38(1):7–10.

91. Panigrahi AK, Saxena A, Acharya SK, et al. Hepatitis G virus in multitransfused thalassaemics from India. J Gastroenterol Hepatol 1998;13(9):902–6.

92. Abraham P, John GT, Raghuraman S, et al. GB virus C/hepatitis G virus and TT virus infections among high risk renal transplant recipients in India. J Clin Virol 2003;28(1):59–69.

93. Kapoor S, Gupta RK, Das BC, et al. Clinical implications of hepatitis G virus (HGV) infection in patients of acute viral hepatitis & fulminant hepatic failure. Indian J Med Res 2000;112:121–7.

94. Asim M, Singla R, Gupta RK, et al. Clinical & molecular characterization of human TT virus in different liver diseases. Indian J Med Res 2010;131:545–54.

95. Uppal Y, Garg S, Mishra B, et al. Prevalence of reproductive morbidity among males in an urban slum in north India. Indian J Comm Med 2007;32(1):54–7.

96. Chowdhury A, Santra A, Chakravorty R, et al. Community-based epidemiology of hepatitis B virus infection in West Bengal, India: prevalence of hepatitis B e antigen negative infection and associated viral variants. J Gastroenterol Hepatol 2005;20(11):1712–20.

97. Bhagyalaxmi A, Lala MK, Jain S, et al. HBsAg carrier status in urban population of Ahmedabad city. Indian J Med Res 2005;121:203–4.

98. Singh J, Bhatia R, Khare S, et al. Community studies on prevalence of HBsAg in two urban populations of southern India. Indian Pediatr 2000;37(2):149–52.

99. Kurien T, Thyagarajan SP, Jeyaseelan L, et al. Community prevalence of hepatitis B infection and modes of transmission in Tamil Nadu, India. Indian J Med Res 2005;121:670–5.

100. Nanu A, Sharma SP, Chatterjee K, et al. Markers of transfusion-tranmissible infections in north Indian voluntary and replacement blood donors: prevalence and trends 1989–1996. Vox Sang 1997;73:70–3.

101. Pahuja S, Sharma M, Baitha B, et al. Prevalence and trends of markers of hepatitis C virus, hepatitis B virus and human immunodeficiency virus in Delhi blood donors. A hospital based study Jpn J Inf Dis 2007;60:689–91.

102. Meena M, Jindal T, Hazarika A. Prevalence of hepatitis B virus and hepatitis C virus among blood donors in a tertiary care hospital in India: a five-year study. Transfusion 2011;51:198–202.
103. Das BK, Gayen BK, Aditya S, et al. Seroprevalence of Hepatitis B, Hepatitis C and human immunodeficiency virus among healthy voluntary first-time blood donors in Kolkata. Ann Trop Med Public Health 2011;4:86–90.
104. Elavia AJ, Banker DD. Prevalence of HBsAg and its subtypes in high risk subjects and voluntary blood donors in Bombay Indian. J Med Res 1991;93:280–5.
105. SatoskarA, Ray V. Prevalence of hepatitis B surface antigen (HBsAg) in blood donors from Bombay. Trop Geogr Med 1992;44:119–21.
106. Nijhawan S, Rai RR, Sharma D, et al. HBsAg prevalence in blood donors in Jaipur. Indian J Gastroenterol 1997;16:162.
107. Singhvi A, Pulimood RB, John TJ, et al. The prevalence of markers for hepatitis B and human immunodeficiency viruses, malarial parasites and microfilaria in blood donors in a large hospital in south India. J Trop Med Hyg 1990;93:178–82.
108. Singh K, Bhat S, Shastry S. Trend in seroprevalence of Hepatitis B virus infection among blood donors of coastal Karnataka, India. J Infect Dev Ctries 2009;3(5):3376–9.

HIV Testing in India

Srikanth Tripathy, MBBS, MD[a],*, Michael Pereira, MSc[a],
Sriram Prasad Tripathy, MD[b]

KEYWORDS

- HIV testing • India • National AIDS Control Organization • HIV surveillance

KEY POINTS

- The National AIDS Control Organization (NACO) has initiated programs for HIV/AIDS control in India.
- Algorithms for HIV testing have been developed for India.
- NACO programs have resulted in HIV situation improving over the last decade.

INTRODUCTION

India has a large number of people living with human immunodeficiency virus (HIV)/acquired immunodeficiency syndrome (AIDS) (PLWHA). With an estimated 2.4 million PLWHA, India currently has the world's third largest number of HIV cases.[1] Indian families affected by HIV/AIDS could spend approximately 49% of their income on the treatment of an HIV-infected individual.[2] In response, India has undertaken a massive prevention and treatment program targeting high-risk populations in India. The Government of India (GOI) has initiated free antiretroviral treatment (ART), and as of January 2011, approximately 393,632 HIV-infected adults and children were receiving ART at 293 centers in the country.[3] Global partners are also supporting the country's efforts to control the epidemic. In the midst of these actions, however, there remain important challenges to adequately scale up the HIV/AIDS response to meet the potential increase in the epidemic in the future. These challenges include, but are not limited to, an adequate health workforce, responsive infrastructure (including laboratory capabilities), comprehensive monitoring, and adequate and sustainable financing.

THE INDIAN EPIDEMIC

India has from the beginning of the global epidemic maintained vigilance against HIV infection. Screening risk groups in the early 1980s provided the first evidence of

The authors have nothing to disclose.
[a] National AIDS Research Institute, 73 G Block, MIDC, Bhosari, Pune 411026, India; [b] The Indian Council of Medical Research 2, Radhika Vaibhav, Jagtapnagar, Wanawadi, Pune 411040, India
* Corresponding author.
E-mail address: stripathy@nariindia.org

Clin Lab Med 32 (2012) 175–191
http://dx.doi.org/10.1016/j.cll.2012.04.014
0272-2712/12/$ – see front matter © 2012 Published by Elsevier Inc.

labmed.theclinics.com

indigenous transmission of HIV in commercial sex workers (CSWs) in Chennai, India in May 1986.[4] Since then, efforts have been made continuously to evolve effective control measures initially directed at prevention of infection, reducing the transmission of HIV and the management and care of HIV-infected persons, and now fully directed toward successful treatment of patients with ART.

HIV/AIDS Scenario in India

Since the first report of HIV infection in CSWs in Tamil in 1986, HIV has now spread to all the states in India. The prevalence of HIV among adults (aged 15–49 years) is less than 1%, but with a population of more than 1.2 billion, India has the world's third largest number of PLWHA, with an estimated 2.4 million living with HIV infection in India by the end of 2011.[4] In six high-HIV prevalence states—Andhra Pradesh (0.44%), Karnataka (0.42%), Maharashtra (0.5%), Manipur (0.56%), Nagaland (1.07%), and Tamil Nadu (0.13%)—the HIV epidemic is classified as a concentrated one. Overall, in India, the HIV prevalence in antenatal clinic (ANC) attendees availing the services of integrated counseling and testing centers (ICTCs) is around 0.27% and HIV prevalence among clinic patients with sexually transmitted infections (STIs) is greater than 5%.[1]

The prevalence of HIV remains the highest among CSWs and their clients, men who have sex with men (MSM), intravenous drug users (IDUs), truck drivers, and patients with STIs, whose behavior puts them at high risk for contacting HIV. Up to about 70% of 15,000 sex workers in Mumbai are HIV positive. Data on MSM and transgendered persons in Mumbai found that 17% of men and 68% of transgendered people were HIV positive. Twenty-two percent of MSM were married, and 44% had visited female CSWs.[5] The IDU epidemic is perceived as a problem mainly in the northeastern states, with an HIV prevalence of more than 70% in sentinel surveillance sites during the past years.[6] However, selected surveys point out the increasing evidence of IDU in other parts of India, including border areas.

A study conducted in India showed that among 4648 drug users interviewed in 14 cities across the country, 43% had injected drugs.[7,8] By 2001, an estimated 15% to 35% of truck drivers nationwide were HIV positive.[9] HIV infection rates among STI patients were 19.6% in Andhra Pradesh and 13% in Manipur.[10]

In India, infection may be due to both HIV-1 and the less pathogenic HIV-2. HIV-1 subtype C is predominant, while HIV-1 A/C recombinants have been described in Maharashtra. In the northeastern states, other subtypes are present, including subtype B′ (similar to the subtype found in Thai IDUs), E, C, and B′/C recombinants.[11,12]

The 2008–2009 HIV estimates highlight an overall reduction in adult HIV prevalence and HIV incidence (new infections) in India. Adult HIV prevalence at the national level has declined from 0.41% in 2000 to 0.31% in 2009.[1] The estimated number of new annual HIV infections has declined by more than 50% over the past decade.[1]

The 2008–2009 India HIV estimates—developed by National AIDS Control Organization (NACO) with support from National Institute of Medical Sciences, National Institute of Health and Family Welfare, UNAIDS, and World Health Organization (WHO)—indicated that India had approximately 0.12 million new HIV infections in 2009, as against 0.27 million in 2000. The estimated adult HIV prevalence in India was 0.32% in 2008 and 0.31% in 2009 (**Table 1**).[1] Among the states in India, Manipur has shown the highest estimated adult HIV prevalence of 1.40%, followed by Andhra Pradesh (0.90%), Mizoram (0.81%), Nagaland (0.78%), Karnataka (0.63%), and Maharashtra (0.55%) (**Table 2**).[1]

Table 1	
HIV prevalence in India	
Category	Estimate (2009)
Total population (in 2009)	1.2 billion
HIV prevalence	
Men	0.38%
Women	0.25%
Both sexes	0.32%
PLHA (adults and children)	2.39 million
Children (younger than 15 years)	3.5%

Data from National AIDS Control Organization, Department of AIDS Control, Ministry of Health and Family Welfare. Government of India. Annual Report 2010–2011. Available at: http://nacoonline.org. Accessed April 23, 2012.

HIV-Infected Subjects Started on Free ART in India

By January 2012, a total of 486,173 HIV-infected subjects have been started on ART in India. The large-scale testing for HIV infection has resulted in the detection of a significant number of HIV subjects who are eligible for ART and can thus start on ART medication that can prevent the morbidity and mortality associated with advanced HIV infection.

Current Status of HIV Infection in India

India is a low-income country with a current population of about 1.2 billion. The HIV epidemic level is a concentrated one, with a substantially higher prevalence among

Table 2	
Adult HIV prevalence in states of India	
State in India	Adult Prevalence (%)
Manipur	1.40
Andhra Pradesh	0.90
Mizoram	0.81
Nagaland	0.78
Karnataka	0.68
Maharashtra	0.55
Goa	>0.31
Chandigarh	
Gujarat	
Punjab	
Tamil Nadu	
Delhi	0.28–0.30
Odisha	
West Bengal	

Data from National AIDS Control Organization, Department of AIDS Control, Ministry of Health and Family Welfare. Government of India. Annual Report 2010–2011. Available at: http://nacoonline.org. Accessed April 23, 2012.

Table 3	
HIV prevalence in high-risk groups in India (2008–2009)	
Category	**Percent Positive**
ANC attendees	0.48
STD clinic attendees	2.46
IDU	9.19
MSM	7.30
FSW	4.94
Migrants	2.3
Truckers	1.60

Data from National AIDS Control Organization, Department of AIDS Control, Ministry of Health and Family Welfare. Government of India. Annual Report 2010–2011. Available at: http://nacoonline.org. Accessed April 23, 2012.

selected high-risk groups (HRGs) than in the general population. Distribution of infection in the country is uneven; in many states, the prevalence is low. In six states—Andhra, Karnataka, Maharashtra, Manipur, Nagaland, and Tamil Nadu—the prevalence is high and these states have received greater focus of attention compared to the rest. The country has 609 districts; in 156 districts (Category A), the prevalence of HIV infection in attendees in ANCs is greater than 1%. In an additional 39 districts (Category B), HIV prevalence in ANCs is less than 1% but prevalence in HRGs is greater than 5%. These 195 districts have received greater attention for the provision of HIV control measures than the rest of the districts. Based on the HIV sentinel surveillance conducted in 2008–2009, it was estimated that India has about 2.39 million HIV-infected persons with an adult HIV prevalence of about 0.31%.[1] Nearly all of the PLWHA are adults and adolescents. Children comprise only about 3.5% of those infected.

Transmission is largely sexual, and mostly heterosexual with a small proportion due to MSM. In addition, there is a sizable population of HIV-infected IDUs in four large cities—Chennai, Mumbai, Delhi, and Chandigarh—and in two states in the northeast—Manipur and Nagaland. The rates of prevalence in the categories of HRGs and general population (antenatal clinic attendees) are indicated in **Table 3** and **Table 4**.[1]

National Response to the Epidemic and Public Health Measures

The HIV control activities in India are executed under the guidance of NACO under the Ministry of Health and Family Welfare. The apex body has organized three successive national AIDS control programs: NACP I, II, and III. NACO formulates policies and plans, monitors, executes, coordinates, and evaluates all aspects of AIDS management in India. The current 5-year program, NACP III, started in 2007. High priority is accorded to measures to promote, prevent, and care, with the objectives of reducing HIV transmission rates, providing care and treatment, and reducing mortality due to AIDS. The State AIDS Control Society (SACS) in each state has the responsibility to administer and monitor the activities in each district. The program is ably assisted and strengthened by outputs from many nongovernmental organizations (NGOs)—WHO, UNAIDS, UNICEF—and other international organizations such as the Bill and Melinda Gates Foundation.

There is evidence that in India, the epidemic has peaked and is declining slowly.[10] NACP III has set 2011 as the year for halting and reversing the epidemic

Table 4
HIV testing in ANC clinics April–December 2010

State/Union Territory	Number Tested	% HIV-Positive
All India	4,790,802	0.27
Andhra Pradesh	621,724	0.44
Arunachal Pradesh	7181	0.04
Assam	108,036	0.06
Bihar	115,277	0.24
Chattisgarh	46,647	0.25
Goa	8854	0.47
Gujarat	374,903	0.18
Haryana	63,818	0.13
Himachal Pradesh	26,224	0.06
Jammu and Kashmir	23,659	0.06
Jharkhand	39,794	0.18
Karnataka	536,243	0.42
Kerala	82,675	0.07
Madhya Pradesh	115,289	0.13
Maharashtra	578,444	0.5
Manipur	32,801	0.56
Meghalaya	8618	0.86
Mizoram	14,315	0.73
Nagaland	10,333	0.07
Odisha	12,940	0.16
Punjab	85,560	019
Rajasthan	222,277	0.12
Sikkim	4774	0.02
Tamil Nadu	682,568	0.13
Tripura	7988	0.09
Uttar Pradesh	294,988	0.11
Uttarakhand	27,635	0.14
West Bengal	159,141	0.12
Andaman and Nicobar Islands	4472	0.0
Chandigarh	15,547	1.0
Dadra & Nagar Haveli	1735	0.06
Daman & Diu	1143	0.17
Delhi	122,055	0.22
Puducherry	21,779	0.11

Data from National AIDS Control Organization, Department of AIDS Control, Ministry of Health and Family Welfare. Government of India. Annual Report 2010–2011. Available at: http://nacoonline.org. Accessed April 23, 2012.

in India. It is targeted to reduce new infections by 60% in high-prevalence states and 40% in vulnerable states.

The Evolution of the HIV/AIDS Program in India

Since the first cases of AIDS were reported in India, the GOI and society have addressed the epidemic with increasing concern and resources. The Ministry of

Health and Family Welfare constituted the National AIDS Committee in 1986. The Committee brought together various ministries, NGOs, and private institutions for effective coordination of program implementation. The Committee acts as the highest-level body to oversee the performance of the Program, to provide overall policy directions, and to forge multisectoral collaboration.[10]

Phase I of the National AIDS Control Program

With the support of the World Bank (WB) and WHO, the GOI drafted a detailed 5-year (1992–1997) National Strategic Plan for the Prevention and Control of HIV/AIDS Phase I, the establishment of NACO in India with the activities focused on preventing transmission of HIV through blood and blood products, control of hospital infections, increasing awareness of the dangers of unsafe sexual behaviors with multiple partners, and sharing of needles for injecting drugs and strengthening of clinical services for both STIs and HIV/AIDS. The formation of the state AIDS societies helped in decentralization of administration and finance for more focused program implementation at the local level.

Phase II of the National AIDS Control Program

Phase II of the National AIDS Control Program (NACP-II) began in 1999. It is a completely centrally sponsored scheme implemented in 35 states and Union Territory (UT)s by the state AIDS control societies and municipal corporations in the cities. NACO assumed the responsibility for activities such as epidemiological surveillance for STIs and HIV/AIDS, training and capacity building, operational research, and monitoring and evaluation. In 2002, the GOI finalized and released the National AIDS Control Policy and the National Blood Safety Program.

Phase III of the National AIDS Control Program

In 2005, NACO developed the Third National AIDS Program Implementation Plan (2006–2011) based on the lessons learned and achievements made in Phases I and II and wide-ranging consultations/discussions with working groups, e-forums, civil society organizations, PLHA networks, NGOs/Community Based Organizations (CBO)s, national expert groups, development partners, and the WB team. The primary goal of Phase III of the National AIDS Control Program (NACP-III) was to halt and reverse the epidemic in India in 5 years time by integrating programs for prevention, care, support, and treatment and reduce the rate of incidence by 60% in the first year of the program in high-prevalence states to obtain the reversal of the epidemic, and by 40% in the vulnerable states to stabilize the HIV epidemic. In NACP-III there was further decentralization of its organizational structure to implement programs at the district level.

HIV Sentinel Surveillance

Conducting HIV sentinel surveillance (HSS) in India was a massive undertaking. In 1994, HSS was conducted in 55 sites and expanded to 1361 sites in 2010.[1] NACO is a government institution established in 1992. To estimate the prevalence of HIV, NACO conducts sentinel surveillance throughout the country. The system uses anonymous unlinked sample screening for HIV antibodies to estimate the prevalence of HIV in various states and population groups. Surveys are conducted annually, and survey sites include sexually transmitted disease (STD) clinics, antenatal clinics, sites that target IDUs, and those that target MSM. HIV testing is offered by government institutions and by private hospital-based or independent clinical laboratories. There is no national information system that collects HIV testing information from clinical laboratories in the private sector, so prevalence estimates are based solely on the sentinel surveillance mechanism.

HSS is conducted annually for a period of 3 months in different population groups called sentinel groups, including ANC attendees, STD patients (bridge population), and HRGs (female CSWs, MSM, eunuchs/transgender, long-distance truck drivers, single male migrants, and IDUs) via an unlinked anonymous testing (UAT) strategy. Sample collection is done by consecutive sampling methodology in which samples are consecutively collected for a period of 3 months in persons aged 15 to 49 years. A sample size of 400 in ANC attendees and 250 in STD patients are collected. In HRGs a sample size of 250 or "take all approach" is used. Until the 2007 round of HSS, venous blood was collected for HIV testing from all sentinel groups. However, in the 2008 round of HSS, dried blood spot (DBS) testing was implemented for collection of blood from HRGs. DBS are collected after UAT with informed consent for high-risk individuals aged 18 to 49 years. For participants between the ages of 15 and 17 years, consent from the participant and informed consent from the guardian/caregiver is obtained. In the last concluded round of HSS in India (HSS 2010), a new sampling methodology called random sampling methodology was used in HRGs, in which a random list of HRI was selected out of the master list by random sampling.[13]

For HIV testing in surveillance, the two test strategies as recommended by NACO are used. The serum samples are first tested either by enzyme-linked immunosorbent assay (ELISA) or rapid tests with high sensitivity. A positive sample is confirmed by a second test of high specificity, and is based on a different antigen preparation and/or different test principle, from the first test. The DBS samples are tested by two ELISAs. A DBS sample found positive by the first ELISA is retested by a second ELISA of higher specificity, based on a different antigen preparation and/or different test principle, from the first test.[14]

HIV testing in antenatal clinics

With the support of UNICEF, NACO launched the national prevention of parent-to-child transmission (PPTCT) program. The key components included antenatal care, HIV counseling and testing, safe delivery practices, administering nevirapine (NVP) to the mother and infant, and counseling for infant feeding options. The Program covers 286 institutions including nationwide private and government medical colleges and all the districts in the six high-prevalence states of India. A summary of data collected during the period from April to December 2010 is given in **Table 4**. The HIV testing acceptance rate was good (86%). The overall HIV prevalence in ANC clinics is approximately 0.27% with statewise variation.

HIV testing in tuberculosis patients

HIV is the most important known risk factor that promotes progression to active TB in people with *Mycobacterium tuberculosis* infection. A study conducted in Pune, India showed that the seroprevalence of HIV among TB patients increased from 10 % in 1995 to 28.75 % in 2000.[15,16] Similar studies done in Tamil Nadu also demonstrated a rise in the seroprevalence of HIV in tuberculosis patients.[17,18] The sentinel surveillance report from NACO indicated a high HIV prevalence of 9.2% in tuberculosis patients in the high-prevalence states of India in 2004.[19] A study from Delhi reported a HIV prevalence of 8.3% among tuberculosis patients during 2003–2005; however, the same hospital had reported a prevalence of 0.4% in 1995–1999 and 9.4% in 2000–2002.[20–22] As per the national estimates, the HIV prevalence among TB patients in India was 4.85% in 2007. This was four times higher than previous estimates, and suggests that tuberculosis patients may be used as an efficient source for HIV case-finding in India.[23]

HIV testing in blood banks

Following a report of transfusion-associated HIV transmission was reported from Vellore in Tamil Nadu in 1987, the routine HIV testing of blood was initiated in 1988.[24] HIV screening in blood banks in India became mandatory in 1989.[25] In 2009, of the estimated 120,000 new HIV infections in the country, transfusion of blood or blood products accounted for 1% of the infections.[1] To reduce the transfusion-associated HIV infection stringent quality control parameters have been defined. For monitoring of blood banks, Blood Transfusion Councils have been established at national and state levels. Currently there are 1127 blood banks in the country.[1] HIV testing in blood banks is carried out following the national strategies/algorithms.

HIV TESTING AND COUNSELING

NACO has been expanding Voluntary Counseling and Testing Centers (VCTCs) since 1998. Significant progress has been made during 2003–2004 with the technical support of WHO and UNAIDS. Seven hundred and nine VCTCs have been established nationwide (655 in NACO and 74 in other GOI settings). All districts in the six high-prevalence states have at least one VCTC. Between April and December 2010, more than 11.1 million were provided pretest counseling for HIV and 10.6 million were tested for HIV, with overall HIV seropositivity being 1.96%.[1] Although the availability of VCTC increased under the project, the number of trained counselors is insufficient. NACO is planning to expand VCTC to the subdistrict level in all states to improve the accessibility of services. A monitoring and supervision system for the performance and quality of VCTC has now been established. Although NACO is scaling up training and improving the quality of HIV testing and counseling in the public sector, the quality is very limited or unknown in the private sector with no regulating mechanism in place.

Objectives of HIV Testing

The objectives of HIV testing include the following: safety of donated blood, blood products, sperms, organs, and tissues; diagnosis of HIV infection in clinically suspected individuals; voluntary testing, after counseling; sentinel surveillance to monitor epidemiologic trends; and research. Client-initiated HIV testing and counseling, also known as Voluntary Counseling and Testing (VCT), involves individuals actively seeking HIV testing and counseling at a facility that offers these services. VCT is conducted in a wide variety of settings including health facilities, stand-alone facilities outside health institutions, through mobile services, in community-based settings, and even in homes if required.

Declining Trends of Adult HIV Prevalence

The adult HIV prevalence at the national level has continued its steady decline from estimated level of 0.41% in 2000 through 0.36% in 2006 to 0.31% in 2009. All the high-prevalence states show a clear declining trend in adult HIV prevalence. HIV has declined notably in Tamil Nadu to reach 0.33% in 2009. However, the low prevalence states of Chandigarh, Orissa, Kerala, Jharkhand, Uttarakhand, Jammu and Kashmir, Arunachal Pradesh, and Meghalaya show rising trends in adult HIV prevalence in the last 4 years.

Based on sentinel surveillance data, HIV prevalence in the adult population can be broadly classified into the three groups of states and union territories in the country:

1. High HIV prevalence states in which prevalence of HIV infection is 1% or higher in antenatal women
2. Moderate HIV prevalence states in which prevalence of HIV infection is 5% or higher among HRGs, but lower than 1% in antenatal women
3. Low HIV prevalence states in which the prevalence of HIV infection is lower than 5% in any of the HRGs and lower than 1% among antenatal women.

The PPTCT Program was started in the country in the year 2002. Currently, there are more than 5233 ICTCs in the country, most of these in government hospitals, that offer PPTCT services to pregnant women. About 10% pregnancies in the country are covered under PPTCT. In the year 2011, 2.1 million pregnant women accessed this service. Of these, more than 16,500 pregnant women were HIV positive. To provide universal access to these services, further scaleup is planned up to the level of Community Health Center and the Primary Health Center, as well as private sector by forging public–private partnerships.

Under NACP-III, VCTCs and facilities providing PPTCT services are remodeled as a hub or ICTC to provide services to all clients under one roof. An ICTC is a place where a person is counseled and tested for HIV, of his own free will or as advised by a medical provider. The main functions of an ICTC are:

1. Conducting HIV diagnostic tests
2. Providing basic information on the modes of HIV transmission, and promoting behavioral change to reduce vulnerability
3. Link people with other HIV prevention, care, and treatment services.

Ideally, a health facility should have an ICTC for all groups of people. However, an ICTC is located in hospitals or facilities that serve specific categories such as pregnant women. Accordingly, an ICTC could be located in the Obstetrics and Gynaecology Department of a medical college or a district hospital or in a maternity home where the majority of clients who access counseling and testing services are pregnant women. The justification for such a center is the need for providing medical care to prevent HIV transmission from infected pregnant women to their infants. Similarly an ICTC could be located in a TB microscopy center or in a TB sanatorium, where the majority of clients would be TB patients. The availability of HIV counseling and testing can help patients to diagnose their status for accessing early anti-HIV treatment.

The challenge before NACO is to make all HIV-infected people in the country aware of their status so that they adopt a healthy lifestyle, access life-saving care and treatment, and help prevent further transmission of HIV. Thus, counseling and testing services are important components of prevention and control of HIV/AIDS in the country.

In 2006, more than 2.1 million clients accessed counseling and testing services in the ICTC throughout the country. Under NACP-III, the target is to counsel and test 22 million clients annually by the year 2012.

Access to HIV testing and counseling is a key strategy in the prevention and control of the HIV/AIDS epidemic. By knowing their HIV status, infected individuals can access HIV-specific care and treatment, undertake interventions to reduce mother-to-child transmission, and reduce their risk of transmitting the virus to others. However, uptake of HIV testing and knowledge of HIV status is low in most countries worldwide.[1]

Objectives of HIV Testing

The following are objectives of HIV testing:

1. Safety of donated blood, blood products, sperms, organs, and tissues
2. Diagnosis of HIV infection in clinically suspected individuals

3. Voluntary testing, after counseling
4. Sentinel surveillance to monitor epidemiologic trends
5. Research.

Client-initiated HIV testing and counseling, also known as Voluntary Counseling and Testing (VCT), involves individuals actively seeking HIV testing and counseling at a facility that offers these services. VCT usually emphasizes individual risk assessment and management by counselors, addressing issues such as the desirability and implications of taking an HIV test, and the development of individual risk reduction strategies.

Provider-initiated HIV testing and counseling (PITC) refers to HIV testing and counseling that is recommended by health care providers to persons attending health care facilities as a standard component of medical care. The major purpose of such testing and counseling is to enable specific clinical decisions to be made and/or specific medical services to be offered that would not be possible without knowledge of the person's HIV status. PITC is neither mandatory nor compulsory.

The National AIDS Control Program of India initiated VCT and PPTCT programs in 1992. Operational guidelines for VCT and PPTCT were designed in 2001 and revised in 2004. In 2006, VCT and PMTCT were merged under the heading of Integrated Counseling and Testing Centers (ICTC)—HIV testing at ANC and outpatient departments at hospitals.

The national ART program has expanded from eight operational centers in April 2004 to 101 centers in December 2006. A total of 68,461 patients were started on ART at these centers by 2006. Currently, more than 387,205 patients are receiving free ART from these ART centers in India.

Excluding pregnant women, 55% of HIV testing was client initiated and 25% provider initiated in 2006. The consent rate at ICTCs has increased from 62% in 2002 to 86% in 2006. The HIV-positive yield decreased from 22% in 2002 to 5.7% in 2006.

TB–HIV cross referral exists in 14 states. HIV testing of TB patients has doubled from 2005 to 2006. Earlier, HIV testing was recommended only for TB patients who do not respond to TB treatment but current guidelines recommend HIV testing for all TB patients.

The management of HIV/AIDS depends not only on drugs, but also on prevention, which continues to be the mainstay of the response to the HIV epidemic, because, without effective prevention, more people will require treatment. HIV testing is integral to prevention, treatment and care efforts. Early knowledge of one's HIV status is important to curb the spread of the disease. Awareness of their HIV status also links those with HIV to medical care and services that may reduce morbidity and mortality and improve the quality of life.

The UNAIDS/WHO further recommend the following four types of testing:

1. VCT, which is client initiated testing
2. Diagnostic HIV testing, which is indicated whenever a person shows signs or symptoms that are consistent with HIV-related disease, to help in clinical diagnosis and management
3. Routine HIV testing, which is offered by health care providers to all patients for various reasons
4. Mandatory testing of all blood that is destined for transfusion or for manufacture of blood products.

All types of testing should be clearly distinguished and practitioners both in the public and the private health care sector should be aware of them. A study conducted in India among private providers concluded that some physicians had inadequate knowledge about the diagnostic tests: fewer than half gave their patients any advice or information before testing, while few laboratories reported adequate patient counseling before testing.

Counseling is vital in the management of HIV patients. Pretest counseling is essential, because it ensures that an individual has sufficient information to make an informed decision about having an HIV test done. It also provides patients with the skills to cope if they test positive and informs them about available support systems, thereby making them confident to take the test.

The HIV counseling and testing services in India were started in the year 1997, have been scaled up in the recent years. Today, there are more than 4000 Counseling and Testing Centers located at all levels of the public health-care system.

An ICTC is a place where a person is counseled and tested for HIV, of his or her own free will or as advised by a medical provider. HIV testing is a key component of HIV control efforts. Broadening access to HIV testing and counseling is important for effective HIV prevention and treatment approaches. HIV counseling and testing services are inadequate in the majority of low- and middle-income countries worldwide. Timely diagnosis of HIV infection is critical for effective medical management because individuals who are diagnosed late respond poorly to therapy and are at increased risk of death. It also offers an opportunity for reducing HIV transmission during the asymptomatic period. In 2006–2007 in India, 3.3% of men and 3% of women in the 15- to 49-year-old age group, and 34.2% of female CSWs, 3% to 67% of MSM, and 3% to 70% of IDUs across various locations were estimated to have received an HIV test in the past 12 months and knew the result of the test.

Linkages between VCTC and HIV prevention, care, and support services helps the individual in the following ways:

1. Early access to medical care, preventive therapy for TB, other opportunistic infections, and even ART
2. STI prevention and treatment
3. Peer support, including access to HIV support groups
4. Additional counseling to promote behavior change and to accept and cope with serostatus
5. Community support to mainstream HIV/AIDS.

HIV testing of any clients, referred from hospitals or voluntary walk-in, is always undertaken after pretest HIV counseling and obtaining client's written informed consent.

HIV Testing in India's Private Medical Sector

The diverse and largely unregulated private medical sector contains nearly 80% of India's practicing physicians and varies greatly in terms of its organization and the care it delivers.[26] Private providers are the preferred source of care for the population regardless of income status, and their role in the diagnosis and management of HIV-infected individuals is significant.[27]

Counseling in HIV: Policy and Practice

The exceptional nature of HIV/AIDS has prompted debate regarding the necessity and the enormous challenges of regulating patient–provider communication around HIV testing.[28–30] Counseling before and after an HIV test is one example of a prescribed code for practitioner–patient communication. Included in the WHO and UNAIDS

(UNAIDS 2004) policies, HIV counseling guidelines have been adopted by many countries including India.[31] India's NACO policies require that physicians conduct HIV testing on a voluntary basis with appropriate pre- and post-test counseling. Physicians are to maintain patient confidentiality and results are to be given out to the members of the patient's family with his or her consent. The guidelines further state that the person should be encouraged to share this information with the family so as to obtain proper home-based care and emotional support from the family members. Attending physicians are encouraged to disclose the HIV status to the spouse or sexual partner of the person with proper counseling.[32] Disclosure of a positive result should ideally be accompanied by supportive information about treatment and coping strategies for the physical, psychological, and financial burden that a patient might face.[32,33]

Issues in HIV Testing and Diagnosis

It is important for every nation to have effective, voluntary counseling and testing services for HIV infection. Benefits include early management of HIV infection and thus improvement in quality of life, and the primary and secondary prevention of HIV infection. Only a small fraction of persons living with HIV are aware of their infection, and of those who do receive clinical testing, many may not have been provided with adequate counseling. Hence, it is essential to make more efforts to ensure that the majority of HIV testing in India is accompanied by adequate pretest and post-test HIV counseling.

Issues Related to Quality Control in HIV Testing/Accreditation

The laboratories in India to take part in quality-assurance and quality-control exercises for HIV testing. HIV test results could be inaccurate for several reasons if quality control measures are not put into place, and these could be: test kits are used after the expiration dates; kits are not stored at the correct temperature; electricity is shut down at night; air-conditioning for the testing equipment is erratic; poor-quality water is used; and tubes, tips, and other equipment are recycled. Makeshift laboratories may have scant respect for quality control or assurance and thus, patients would not necessarily be sure of their test results, especially when these laboratories do not provide patients with an opportunity to discuss their lifestyles and risk histories with a counselor who could then help them place the result within that context.

HIV TESTING METHODOLOGIES IN INDIA

Unlike other infectious diseases, HIV/AIDS is a difficult disease to deal with. Many issues ethical, moral, legal, and psychological issues are associated with an HIV-positive status of an individual. Therefore persons who deal with HIV status of an individual must be well versed with the aforementioned issues along with testing strategies and algorithms, protocols, reason for using the test kits, correct way of communicating the result to the individual, counseling, and maintaining confidentiality. HIV testing is done for the following purposes:

1. To ensure safety of blood and blood products
2. To know the efficacy of targeted intervention programs conducted in HRGs
3. To monitor the trends of HIV epidemic in the country
4. To diagnose clinically suspected cases
5. To detect asymptomatic persons practicing high-risk behavior
6. For prevention, management and treatment of HIV and related infections

7. To bring behavior change persons test positive and prevent transmission of infection by counseling.

There are a variety of tests available for the detection of HIV infection. ELISA is a commonly used screening test for the detection of HIV antibodies. In India, ELISA is routinely performed as a screening test in blood banks and tertiary care hospitals that receive large number of samples for HIV testing because the test is easy to perform, cheap, sensitive, and specific.

Rapid HIV tests give results in 30 minutes. A multicentric study conducted in India has shown that the rapid tests are as sensitive and specific as that of ELISA. These tests have been recommended for use in ICTCs, PPTCTs, and emergency situations as screening as well as supplemental/confirmatory tests following national strategies and algorithms of testing. HIV antibodies are commonly detected in serum, blood, or plasma. Detection of HIV in oral fluids or urine is not commonly done in India.

Selection of good quality HIV test kits is an important part of HIV testing. Each test kit manufacturer claims to have high sensitivity, specificity, and predictive values for its kits. Many factors such as condition of the laboratory, technical expertise, and population being tested affect the performance of the test kit. Hence, before being available for testing purposes, these kits are evaluated per the directives of Drug Controller of General of India. National Institute of Biologicals (NIB, Noida, Uttar Pradesh, India), a statutory body, has been entrusted with the responsibility of evaluating and approving these kits before they are distributed to the government and private sector. After approval is obtained from NIB, each lot of test kits is evaluated by the National Reference Laboratories before their use in government testing laboratories. Sensitivity, specificity, efficiency, positive predictive value, and negative predictive value are the parameters evaluated to assess the performance character-istics of test kits.

WHO/GOI have evolved strategies/algorithms for the detection of HIV infection in different population groups. These strategies use different categories of tests in different permutations and combinations. Different strategies/algorithms used in HIV testing are as follows[34]:

- **Strategy/algorithm I:** In this strategy, serum is tested for HIV by ELISA/rapid. If the test result is negative, the sample is considered as negative for HIV. If positive, the sample is considered as HIV positive. This strategy/algorithm is used to assess donation safety of blood, blood products, and tissues. The unit of blood found to be HIV positive is discarded. If consent was obtained from the donor, the test result is given to the donor with a referred to ICTC for counseling and confirmation of the test result.
- **Strategy/algorithm II:** This strategy is used in sentinel surveillance; if the first test is negative the sample is considered as negative. But if the first test is positive, the sample is tested by a second test different from the first test.
- **Strategy/algorithm IIB:** This algorithm uses two to three different test kits. The sample is considered as negative if the test result is negative and positive if two serial tests of different test principle or having different antigens give a positive result. However, if the first test is positive and the second test is negative, a third test is employed to confirm the result. If the result of the third test is positive, the sample is considered as indeterminate and repeat testing is done after 2 to 4 weeks. If the third test result is negative, the sample is considered as HIV negative. This algorithm is used for the diagnosis of symptomatic clinically suspected AIDS cases.

- **Strategy/algorithm III:** This strategy is similar to strategy IIB; however, a third consecutive test is required to confirm the results first two tests before being reported as HIV positive. The first test used should have the highest sensitivity and the second and third tests the highest specificity. All three tests either have different test principles or different antigens. This strategy is used for the diagnosis of HIV infection in asymptomatic individuals at PPTCTs and ICTCs.

In both strategies (IIB and III) guidelines of counseling, informed consent, and confidentiality are followed strictly.[34] HIV testing methodologies are based on national programs. Based on the purpose, different testing methodologies are being used. Detection of antibodies to HIV in the blood of an HIV-infected person is the most common method of diagnosis of HIV infection. The HIV testing methodologies used in India for various purposes are described in the following subsections.

ICTCs

In an ICTC setting, rapid HIV tests are used for HIV testing per NACO recommendation, which provide results within 30 minutes after the test. Rapid test kits that detect greater than 99.5% of all HIV-infected patients and give false-positive results in fewer than 2% of all those who are tested are recommended for use. The testing will be done free of cost for all persons in all ICTCs situated in government hospitals and in all stand-alone ICTCs supported by NACO. If the result of one test is negative then the person is declared as HIV negative. The test may be negative during the window period and testing is repeated after 12 weeks. When the result of one test is positive, then the same blood is tested by two additional tests using kits with different antigens/principles. In an HIV-positive person all the three tests will be positive. In an emergency situation such as a women in labor with unknown HIV status, basic information on HIV/AIDS and testing is provided to the individual and a single HIV test is performed to determine the HIV status of the women and need for ART to prevent mother-to-child transmission. A repeat testing is conducted subsequently to confirm the HIV status.

Diagnosis of HIV in the Newborn

Detection of HIV antibodies in infant blood sample cannot be used for diagnosis of HIV infection and are not useful because maternal antibodies may be present in the newborn for up to 18 months. Therefore, molecular diagnostic tests such as DNA or RNA polymerase chain reaction (PCR) are used in the diagnosis of HIV infection in newborns. These tests are done twice, once at 6 weeks and again at 6 months of age but the results need to be confirmed by conducting serologic testing of the infant when the child is 18 months of age.

COST OF HIV TESTING IN INDIA

A study conducted in 2005 in Andhra Pradesh showed that the cost of complete VCT services to each HIV-positive and negative person was Rs123.5 (US$2.54) and Rs59.2 (US$1.22), respectively.[35]

QUALITY ASSURANCE/QUALITY CONTROL IN HIV TESTING

Quality Assurance and Quality Control are an integral part of HIV testing. NACP III has focused on the assurance of quality in kit evaluation and assessment of HIV testing services through implementation of an External Quality Assessment Scheme (EQAS). In 2000, NACO launched the National External Quality Assessment Scheme (NEQAS) to ensure standard quality of the HIV tests being performed in the program.

Internal Quality Control Procedures

NACO in the NACP III program has recommended use of known controls, both positive and negative, on a day-to-day basis. The responsibility of preparation and sending of internal QC samples to State Reference Laboratories (SRLs) has been given to National Reference Laboratories (NRLs). The SRLs further aliquot these samples and send them to the peripheral testing centers.

EQAS

Under the NEQAS, the HIV testing laboratories have been categorized into four levels: Apex laboratory, NRLs, SRLs, and District level (ICTC and blood banks). Currently there is one Apex laboratory, 13 NRLs, and 118 SRLs.[1] Each NRL monitors the designated states allotted to it and is also responsible for training and supervision SRLs. The ICTC and blood banks are monitored by the designated SRLs. All ICTCs participate in an external quality assessment scheme and have been assigned an SRL. Under EQAS, each ICTC receive coded samples from the reference laboratories twice a year for testing. In addition, ICTCs also send 20% of all positive samples and 5% of all negative samples collected in the first week of every third month for cross-checking to the SRL once every quarter.[36] In blood banks positive and negative controls (from kit and in-house) are to be run with every test as a quality control measure.

In HSS, before the commencement of the survey activity as part of EQAS, proficiency testing is conducted by sending the coded samples from NRLs to respective SRLs because these have been identified as testing centers for HIV testing. During the surveillance period, the SRLs will send all positive samples and 5% negative samples to the respective NRLs for the purpose of cross checking.[14]

REFERENCES

1. National AIDS Control Organization (NACO). Annual report 2010–2011. Delhi (India): Department of AIDS Control, National AIDS Control Organization, Ministry of Health and Family Welfare, Government of India. Available at: http://nacoonline.org. Accessed October 23, 2011.
2. Duraisamy P, Ganesh AK, Homan R, et al. Costs and financial burden of care and support services to PLHA and households in South India. AIDS Care 2006;18:121–7.
3. National AIDS Control Organization (NACO). List of ART centres as on January 2011. Delhi (India): Department of AIDS Control, National AIDS Control Organization, Ministry of Health and Family Welfare, Government of India. Available at: http://www.nacoonline.org. Accessed June 7, 2011.
4. Simoes EA, Babu PG, John TJ, et al. Evidence for HTLV-III infection in prostitutes in Tamil Nadu (India). Indian J Med Res 1987;85:335–8.
5. Ekstrand M, Garbus L, Marseille E. HIV/AIDS in India. Country AIDS Policy Analysis Project. UCSF. San Francisco (CA): AIDS Policy Research Center, University of California; 2003.
6. Eicher AD, Crofts N, Benjamin S, et al. A certain fate: Spread of HIV among young injecting drug users in Manipur, north-east India. AIDS Care 2000;12:497–504.
7. United Nations Office on Drugs and Crimes (UNODC) and Ministry of Social Justice and Empowerment (MSJE). Rapid assessment survey of drug abuse in India. New Delhi (India): UNDCP Regional Office for South Asia and Ministry of Social Justice and Empowerment, Government of India; 2002.
8. Dorabjee J, Samson L. A multicentre rapid assessment of injecting drug use in India. Int J Drug Policy 2000;11:99–112.

9. UNAIDS. India: illustrative menu of partnership options in India. January 2002. Available at: http://www.unaids.org/partnership/pdf/INDIAinserts.pdf. Accessed May 23, 2012.

10. National AIDS Control Organization (NACO). Facts and figures: observed HIV prevalence levels state wise: 1998–2004. Delhi (India):.National AIDS Control Organization, Ministry of Health and Family Welfare, Government of India; 2005.

11. Tripathy SP, Kulkarni SS, Jadhav SD, et al. Subtype B and subtype C HIV type 1 recombinants in the northeastern state of Manipur, India. AIDS Res Hum Retroviruses 2005;21(2):152–7.

12. Sahni AK, Gupta RM, Nagendra A, et al. Identification of human Immunodeficiency virus type-1: subtyes by Heteroduplex Mobility Assay. MJAFI 2007;63:249–52.

13. National AIDS Control Organization (NACO). HIV sentinel surveillance: operational manual for HRG sentinel sites. Department of AIDS Control. Delhi (India): National AIDS Control Organization, Ministry of Health and Family Welfare, Government of India; 2010.

14. National AIDS Control Organization (NACO). Operational guidelines for HIV sentinel surveillance. Delhi (India): National AIDS Control Organization, Ministry of Health and Family Welfare, Government of India; 2008.

15. Paranjape RS, Tripathy SP, Menon PA, et al. Increasing trend of HIV seroprevalence among pulmonary tuberculosis patients in Pune, India. Indian J Med Res 1997;106: 207–11.

16. Tripathy S, Joshi DR, Mehendale SM, et al. Sentinel survelliance for HIV infection in tuberculosis patients in India. Indian J Tuberc 2002;49:17–20.

17. Ramachandran R, Datta M, Subramani R, et al. Seroprevalence of human immunodeficiency virus (HIV) infection among tuberculosis patients in Tamil Nadu. Indian J Med Res 2003;118:147–51.

18. Rajasekaran S, Uma A, Kamakshi S, et al. Trend of HIV infection in patients with tuberculosis in rural south India. Indian J Tuberc 2000;47:223–6.

19. National AIDS Control Organization (NACO). Annual report 2002–2004. Delhi (India): National AIDS Control Organization, Ministry of Health and Family Welfare, Government of India; 2004.

20. Piramanayagam P, Tahir M, Sharma SK, et al. Persistently high HIV seroprevalence among adult tuberculosis patients at a tertiary care centre in Delhi. Indian J Med Res 2007;125:163–6.

21. Sharma SK, Saha PK, Dixit Y, et al. HIV seropositivity among adult tuberculosis patients in Delhi. Indian J Chest Dis Allied Sci 2000;42:157–60.

22. Sharma SK, Aggarwal G, Seth P, et al. Increasing HIV seropositivity among adult tuberculosis patients in Delhi. Indian J Med Res 2003;117:239–42.

23. Dewan PK, Gupta D, Williams BG, et al. National estimate of HIV seroprevalence among tuberculosis patients in India. Int J Tuberc Lung Dis 14(2):247–9.

24. John TJ, Babu PG, Pulimood BR, et al. Prevalence of human immunodeficiency virus infection among voluntary blood donors. Indian J Med Res 1989;89:1–3.

25. Dasgupta PR, Jain MK, John TJ. Government response to HIV/AIDS in India. AIDS 1994;6(Suppl):S83–S90.

26. Bhat R. Regulating the private health care sector: the case of the Indian Consumer Protection Act. Health Policy Plan 1996;11:265–79.

27. Raghuram S, Iyer A, Sen G. Health sector changes and health equity in the 1990s. In: Raghuram S, editor. Health and equity—effecting change. Bangalore (India): Humanist Institute for Cooperation (HIVOS); 2000.

28. De Cock KM, Johnson AM. From exceptionalism to normalization: a reappraisal of attitudes and practice around HIV testing. BMJ 1998;316:290–3.

29. Pochard F, Grassin M, Le Roux N, et al. Medical secrecy or disclosure in HIV transmission: a physician's ethical conflict. Arch Inter Med 1998;158:1716–9.
30. Pinching AJ, Higgs R, Boyd KM. The impact of AIDS on medical ethics. J Med Ethics 2000;26:3–8.
31. Coovadia HM. Access to voluntary counseling and testing for HIV in developing countries. Ann N Y Acad Sci 2000;918:57–63.
32. National AIDS Control Organization (NACO). National AIDS prevention and control policy. New Delhi (India): National AIDS Control Organization, Ministry of Health and Family Welfare, Government of India; 2003.
33. UNAIDS/WHO. UNAIDS/WHO Policy Statement on HIV Testing, June 2004. Joint United Nations Programme on HIV/AIDS. Available at: http://www.who.int/hiv/pub/vct/statement/en/. Accessed May 23, 2012.
34. National AIDS Control Organization (NACO), Ministry of Health AND Family Welfare. Guidelines on HIV testing. New Delhi (India): National AIDS Control Organization, Ministry of Health and Family Welfare, Government of India; 2007.
35. Dandona L, Sisodia P, Ramesh YK, et al. Cost and efficiency of HIV voluntary counselling and testing centres in Andhra Pradesh, India. Natl Med J India. 2005; 18(1):26–31.
36. National AIDS Control Organization (NACO). Operational guidelines for integrated counselling and testing centres. New Delhi (India): National AIDS Control Organization, Ministry of Health and Family Welfare, Government of India; 2007.

Screening for Cervical Cancer and Human Papilloma Virus Indian Context

Kedar K. Deodhar, MD, FRCPath

KEYWORDS

- Cervical cancer • Screening • Visual inspection with acetic acid
- Human papilloma virus testing

KEY POINTS

- Cervical cancer remains the most common fatal cancer in Indian women.
- The primary underlying cause of cervical cancer is persistent infection with human papilloma virus (HPV); HPV 16 and 18 account for nearly 70% of all cervical cancers worldwide.
- Cytology-based cervical screening programs have been very effective, but require establishing an infrastructure and quality control mechanisms, which can be a challenge.
- Cervical screening by visual inspection with acetic acid (VIA) and visual inspection with Lugol's iodine (VILI) are acceptable alternatives for low-resource settings.
- Primary screening for cervical cancer with HPV testing is attractive but cost could be the limiting factor. A less expensive HPV test holds promise.

INTRODUCTION

Cervical cancer is the third most common cancer in women, and the seventh overall, with an estimated 530,000 new cases in 2008. More than 85% of the global burden occurs in developing countries, where it accounts for 13% of all female cancers. Overall, the mortality/incidence ratio is 52%, and cervical cancer was responsible for 275,000 deaths in 2008, approximately 88% of which occurred in developing countries: 53,000 in Africa, 31,700 in Latin America and the Caribbean, and 159,800 in Asia.

In India, cervical cancer remains the most common cancer in women, with carcinoma of the breast a close second. Estimated incidence in Indian women (age-standardized ratio [ASR]) for cervical cancer is 27 per 100,000 and 22.9 per 100,000 for carcinoma of the breast. In India an estimated 134,420 new cases and

The author has nothing to disclose.
Department of Pathology, Tata Memorial Hospital, Dr. E. Borges Road, Parel, Mumbai 400012, Maharashtra, India
E-mail address: kedardeodhar@hotmail.com

Clin Lab Med 32 (2012) 193–205
http://dx.doi.org/10.1016/j.cll.2012.04.003
0272-2712/12/$ – see front matter

labmed.theclinics.com

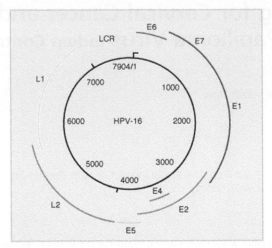

Fig. 1. HPV genome.

72,825 deaths due to cervical cancer were recorded in 2008, contributing to greater than 23% mortality in women.[1]

According to a recent study of cancer mortality in India by Dikshit and colleagues, the most common fatal cancers in Indian women are cervical (17.1%), stomach (14.1%), and breast (10.2%).[2] Of note, cervical cancer is the most preventable cancer, and significant declines have occurred in high-income countries (HICs), where screening programs have been ongoing for the last three decades.

ETIOLOGY

The primary underlying cause of cervical cancer is persistent infection with human papilloma virus (HPV), a common virus that is sexually transmitted. The causal relationship has been generally accepted from molecular epidemiology studies, case-control studies, cohort studies using cervical intraepithelial neoplasia (CIN) 2 and 3 as the endpoints, and screening studies.[3,4]

HPV

Zur Housen in the late 1970s suggested that there might be an association between HPV and cervical carcinoma.[5] Papilloma viruses are part of papillomaviradae family **(Fig. 1)**.[6]

The viral genome can be divided into three regions: the upstream regulatory region (URR), also known as long central region (LCR); the early region; and the late region. The URR is the noncoding region of the viral genome and is important in viral replication. Both the early region and late region contain a series of open reading frames (ORFs), which lack stop codons and are potentially translated into proteins. The early region ORFs encode for protein required for viral replication and maintenance of high viral copy number in infected cells. Six different ORFs, designated as E1, E2, E4, E5, E6, and E7, have been identified in the early regions of HPV.

The late region of HPV is downstream of the early region and contains two ORFs, which encode L1 and L2 that encode capsid proteins. The L1-encoded protein is the major capsid protein and is highly conserved among papillomaviruses of all species.[6]

Most HPV infections resolve spontaneously; those that persist may lead to development of cervical cancer. More than 100 subtypes of HPV have been recognized.

HPV-Induced Carcinogenesis

Two viral oncoproteins, E6 and E7, are known to play a major role in HPV-mediated cervical carcinogenesis. In vitro experiments showed that rodent fibroblasts are transformed or fully immortalized by expression of HPV 16 E6 and E7 protein. These rodent cells acquire the ability to grow in an anchorage-independent manner and are tumorigenic. HPV E6 and E7 are able to immortalize human keratinocytes, which are the natural host cells for HPV.[7,8]

E6 and E7 brings about the neoplastic changes by interacting with tumor suppressor protein TP53 and tumor suppressor gene *pRB*. Both interactions cause rapid degradation of the cellular proteins via the ubiqutin pathway. Normally, TP53 safeguards the integrity of the genome by bringing about cell cycle arrest and apoptosis. Retinoblastoma protein (pRB) controls the correct G1/S transition of the cell cycle. Disruption of both of these normal control mechanisms leads to uncontrolled cell proliferation and tumorigenesis.[9–13]

More than 100 types of HPV are recognized. The types of HPV that are considered as carcinogenic are 16,18, 31,33, 35, 39, 45, 51, 52, 56, 58, 59, and 68. The others, such as types 26, 53, 66, 67, 70, 73, and 82, are considered possibly carcinogenic.[11] HPV 16 and 18 account for nearly 70% of all cervical cancers worldwide.[14,15] Interestingly, HPV types 16, 18, and 45 were the most common HPV types in cervical adenocarcinomas.[15]

Cross-sectional studies of the prevalence of HPV show that HPV DNA in high-grade squamous intraepithelial neoplasia (HSIL) was found to be associated in 85% of the cases. HPV 16 accounts for 45% of all high-grade lesions (CIN 2/3).[16]

Several contributory factors can aid persistence of HPV infection, which include immunosuppression[17] or HIV infection,[18] high parity,[19] oral contraceptive use,[20] smoking,[21] and certain sexually transmitted diseases such as *Chlamydia* infection.[22]

SCREENING EFFORTS: CYTOLOGY, VISUAL INSPECTION WITH ACETIC ACID, VISUAL INSPECTION WITH LUGOL'S IODINE, AND HPV SCREENING
Conventional Cervical Cytology

Screening using conventional cervical cytology, that is, the Papanicolaou test (Pap smear), is the most effective cancer reduction program ever devised. The aim of any cancer screening program is to reduce the mortality associated with that disease. In the natural history of cervical cancer, significant precancerous lesions (CIN 2/3) can take 10 to 15 years to develop into an invasive carcinoma. Hence, after detection, appropriate treatment can be offered to the patient to treat CIN 2/3, thus minimizing the chances of development of the cancer.

Cervical screening by cytology has succeeded in reducing the death rate from carcinoma of the cervix. Although screening using the Pap smear has not been tested in a randomized clinical trial in developed countries, the marked differences in the incidence and mortality figures for cervical cancer before and after the introduction of screening has been interpreted as robust evidence of the effectiveness of such a program. The first screening clinics were started in 1940 in the United States. The mortality rate from cervical cancer was dramatically reduced by 70% in Kentucky.[23] Among the Scandinavian countries, in Iceland the death rate fell by 80%; in Norway, where the screening was lowest, the death rate fell by 10%.[24] It was also noted that frequent screening is more effective; that is, there was a direct correlation between the intensity of screening and decrease in mortality. A similar correlation was observed in high- and low-screening regions of Scotland.[25]

Obtaining a cervical smear is a simple, painless, outpatient procedure. A few cells are scraped from the cervical epithelium using a wooden spatula or brush and then are smeared on a glass slide. The slide is then quickly fixed in appropriate fixative, stained, and then screened/read by a cytologist. It is reported in standard formats. The majority of the centers use The Bethesda System 2001 diagnostic categories; whereas in the United Kingdom, similar (but not identical) diagnostic terminologies are used as per guidelines by the National Health Service cervical screening program. (Diagnostic categories used in The Bethesda System are given in brief in Appendix 1). A successful cervical screening program mandates the need for appropriately trained personnel, laboratory infrastructure with stringent quality control measures, and an efficient system or communicating the results to the referring physician.

Large population-based cytology screening programs have been in place for several years in HICs/developed countries, for example, Nordic countries, the United Kingdom, the United States, Australia, and New Zealand. Systematic implementation of such programs has over the last few decades led to a drastic reduction in both the incidence of and mortality from cervical cancer.

For conventional Pap tests, estimates of sensitivity and specificity varied greatly in individual studies. A systematic review conducted by Nanda and colleagues stated sensitivity ranged from 30% to 87% and specificity ranged from 86% to 100%. The authors further conclude that most studies of conventional Pap tests are severely biased; the best estimate suggests that it is only moderately accurate and does not achieve concurrently high sensitivity and specificity.[26] Although annual testing would be ideal, it may not always be practicable and testing every 3 years is an acceptable compromise without any significant loss of protective efficacy.

The success of such a program depends on the wider coverage of the population. Well-organized screening programs with systematized call–recall mechanisms and stringent follow-up have proved to be the most effective.

Liquid-Based Cytology

The last decade has seen the emergence of liquid-based cytology (LBC) as an alternative to conventional Pap testing. In this method, cervical cells are collected using a traditional sampling device into a vial containing preservative solution, and are rinsed into it instead of smeared on a slide. A thin monolayer smear is then prepared by an automatic or semiautomatic technique. This has the advantage of eliminating background blood and inflammatory cells, giving a clean slide to interpret. The main advantage of LBC is reduction in inadequate smears. It also allows reflex testing for HPV with the same sample. However, it has not been shown to perform better than the conventional Pap test in terms of relative sensitivity and positive predictive value for detection of cervical precancer.[27] The relatively high cost of establishing the setup is the limitation.

India lacks a national screening program for cervical cancer. Cytology screening in this country is conducted at few centers as field programs under a research setting, but it is largely opportunistic and restricted mainly to the urban metros. Inadequacy of a uniform infrastructure leading to poor coverage of at-risk women, suboptimal follow-up/treatment of screen-positive women, and suboptimal quality assurance measures are some of the barriers to having a well established screening program.

A critical evaluation of the limitations of cytology as a screening test led to a search for alternative screening techniques based on visual inspection of the cervix, that is, visual

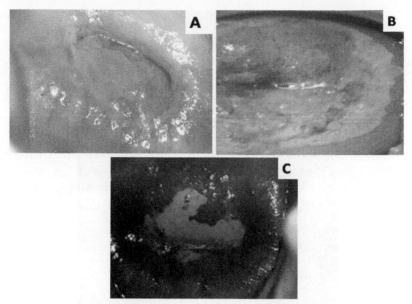

Fig. 2. (*A*) Colposcopic image of squamous metaplasia. (*B*) Colposcopic image, VIA positive. (*C*) Colposcopic image, VILI positive. (*Courtesy of* Dr Sharmila Pimple, Department of Preventive Oncology, Tata Memorial Hospital, Mumbai.)

inspection with acetic acid (VIA), visual inspection with Lugol's iodine (VILI), and HPV DNA testing.

Visual Inspection Tests: VIA and VILI

Visual inspection of the cervix has reemerged as a screening tool for low- and middle-income group countries (LMICs), despite its limited specificity, because it is economical and provides immediate results. It involves examination of the cervix using a naked eye examination with a speculum and a bright halogen focus lamp after applying 4% acetic acid. VIA results are reported 1 minute after the application as per the criteria mentioned in the International Agency for Research on Cancer (IARC) manual.[28] VIA is negative when no acetowhite lesions or ill defined, scattered, or geographic acetowhite areas away from the squamocolumnar junction (SCJ) are detected. VIA is positive when dense, opaque, well defined acetowhite lesions touching the squamocolumnar junction or cervical growth turning acetowhite are seen (**Fig. 2**). This is a simple technique and can be performed by nurses after adequate training. The positive cases can then be referred for colposcopy, directed biopsy, and further appropriate therapy (either cryotherapy or loop electrosurgical excision procedure). VILI involves naked eye examination of the cervix after application of Lugol's iodine. The results are reported immediately. A positive result involves mustard yellow area on the cervix close to the SCJ or on the os or on a cervical growth (see **Fig. 2**; **Fig. 3**).

The test characteristics of VIA have been evaluated in several cross-sectional studies in LMICs. These studies together have involved more than 150,000 women and have shown promising results that support its use as an alternative to conventional cytology. The sensitivity of VIA to detect high-grade precursor lesions and invasive cervical cancer has varied from 49% to 96% and the specificity from 49% to 98%.[29–31]

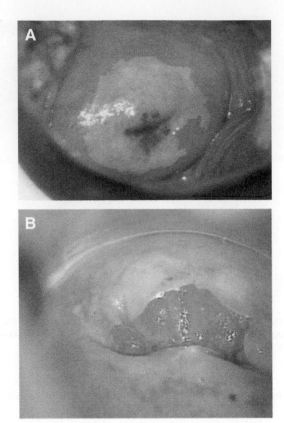

Fig. 3. (*A*) Colposcopic image of CIN 2. (*B*) Colposcopic image of CIN 2/3. (*Courtesy of* Dr Sharmila Pimple, Department of Preventive Oncology, Tata Memorial Hospital, Mumbai.)

The specificity values of VILI varied over a similar range as VIA, between 73.0% and 91.6%. The overall pooled sensitivity for VILI (91.2%; confidence interval [CI] 87.8%–94.6%) was statistically significantly higher than for VIA. On the other hand, the pooled specificity of VILI (84.5%; CI 81.3%–87.8%) was not significantly different from that of VIA.[32,33] A large cluster randomized trial in southern India showed that a single round of screening with VIA reduces cervical cancer incidence and mortality by 25% and 35%, respectively.[34]

Cost-effectiveness studies based on data from India, Kenya, Peru, South Africa, and Thailand indicate that the most cost-effective strategies for cervical screening are those approaches requiring the fewest visits, leading to improved follow-up testing and treatment. The analyses report that screening women once in their lifetime, at the age of 35 years, with a one- or two-visit screening strategy involving VIA or HPV testing reduced the lifetime risk of cancer by approximately 25% to 36%, and costs less than $500 per year of life saved.[35,36]

HPV Testing

HPV causality for cervical cancer is now firmly established and is considered a necessary cause of the disease. HPV 16 and 18 account for 70% of cervical cancer cases. Testing for HPV thus can be an alternative approach in screening. The main benefit of HPV testing is that it has a high sensitivity and a high negative predictive value. A woman with a negative HPV DNA test is highly unlikely to develop CIN 3 for the next 5 to 10 years.[37] However, many younger woman may have transient HPV infection that is largely self eliminated by a host immune response. A single HPV DNA positive result in a younger woman may not be clinically significant. Thus use of HPV testing is better focused on women aged 30 years and older.[38]

Reviews of the HPV-based screening have shown an improved sensitivity (by 23%–25%) and a reduced specificity (by 6%) compared to conventional cytology, at a cutoff of atypical squamous cells of undetermined significance.[39,40]

HPV testing is currently practiced as an adjunct to cytology (reflex testing after a diagnosis of low-grade abnormality on cytology), or also tested in a trial setting with conventional cytology.[39,41]

In 2000, a large population-based cluster randomized trial was initiated involving more than 130,000 women aged 30 to 59 years from a relatively stable rural population in Osmanabad district (Maharashtra State, India). This study was designed to test the effect of a single round of screening by the HPV DNA test, conventional cervical cytology, or VIA on the incidence of and associated mortality from cervical cancer. The results suggested that VIA was more sensitive, slightly less specific, and significantly less costly than cytology. Also, there was no reduction in the incidence of or mortality from cervical cancer in the group undergoing screening by cytology. HPV testing alone was associated with a significant reduction in the numbers of advanced cervical cancers and deaths from cervical cancer.[42]

Similar results were reported by a large trial in Italy, where the first screening round identified almost double the number of CIN 2+ in the HPV arm as compared to the cytology arm, with an almost equal number of invasive cancers in both arms. In the second screening round (at a 3-year interval), the number of CIN 2+ in the HPV arm was significantly less than in the cytology arm. In the second round, the cytology arm had incident cases of invasive cancers, whereas the HPV arm showed no incident cases.[43,44] Studies suggest that when women older than 30 years are offered HPV-based screening, there is minimal overdiagnosis and that HPV screening is useful even when performed less frequently.[39]

Current HPV DNA detection tests are based on hybridization with signal amplification of HPV DNA. Hybrid Capture 2 by Qiagen Inc. (Gaithersburg, MD, USA),[45] Cervista HPV HR by Hologic (Madison, WI, USA),[46] or genomic amplification using polymerase chain reaction (PCR; Amplicor HPV test by Roche Diagnostics, IN, USA; and Cobas HPV test, by Roche Molecular Systems, Pleasanton, CA, USA)[47,48] are some examples.

A rapid, simple to perform, and cost-effective method, which detects 14 high-risk HPV types, has been described recently (Care HPV) and is showing promise.[49] This method has the benefits of low-cost, simple technology and short reporting period that allows for strategies incorporating the see-and-treat approach.

In further efforts to improve specificity and thereby the costs of overdiagnosis/overtreatment, newer technology using E6 and E7 HPV mRNA is being tested. The APTIMA HPV assay detects the mRNA of 14 high-risk HPV types in LBC specimens. Early results from E6/E7screening and triage trials are now being published. When an RNA test (APTIMA) was compared with the DNA test Hybrid Capture 2, it showed a 5% to 6% gain in specificity for CIN 2+ and CIN 3+ at the same levels of sensitivity, and both assays showed 20% superiority compared to LBC.[50–52] These technologies confer a significant advantage over conventional cytology in both screening and triage situations.

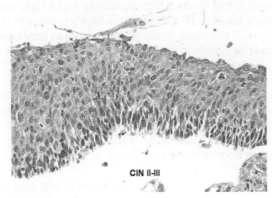

Fig. 4. CIN II–III (H & E histology).

Screening in the Era of HPV Vaccines

As we know, a quadrivalent vaccine (Gardasil by Merck, NJ, USA) containing virus-like particles (VLPs), resembling HPV 6, 11, 16, 18 and a bivalent vaccine (Cervarix by GlaxoSmithKline Biologicals, Rixensart, Belgium) containing VLPs resembling HPV 16 and 18 have been developed. The vaccines essentially contain purified L1 proteins for these types of viruses. They were evaluated in clinical trials and are now licensed in more than 100 countries, including India. The quadrivalent vaccine uses aluminum hydroxyphosphate sulfate (225 μg) as an adjuvant, whereas the bivalent vaccine uses aluminum hydroxide (500 μg) with 50 μg of 3 deacyclated monophosphoryl lipid A (ASO$_4$) as an adjuvant. Both vaccines are found to be effective and safe.[53–55] Generally a schedule of three doses is recommended. The cost of the vaccines is a limiting factor for their wider use in developing countries. Even if these are widely available, does that eliminate the need for cervical cancer screening? The answer is NO. Screening for cervical cancer will need to continue into the foreseeable future. The role of therapeutic HPV vaccines is currently not established.

In a costing exercise in 2005, Lewood and colleagues[56] put forward the cost per case of CIN grade 2/3 or invasive cancer CIN 2/3+ detected. The average total costs per 1000 women eligible for screening were US$3917, US$6609, and US$11779 with VIA, cytology, and HPV respectively, at the prevailing cost. They found screening with VIA to be the least expensive option, but it detected fewer cases of CIN 2/3+.

Tissue Biomarker: p16 *INK4A*

p16 is a cyclin-dependent kinase inhibitor that is overexpressed in cancerous and precancerous cervical tissue. It reflects increased expression of viral E7 oncoprotein, which disrupts the cell cycle regulator (pRb). It has been identified as a biomarker for transforming HPV infection, and is useful for diagnosis of HSIL.[57] Its utility in diagnosing low-grade dysplasia on cervical biopsy, in daily practice, in my opinion, is less clear. In LSIL cytology samples, it has a low sensitivity and acceptable specificity for detection of CIN 2+ lesions.[58] **Fig. 4** shows a CIN 2/3 lesion on histology whereas **Fig. 5** shows diffuse positive p16 staining in CIN 3.

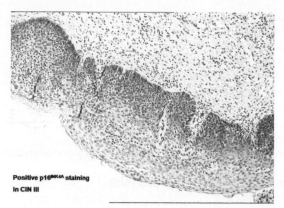

Positive p16^{INK4A} staining
in CIN III

Fig. 5. p16 immunohistochemistry in CIN 3. Note continuous, basal, nuclear, and cytoplasmic staining.

SUMMARY

1. Cytology-based cervical screening programs have stood the test of time but have limitations in establishing the infrastructure and quality control mechanisms.
2. VIA and VILI are acceptable alternatives for low-resource settings.
3. Primary screening for cervical cancer with HPV testing is attractive but cost could be the limiting factor. A less expensive HPV test holds promise.

FUTURE DIRECTIONS

1. Prophylactic HPV vaccines are gaining wider acceptance, but the need for cervical cancer screening remains for the foreseeable future.
2. In low- and middle-income countries, organizing a cervical screening program is a challenge. Hence, VIA, VILI, and low-cost HPV DNA testing (alone or in combination) can emerge as primary screening modalities.

APPENDIX 1

The Bethesda System 2001 (diagnostic categories in cervical cytology)

Specimen Adequacy

General Categorization (optional)

- Negative for intraepithelial lesion or malignancy
- Epithelial cell abnormality
- Others.

Interpretations/Results

Negative for intraepithelial lesion or malignancy

Organisms
Other non-neoplastic findings.

Epithelial cell abnormality

Squamous cell

- Atypical squamous cells (ASC)
  - Of undetermined significance (ASCUS)
  - Cannot exclude HSIL (ASC-H)
- Low-grade squamous intraepithelial lesion (LSIL)
- High-grade squamous intraepithelial lesion (HSIL)
- Squamous cell carcinoma.

Glandular cell
- Atypical glandular cells (AGCs) specify endocervical, endometrial, or not otherwise specified
- Atypical glandular cells, favor neoplastic (specify endocervical or not otherwise specified)
- Endocervical adenocarcinoma in situ (AIS)
- Adenocarcinoma.

Other
- Endometrial cells in a woman greater than equal to 40 years age.

Automated Review and Ancillary Techniques
Educational Notes and Suggestions (Optional)

ACKNOWLEDGMENTS

I sincerely thank Dr S. Shastri Professor and Head Department of Preventive Oncology, Tata Memorial Hospital, Parel, Mumbai for his critical evaluation of the manuscript.

REFERENCES

1. Globocan 2008 (IARC). Section of Cancer Information. Available at: http://www.globocan.iarc.fr/factsheet.asp. Accessed May 6, 2012.
2. Dikshit R, Gupta PC, Ramasundarahettige C, et al. Cancer mortality in India: a nationally representative survey. Lancet 2012;379(9828):1807–16..
3. Bosch FX. Human papillomavirus: science and technologies for the elimination of cervical cancer. Expert Opin Pharmacother 2011;12:2189–204.
4. Bosch FX, Lorincz A, Munoz N, et al. The causal relation between human papilloma virus and cervical cancer. J Clin Pathol 2002;55:244–65.
5. Zur Housen H. Human papilloma viruses and their possible role in squamous cell carcinomas Curr Top Microbiol Immunol 1977;78:1–30.
6. Kurman RJ, editor. Blaustein's pathology of the female genital tract. 5th edition. New York: Springer; 2002. p. 260–4.
7. Crook T, Morgenstern JP, Crawford L, et al. Continued expression of HPV 16 E6 protein is required for maintenance of the transformed phenotype of cells cotransformed by HPV 16 plus EJ-ras. Embo J 1989;8:513.
8. Phelps WC, Yee CL, Munger K, et al. The human papilloma virus type 16 E7 gene encodes the transactivation and transforming functions similar to those of adenovirus EIA. Cell 1988;58:539–47.
9. Dyson N, Howley PM, Munger K, et al. The human papilloma virus 16 E7 oncoprotein is able to bind to the retinoblastoma gene product. Science 1989;243:934–7.
10. Scheffner M, Huibregtse JM, Vierstra RD, et al. The HPV 16 E6 and E6–AP complex functions as a ubiquitin protein ligase in the ubiquitination of P53. Cell 1993;75:495–505.
11. Bouvard V, Bann R, Straif K, et al. A review of human carcinogens. Part B: Biological agents. Lancet Oncol 2009;10:321–2.

12. Duensing S, Munger K. Mechanisms of genomic instability in human cancer: insights from studies with human papillomavirus oncoproteins. Int J Cancer 2004;109:157–62.
13. Sahasrabudhhe VV, Luhn P, Wentzensen N. Human papillomavirus and cervical cancer: biomarkers for improved prevention efforts. Future Microbiol 2011;6: 1083–98.
14. Munoz N, Bosch FX, Castellsague X, et al. Against which human papillomavirus types shall we vaccinate and screen? The international perspective. Int J Cancer 2004;111: 278–85.
15. de Sanjose S, Quin WG, Alemany L, et al. Human papillomavirus genotype attribution in invasive cervical cancer: a retrospective cross sectional worldwide study. Lancet Oncol 2010;11:1048–56.
16. Smith JS, Lindsay I, Hoots B, et al. Human paillpomavirus type distribution in invasive cervical cancer and high grade cervical lesions: a meta-analysis update. Int J Cancer 2007; 121:621–32.
17. Birkeland SA, Storm HH, Lamm LU, et al. Cancer risk in the renal transplant patients in the Nordic countries,1964–1986. Int J Cancer 1995;60:183–9.
18. Frisch M, Biggar RJ, Goedert JJ. Human papilloma virus-associated cancers in patients with human immunodeficiency virus infection and acquired immunodeficiency syndrome. J Natl Cancer Inst 2000;92:1500–10.
19. Munoz N, Franceschi S, Bosetti C, et al. For the IARC multicentric cervical cancer study group. The role of parity and human papilloma virus in cervical cancer. The IARC multicentre case control study. Lancet 2002;359:1093–101.
20. Moreno V, Bosch FX, Munoz N, et al. Multicentric cervical cancer study group. Effect of oral contraceptives on risk on cervical cancer in women with papilloma virus infection: the IARC multicentric case control study. Lancet 2002;30:359:1085–92.
21. Wyatt SW, Lancaster M, Bottorff D, et al. History of tobacco use among Kentucky women diagnosed with invasive cervical cancer 1997–1998. J Ky Med Assoc 2001; 99:537–9.
22. Smith JS, Munoz N, Herrero R, et al. Evidence of *Chlamydia trachomatis* as a human papilloma virus cofactor in the aetiology of the invasive cervical cancer in Brazil and the Philippines. J Infect Dis 2002;185;324–31.
23. Christopherson WA, Scott MA. Trends in mortality from uterine cancer in relation to mass screening Acta Cytol 1977;21:5–9.
24. Laara E, Day NE, Hakama M. Trends in mortality from cervical cancer in the Nordic countries: association with organized screening programmes. Lancet 1987;1: 1247–9.
25. MacGregor JE, Teper S. Mortality from carcinoma of cervix uteri in Britain. Lancet 1978;2:774–6.
26. Nanda K, McCrory DC, Myers ER, et al. Accuracy of the Papanicolaou test in screening for and follow up of cervical cytologic abnormalities: a systematic review. Ann Intern Med 2000;132:810–9.
27. Siebers AC, Klinkhamer PJ, Grefte JM, et al. Comparison of liquid-based cytology with conventional cytology for detection of cervical cancer precursors: a randomized controlled trial. Jama 2009;302:1757–64.
28. Sankaranarayanan R, Wesley R. A practical manual on visual screening for cervical neoplasia. IARC Technical Publication No. 41. Lyon (France): International Agency on Research on Cancer, IARC Press; 2003.
29. Sankaranarayanan R, Basu P, Wesley RS, et al. Accuracy of visual screening for cervical neoplasia: results from an IARC multicentre study in India and Africa. Int J Cancer 2004;110:907–13.

30. Sankaranarayanan R, Wesley R, Thara S, et al. Test characteristics of visual inspection with 4% acetic acid (VIA) and Lugol's iodine (VILI) in cervical cancer screening in Kerala, India. Int J Cancer 2003;106:404–8.

31. Sankaranarayanan R, Gaffikin L, Jacob M, et al. A critical assessment of screening methods for cervical neoplasia. Int J Gynaecol Obstet 2005;89(Suppl 2):S4–12.

32. Mahe C, Gaffikin L. Screening test accuracy studies: how valid are our conclusions? Application to visual inspection methods for cervical screening. Cancer Causes Control 2005;16:657–66.

33. Sauvaget C, Jean-Marie Fayette A, Muwonge R, et al. Accuracy of visual inspection with acetic acid for cervical cancer screening Int J Gynecol Obstet 2011;113:14–24.

34. Sankaranarayanan R, Esmy PO, Rajkumar R, et al. Effect of visual screening on cervical cancer incidence and mortality in Tamil Nadu, India: a cluster randomized trial. Lancet 2007;370:398–406.

35. Goldie SJ, Gaffikin L, Goldhaber-Fiebert JD, et al. Cost effectiveness of cervical screening in five developing countries. N Engl J Med 2005;353:2158–68.

36. Legood R, Gray AM, Mahe C, et al. Screening for cervical cancer in India: how much will it cost? A trial based analysis of the cost per case detected. Int J Cancer 2005;117:981–7.

37. Dillner J, Rebolj M, Birembaut P, et al. Long term predictive values of cytology and human papillomavirus testing in cervical cancer screening: joint European cohort study. BMJ 2008;337:A1754.

38. Meijer CJ, Berkhof J, Castle PE, et al. Guidelines for human papilloma virus DNA test requirements for primary cervical cancer screening in women 30 yrs and older. Int J Cancer 2009;124:516–20.

39. Cuzick J, Arbyn M, Sankaranarayanan R, et al. Overview of human papillomavirus-based and other novel options for cervical cancer screening in developed and developing countries. Vaccine 2008;26(Suppl 10):K29–41.

40. Arbyn M, Sasieni P, Meijer CJ, et al. Clinical applications of HPV testing: a summary of meta-analyses. Vaccine 2006;24(Suppl 3):S3/78–89.

41. Ronco R, Giorgi-Rossi PJ, Carozzi F, et al. Results at recruitment from a randomized controlled trial comparing human papillomavirus testing alone with conventional cytology as the primary cervical cancer screening test. J Natl Cancer Inst 2008;100:492–501.

42. Sankaranarayanan R, Nene BM, Shastri SS, et al. HPV screening for cervical cancer in rural India. N Engl J Med 2009;360:1385–94.

43. Ronco G, Brezzi S, Carozzi F, et al. The New Technologies for Cervical Cancer Screening randomised controlled trial: an overview of results during the first phase of recruitment. Gynecol Oncol 2007;107(Suppl 1):S230–2.

44. Ronco G, Giorgi-Rossi P, Carozzi F, et al. Efficacy of human papillomavirus testing for the detection of invasive cervical cancers and cervical intraepithelial neoplasia: a randomised controlled trial. Lancet Oncol 2010;11:249–57.

45. Eder PS, Lou J, Huff J, et al. The next generation hybrid capture high risk HPV DNA assay on a fully automated platform J Clin Virol 2009;45(Suppl 1):S85–92.

46. Bartholomew DA, Luff RD, Quigley NB, et al. Analytical performance of Cervista[R] HPV 16/18 genotyping test for cervical cytology samples J Clin Virol 2011;51:38–43.

47. De Francesco MA, Gargiulo F, Schreiber C, et al. Comparison of the AMLICOR human papilloma virus test and the hybrid capture 2 assay for detection of high risk human papilloma virus in women with abnormal PAP smear. J Virol Methods 2008;147:10–7.

48. Stoler MH, Wright TC Jr, Sharma A, et al. High risk human papilloma virus testing in women with ASC-US cytology: results from the ATHENA HPV study. Am J Clin Pathol 2011;135:468–75.

49. Qiao YL, Sellors JW, Eder PS, et al. A new HPV-DNA test for cervical-cancer screening in developing regions: a cross-sectional study of clinical accuracy in rural China. Lancet Oncol 2008;10;929–36.

50. Dockter J, Schroder A, Hill C, et al. Clinical performance of the APTIMA HPV assay for the detection of high-risk HPV and high-grade cervical lesions. J Clin Virol 2009; 45(Suppl 1):S55–61.

51. Monsonego J, Hudgens MG, Zerat L, et al. Evaluation of oncogenic human papillomavirus RNA and DNA tests with liquid-based cytology in primary cervical cancer screening: the FASE study. Int J Cancer 2011;129:691–701.

52. Dockter J, Schroder A, Eaton B, et al. Analytical characterization of the APTIMA HPV Assay. J Clin Virol 2009;45(Suppl 1):S39–47.

53. Sankaranarayanan R, Jivarajani P, Joshi S. HPV vaccination in primary prevention of cervical cancer. In: Rajaram S, Chitrathara K, Maheshwari A, editors. Cervical cancer contemporary management. New Delhi: Jaypee; 2012. p. 66.

54. Haupt RM, Sings HL. The efficacy and safety of the quadrivalent human papillomavirus 6/11/16/18 vaccine gardasil. J Adolesc Health 2011;49:467–75.

55. Khatun S, Hussain SMA, Chowdhury S, et al. Safety and immunogenicity profile of human papillomavirus-16/18 ASO4 adjuvant cervical cancer vaccine: a randomized controlled trial in healthy adolescent girls of Bangladesh. Jpn J Clin Oncol 2012;42: 36–41.

56. Legood R, Gray AM, Mahe C, et al Screening for cervical cancer in India: how much will it cost? A trial based analysis of the cost per case detected. Int J Cancer 2005;117:981–7.

57. Pinto AP, Crum CP, Hirsch MS. Molecular markers of early cervical neoplasia. Diagn Histopathol 2010;16:445–54.

58. Valasoulis G, Tsoumpou I, Founta M, et al. The roll of p16 [(INK4A)] immunostaining in the risk assessment of women with LSIL cytology: a prospective pragmatic study. Eur J Gynaecol Oncol 2011;32:150–2.

Type 2 Diabetes in Asian Indians

Shashank R. Joshi, MBBS, MD, DM[a,b,c,*]

KEYWORDS

- Asian Indian • Physical inactivity • Nutrition transition • Epidemiology
- Screening • Thin-Fat phenotype • Prevention

KEY POINTS

- India is a global leader in diabetes, currently with second largest pool of diabetes in the world.
- Asian Indian phenotype is uniquely predisposed to develop type 2 diabetes because of strong familial aggregation as well lifestyle factors of imprudent diet and sedentary physical habit.
- The typical Asian Indian phenotype is the "thin-fat Indian" which means that Asian Indians have higher body fat composition and lesser muscle mass (sarcopenia) than the white or African counterparts.
- Aggressive screening and treatment strategies are advocated in this high-risk diabetic race.
- Prevention is the key for diabetes in Indians, and simple prevention themes like "Eat less, eat on time, eat right, walk more, sleep well, and smile" are needed.

INTRODUCTION

India is the global hub for the rapidly escalating type 2 diabetes epidemic. India recently lost its top rank to China in terms of total number of diabetics, although both nations do not boost the high prevalence of diabetes beyond 20%, as is seen in some rare island communities or Middle Eastern nations. The global diabetes epidemic is caused by better living conditions, which makes humans more sedentary with consumption of higher glycemic load and fat diets. Some races are more predisposed than the others because of some unique genetic and environmental influences. Humans are a migratory race, which often leads to survival instinct, and migration leads to affluence and wealth. Rapidly changing socioeconomic demographics has

The author has nothing to disclose.
[a] Department of Endocrinology, Lilavati Hospital, Bhatia Hospital, B23 Kamal Pushpa, 6, Bandra Reclamation, Bandra (West), Mumbai 400050, Maharashtra, India; [b] Department of Endocrinology, Grant Medical College and Sir J J Group of Hospitals, Sir J J Marg, Mumbai 400008, India; [c] Research Society for Study of Diabetes in India, Mumbai, India
* Department of Endocrinology, Lilavati Hospital, Bhatia Hospital, B23 Kamal Pushpa, 6, Bandra Reclamation, Bandra (West), Mumbai 400050, Maharashtra, India.
E-mail address: Shashank.sr@gmail.com

Clin Lab Med 32 (2012) 207–216
http://dx.doi.org/10.1016/j.cll.2012.04.012
0272-2712/12/$ – see front matter © 2012 Elsevier Inc. All rights reserved.

changed the global landscape of diabetes. The world's 2 most populous nations, India and China, are not only growing by sheer numbers but also are the most rapidly developing nations of the globe. This has led to unique environmental exposures, which are discussed in this review. Asian Indians are original migrants from Africa but uniquely have a hybrid genomic composition of Aryan, Persian, and Dravidian legacies. Asian Indian native to the land are unique to the subcontinent, especially in India, Pakistan, Bangladesh, and parts of Sri Lanka and Nepal. However, many settled in South Africa and East Africa (Kenya, Uganda, and Tanzania); Singapore and Malaysia; Mauritias; Fiji islands; Indonesia; Australia; Europe, especially the United Kingdom and Spain; the United States of America; and Canada. Studies from these migrant Asian communities led to better understanding of diabetes in this unique race, especially in the last century. This century, a lot of original work from natives of India is also now available for better understanding. Many confusing terms have thus come from this, *Southeast Asian* refers to natives of India, Pakistan, and Bangladesh; *Asian Indian* refers to people who reside in India (native) or who migrated to East and South Africa, the United Kingdom, Singapore, Indonesia, and the United States; *East Asian* refers people living in China, Korea, or, Taiwan; and the term *South Asian* is more generic than *Southeast Asian* or *Asian Indian*. This review uses the term *Asian Indian* based on both natives of Indian geography and those from their native land who migrated to the rest of the globe.

INCIDENCE AND PREVALENCE OF DIABETES IN INDIA

True Incidence data in the Asian India community is sparse except from a South African and a South Indian (Chennai) cohort.[1,2] There have only been 5 multicentre studies on the prevalence of diabetes in India. The earliest study reported a prevalence of 2.1% in urban and 1.5% in rural areas.[3] The National Urban Diabetes Survey[4] showed an overall age-standardized prevalence of 12.1% for diabetes and 14% for impaired glucose tolerance (IGT) in 6 large metropolitan cities. The Prevalence of Diabetes in India Study[5] reported diabetes prevalence of 5.9% and 2.7% in small towns and rural areas, respectively.

The first phase of Indian Council of Medical Research - India Diabetes (ICMR-INDIAB) study recently reported a four-states national study to determine the prevalence of diabetes and prediabetes (impaired fasting glucose or IGT) in India.[6] A total of 363 primary sampling units (188 urban, 175 rural), in 3 states (Tamilnadu, Maharashtra, and Jharkhand) and 1 union territory (Chandigarh) of India were sampled using a stratified multistage sampling design to survey individuals age greater than equal to 20 years. The prevalence rates of diabetes and prediabetes were assessed by measurement of fasting and 2-hour postglucose load capillary blood glucose. Of the 16,607 individuals selected for the study, 14,277 (86%) participated, of whom, 13,055 gave blood samples. The weighted prevalence of diabetes (both known and newly diagnosed) was 10.4% in Tamilnadu, 8.4% in Maharashtra, 5.3% in Jharkhand, and 13.6% in Chandigarh. The prevalences of prediabetes (impaired fasting glucose or IGT) were 8.3%, 12.8%, 8.1%, and 14.6%, respectively. Multiple logistic regression analysis showed that age, male sex, family history of diabetes, urban residence, abdominal obesity, generalized obesity, hypertension, and income status were significantly associated with diabetes. Significant risk factors for prediabetes were age, family history of diabetes, abdominal obesity, hypertension, and income status. Based on this study, we estimate that in 2011, Maharashtra will have 6 million individuals with diabetes and 9.2 million with prediabetes, Tamilnadu will have 4.8 million with diabetes and 3.9 million with prediabetes, Jharkhand will have 0.96 million with diabetes and 1.5 million with prediabetes, and Chandigarh will have

0.12 million with diabetes and 0.13 million with prediabetes. Projections for the whole of India would be 62.4 million people with diabetes and 77.2 million people with prediabetes.[6] Eight state study results were also published recently called SITE-Screening for the twin epidemics based on primary care clinic based survey.[7] The SITE study aimed at collecting data on the prevalence of diabetes and hypertension and the underlying risk factors in various outpatient facilities throughout India. This cross-sectional study was planned to be conducted in 8 Indian states, 1 state at a time. It was targeted to enroll about 2000 patients from 100 centers in each state. Each center enrolled the first 10 patients ($\geq$18 years of age, not pregnant, signed consent) per day on 2 consecutive days. *Diabetes* and *hypertension* were defined by the American Diabetes Association (2008) and Joint National Committee's 7th report guidelines, respectively. Patient data—demographics, lifestyle factors, and medical history and laboratory diagnostic results—were collected and analyzed. During 2009 to 2010, a total of 15,662 eligible patients (54.8% men; mean age 48.9 $\pm$ 13.9 years) from 8 states were enrolled. Diabetes was prevalent in 5427 (34.7%) patients, and 7212 (46.0%) patients had hypertension. Diabetes and hypertension were coexistent in 3227 (20.6%) patients. Among those whose disease status was not known at enrolment, 7.2% (793 of 11028) and 22.2% (2408 of 10858) of patients were newly diagnosed with diabetes and hypertension, respectively; additionally, 18.4% (2031of 11028) were classified as prediabetics and 60.1% (6521of 10858) as prehypertensives. A positive association (P<.05) was observed between diabetes/hypertension and older age, familial history of either, a medical history of cardiovascular disorders, alcohol consumption, and diet. Thus, the SITE study shows that a substantial burden of diabetes and hypertension is on the increase in India. Patient awareness and timely diagnosis and intervention hold the key to limiting this twin epidemic.[7]

FETAL ORIGIN AND THRIFTY GENOTYPE HYPOTHESIS FOR DIABETES IN ASIAN INDIANS

The susceptibility to type 2 diabetes may be conferred by evolutionary enrichment of thrifty genes, which long ago enhanced survival during periods of famine but have now created detriment with conditions of plentiful food and sedentary lifestyles.[8] Barker,[9] Hales and Barker,[10] and Yajnik[11] have an alternative explanation that has been recently proposed: the thrifty phenotype hypothesis (subsequently generalized as fetal origins), which links the obesity and type 2 diabetes epidemic to an unfavorable intrauterine environment. This thinking is based on certain observations of an inverse relationship between birth weight and risk of type 2 diabetes in adult populations. Asian Indians, as a group, have small body size, which has been named *Thin-fat Indian*. Women from the rural parts of India are small and are thought to be chronically undernourished because of their low body mass index (BMI). Iron and other nutrient deficiencies are very common in this group. Indian babies are the smallest in the world; one-third are born with low birth weight (<2.5 kg).[11] Thus, it is possible that maternal and fetal undernutrition may contribute to the type 2 diabetes epidemic in Asian countries, especially India. In Asian Indians, type 2 diabetes is diagnosed at least a decade or 2 earlier, and individuals are considerably thinner than their British counterparts.[11] Asian Indians have thinner limbs, which is suggestive of smaller muscle mass. However, despite their thinness, they are centrally obese, with higher waist/hip ratio and higher subscapular/triceps skinfold ratio than their British counterparts.[11] Many studies show that Asian Indians have more body fat for any given BMI compared with whites and black Africans.[12,13] Indians also have higher levels of central obesity (measured as waist circumference, waist/hip ratio, visceral fat, and posterior subcutaneous abdominal fat). This is reflected in higher plasma

Table 1		
Classification of overweight and obesity by BMI for Asian Indians		
	Obesity Class	BMI (kg/m²)
Underweight		<18.5
Normal		18.5–22.9
Overweight		23.0–24.9
Obesity	I	25.0–29.9
	II	30.0–34.9
Extreme obesity	III	≥35

Adapted from Misra A, Chowbey P, Makkar BM, et al; Concensus Group. Consensus statement for diagnosis of obesity, abdominal obesity and the metabolic syndrome for Asian Indians and recommendations for physical activity, medical and surgical management. J Assoc Physicians India 2009;57:163–70, with permission.

nonesterified fatty acid and triglyceride concentrations, hyperinsulinemia with fasting as well as postglucose challenge states, and higher insulin resistance.[14] Thus, Asian Indians have an unusual thin-fat body composition associated with the insulin resistance syndrome, and this is the now popular thin-fat Indian concept. The Asian Indian BMI cut off is a little less than that in the white and African-American counterparts and is now well accepted (Table 1).

The Pune Maternal Nutrition Study[15] has given insight into fetal development in Indian populations. This prospective, population-based, observational research assessed rural Indian women and their offspring. Mothers were short and thin (mean prepregnant height and BMI: 152 cm and 18.1 kg/m², respectively); mean full-term birth weight was only 2.7 kg. Detailed anthropometry of the newborns showed that their body composition differed from white babies born in the United Kingdom. The Indian babies were lighter by almost 2 standard deviations (SDs), and lean tissues such as muscle (mid-upper arm circumference) and abdominal viscera (abdominal circumference) showed a similar deficit. Truncal fat (subscapular skinfolds), however, was relatively spared (–0.5 SD). Thus, although extremely small and thin, the babies had relatively increased adiposity. A similar pattern is seen in urban Indian adults. It has been suggested that increasing maternal parity predicts increasing adiposity in the newborn infant. This may result from maternal nutritional, cardiovascular, or immunologic factors.[15]

NUTRITION ISSUES IN ASIAN INDIAN TYPE 2 DIABETES

India has suddenly undergone a rapid transition from an import-oriented famine-struck nation to a food surplus export oriented country. Recent nutritional and economic transitions have revealed certain trends and patterns in the nutritional transition in India. A hectic, busy lifestyle and the easy availability of convenience or fast foods have led to irregular meals and frequent snacking on energy-dense fast foods, including ready-to-use gravies and soups, packaged salty snacks, ready-made cookies, and commercial fast foods, rather than traditional home-cooked food. Furthermore, consumption of animal foods, sugar (especially sweetened, carbonated beverages), and traditional Indian energy-dense foods has also increased. The diets of all income groups have moved away from whole-grain cereals to other food groups, with greater shifts noted among the urban populations and the higher-income groups.[16]

India progressed toward caloric adequacy in the 1970s and early 1980s, as documented by the National Nutrition Monitoring Bureau[17] and other surveys. The surveys showed a gradual improvement in caloric intake per capita, typified by an increase in consumption of cereal grains, whereas the intake of most other food items, such as milk, oil, and sugar, remained largely unchanged. However, many of these surveys revealed disparities in the intakes of most foods between rural and urban populations and between different socioeconomic groups. Comparison of food consumption patterns shows a gradual reduction in cereal grain consumption between 1975 and 1995 that has not affected the average energy intake. This is largely the result of a progressive increase in the intake of protein and, likely, fats. The latter is caused by a significant increase in the consumption of milk and other dairy products as well as an increase in the intake of animal products (designated flesh foods), fats, and oils. The production of pulses and legumes is also a concern; consequently, their cost and consumption have decreased dramatically. This is somewhat worrisome because pulses and legumes were once a very important source of vegetable proteins in the traditional Indian diet. Trends in the changes in consumption of urban populations are not readily available, although the surveys conducted between the late 1970s and the 1990s show wide differences between the socioeconomic strata in an urban environment. One would have expected these disparities to have widened further over the years, although this is not evident from the data.[17]

Although carbohydrates remain the major source of energy in Indian diets, the percentage of total energy intake derived from carbohydrates has declined (1975–1979, 80.3%; 2001, 75.5%); however, the quality of carbohydrates has changed from the traditional high-fiber carbohydrates to the low-fiber carbohydrates like polished white rice, which has a higher glycemic index. There is also an increase in the percentage of energy coming from dietary fats (1975–1979, 8.9%; 2001, 13.9%). However, the proportion of dietary energy coming from fat still remains less than 15%, which is lower than the recommended dietary allowance of 15% to 30%.[17,18] Consumption of oils, fats, and animal products has increased in almost all the states.[17] Energy intake is lower in urban areas, in spite of higher intake of fats and oils, because of lower cereal consumption compared with rural areas.[16] Reasons for these dichotomous observations of decreased energy intake with increasing prevalence of obesity could be underreporting of dietary consumption data, higher energy intake in comparison with energy expenditure, and increasingly sedentary lifestyles.[16]

REGIONAL DISPARITIES IN INDIA

India is a diverse country covering 28 states and 7 union territories, which makes it a mini continent, as there is a huge geolinguistic disparity, which makes it a very heterogenous population. Regional disparities in type 2 diabetes are common, attributable to the vast variation in culture and dietary habits across regions. In an attempt to understand these variations and disparities, there has been an explosion in type 2 diabetes epidemiology studies in India over the last 20 years.[19] In the large cities of north and south India (Chennai,[19-22] Trivandrum,[23,24] Mumbai,[25] Delhi,[26,27] Jaipur,[28] and Guhawati[29]), in large metropolises,[30] and in industrial populations,[31] type 2 diabetes prevalence among adults (>20 years of age) has ranged from 8% to 15%. Within urban populations, a large heterogeneity of type 2 diabetes prevalence is noted, depending on the socioeconomic stratum studied and sampling response rates. There are few epidemiologic studies in semiurban India,[16] and many in rural populations.[16] In earlier years, there was a very low prevalence of type 2 diabetes in rural populations. However, recent studies from Maharashtra and Andhra Pradesh report very high prevalence rates similar to those in urban Indian populations.

Interestingly, a significant correlation of BMI with type 2 diabetes has been observed in these studies. It has been hypothesized that although there is a significant increase in type 2 diabetes as populations move from rural to semiurban to urban and cosmopolitan habitats, a reverse migration of culture may already be taking place in Indian rural populations. Earlier rural-urban disparities in type 2 diabetes could be caused by a low prevalence of overweight and obesity in rural, compared with urban, subjects.[16]

SEDENTARY HABIT IN ASIAN INDIANS

Numerous studies have indicated the importance of physical inactivity in the development of type 2 diabetes.[32,33] In the Nurses' Health Study,[33] women who reported exercising vigorously had an age-adjusted incidence rate of self-reported, clinically diagnosed type 2 diabetes that was two-thirds as high as that of women who exercised less frequently. The deleterious effect of low levels of physical activity is seen particularly among those subjects who have other risk factors, such as high BMI, hypertension, or familial diabetes. Similarly, among male physicians, the incidence of self-reported type 2 diabetes was negatively related to the frequency of vigorous exercise, and the strength of this relationship was greater in those with higher BMI.[16] For equivalent degrees of obesity, more physically active subjects have a lower incidence of the disease.[33]

Several studies have found that Asian Indians are more sedentary than whites.[34] For example, findings from the Newcastle Heart Project (comprising Asian Indians [n = 105] and Europeans [n = 416]) showed that Asian Indians are less physically active than Europeans. Similarly, another UK study showed that lower physical activity in Asian Indians, Pakistanis, or Bangladeshis, compared with their European counterparts, was inversely correlated with BMI, waist circumference, systolic blood pressure, plasma glucose, and plasma insulin levels.[35] The prevalence of type 2 diabetes and IGT has been shown to be significantly lower in higher quartiles of physical activity in South Indians (ie, 17.0%, 9.7%, and 5.6% for sedentary, moderately heavy, and heavy physical activity, respectively).[36] It is believed that a sedentary lifestyle is an important factor contributing to the development of type 2 diabetes and cardiovascular disease (CVD) in Asian Indians.[16] The Consensus Development Group for formulating the Consensus Physician Activity Guidelines for Asian Indians considered the available physical activity guidelines from International and Indian studies and formulated the following India-specific guidelines.[16,37,38]

A total of 60 minutes of physical activity per day is recommended for healthy Asian Indians in view of the high predisposition to type 2 diabetes and CVD in Asian Indians. This should include at least 30 minutes of moderate-intensity aerobic activity, 15 minutes of work-related activity, and 15 minutes of muscle-strengthening exercises. For children, moderate-intensity physical activity for 60 minutes daily should be in the form of sports and physical activity. This consensus statement also includes physical activity guidelines for pregnant women, the elderly, and those suffering from obesity, type 2 diabetes and CVD in Asian Indians and other components of Maharashtra State. Proper application of guidelines is likely to have a significant impact on the prevalence and management of these cardiometabolic factors in Asian Indians.[37,38]

Studies have looked at a community-based participatory research approach to translate the original Diabetes Prevention Program in the United States into one that is age specific and culture specific for other regions of the world. These studies have evaluated cultural strategies for healthy behaviors, including culture-specific physical activities, knowledge and access to healthy foods, physical activity for youth and their parents, interactive hands-on learning activities for healthy lifestyles, and group formats for adopting healthy behaviors.[16]

BARRIERS TO CLINICAL MANAGEMENT

Sociocultural and religious factors influence health beliefs, diet, and lifestyle management in Asian Indians.[16,39–41] Cultural factors (eg, festivals and holidays) contribute to a greater frequency of missed clinic appointments by Asian Indians compared with whites. Furthermore, poor adherence with type 2 diabetes therapy (insulin or oral agents) is common among Asian Indians during holidays, and glycemic control is unsatisfactory because of religious fasting.[42–44] Asian Indian patients with type 2 diabetes also tend to have a more negative attitude and tend to believe they were made to wait longer in clinics than UK whites do.[45,46] Response to drugs has been suspected to be different in Asian Indians compared with whites, but this phenomenon has not been adequately investigated. Prevalence of associated conditions like dyslipidemia, hypertension, and CVD are also affected by differences in body fat composition, dietary changes, abdominal obesity, and BMI.[16] A recent study showed that self-efficacy is an important factor in determining outcomes.[16] Normal values in Asian Indian population with reference ranges are being worked out.[46,47] These data are sparse too, but soon normative data in this population will emerge. In contrast, an advantageous sociocultural factor seen in Asian Indians is the extended family structure, often helping patients cope better with insulin therapy and morbidities.[16]

ASIAN INDIAN APPROACH TOWARD MANAGEMENT OF PREDIABETES AND TYPE 2 DIABETES

The enormous social and personal cost of type 2 diabetes makes a compelling case for prevention. In view of the evidence and the devastating health impact of cardiometabolic disease, it seems prudent that primary prevention should be a major priority. The greatest hope lies in implementing lifestyle intervention programs on a large scale, targeting multiple nodes in a complex cultural network or system, buttressed by a favorable political and regulatory strategy and initially focused on high-risk persons. Meta-analysis studies[48] looking at type 2 diabetes education and a variety of weight loss methods have found that nutrition interventions have the largest statistically significant effect on metabolic control and weight loss. In addition, these meta-analyses have found that type 2 diabetes education, in general, is effective in improving knowledge, skills, psychosocial adjustment, and metabolic control. Overall, the evidence involving medical nutrition therapy in type 2 diabetes management supports nutritional intervention. Thus, India is one of the epicenters of the diabetes epidemic. It is imperative to universally screen all Asian Indians older than age 40. It is also important to screen Asian Indians older than 20 who have a positive family history or waist circumference more than 90 cm in men or 80 cm in women. Apart from screening for glucose as a vital sign, it is important to screen Asian Indians for hypertension, dyslipidemia, and other various features of metabolic syndrome, including coronary artery disease, nonalcoholic fatty liver, polycystic ovarian syndrome in women, and even hypogonadism in men. Because it is an asymptomatic disease, Asian Indians present with complications. Asian Indians usually manifest with diabetes a decade or 2 earlier compared with their white or African counterparts. Key management strategies must center on lifestyle modification with evidence-based algorithms for pharmacotherapy. However, prevention holds the key. In the last few years, several controversies have erupted in lifestyle areas as well as pharmacotherapies. Prevention is the key for Asian Indians. Diabetes and its complications threaten to bankrupt the growing Indian economy. The keys to prevention are simple messages that work. The current theme for prevention in Asian Indians is "Eat less, eat on time, eat right, walk more (be physically active), sleep well and smile."

REFERENCES

1. Joshi SR. Incidence data on diabetes from India. J Assoc Physicians India 2008;56: 149–51.
2. Mohan V, Deepa M, Anjana RM, et al. Incidence of diabetes and pre-diabetes in a selected urban south Indian population (CUPS-19). J Assoc Physicians India 2008; 56:152–7.
3. Ahuja MMS. Epidemiological studies on diabetes mellitus in India. In: Ahuja MMS, editor. Epidemiology of diabetes in developing countries. New Delhi: Interprint; 1979. p. 29–38.
4. Ramachandran A, Snehalatha C, Kapur A, et al. High prevalence of diabetes and impaired glucose tolerance in India: National Urban Diabetes Survey. Diabetologia 2001;44:1094–101.
5. Sadikot SM, Nigam A, Das S, et al. The burden of diabetes and impaired glucose tolerance in India using the WHO 1999 criteria: Prevalence of Diabetes in India Study (PODIS). Diabetes Res Clin Pract 2004;66:301–7.
6. Anjana RM, Pradeepa R, Deepa M, et al. Prevalence of diabetes and prediabetes (impaired fasting glucose and/or impaired glucose tolerance) in urban and rural India: phase I results of the Indian Council of Medical Research–INdia DIABetes (ICMR-INDIAB) study. Diabetologia. 2011;54:3022–7.
7. Joshi SR, Saboo B, Vadivale M, et al, SITE Investigators. Prevalence of diagnosed and undiagnosed diabetes and hypertension in India—results from the Screening India's Twin Epidemic (SITE) study. Diabetes Technol Ther 2012;14(1):8–15.
8. Neel JV. Diabetes mellitus: a "thrifty" genotype rendered detrimental by "progress"? Am J Hum Genet 1962;14:353–62.
9. Barker DJ. Fetal origins of coronary heart disease. BMJ 1995;311:171–4.
10. Hales CN, Barker DJ. Type 2 (non-insulin-dependent) diabetes mellitus: the thrifty phenotype hypothesis. Diabetologia 1992;35:595–601.
11. Yajnik CS. Early life origins of insulin resistance and type 2 diabetes in India and other Asian countries. J Nutr 2004;134:205–10.
12. Banerji MA, Faridi N, Atluri R, et al. Body composition, visceral fat, leptin, and insulin resistance in Asian Indian men. J Clin Endocrinol Metab 1999;84:137–44.
13. Deurenberg P, Deurenberg-Yap M, Guricci S. Asians are different from Caucasians and from each other in their body mass index/body fat per cent relationship. Obes Rev 2002;3:141–6.
14. McKeigue PM, Shah B, Marmot MG. Relation of central obesity and insulin resistance with high diabetes prevalence and cardiovascular risk in South Asians. Lancet 1991;337:382–6.
15. Joshi NP, Kulkarni SR, Yajnik CS, et al. Increasing maternal parity predicts neonatal adiposity: Pune Maternal Nutrition Study. Am J Obstet Gynecol 2005;193:783–9.
16. Joshi SR, Mohan V, Joshi SS, et al. Transcultural diabetes nutrition therapy algorithm: the Asian Indian application. Curr Diab Rep 2012;12(2):204–12.
17. National Nutrition Monitoring Bureau. Report of Second Repeat Surveys in Rural Area in NNMB States. NNMB Technical Report Number 18. Hyderabad, India, 1999.
18. National Institute of Nutrition. Dietary guidelines for Indians: a manual. National Institute of Nutrition, Indian Council of Medical Research. Hyderabad, India, 1998.

19. Verma NP, Mehta SP, Madhu S, et al. Prevalence of known diabetes in an urban Indian environment: the Darya Ganj diabetes survey. Br Med J (Clin Res Ed) 1986; 293:423–4.

20. Mohan V, Deepa M, Deepa R, et al. Secular trends in the prevalence of diabetes and impaired glucose tolerance in urban South India—the Chennai Urban Rural Epidemiology Study (CURES-17). Diabetologia 2006;49:1175–8.

21. Mohan V, Mathur P, Deepa R, et al. Urban rural differences in prevalence of self-reported diabetes in India—the WHO-ICMR Indian NCD risk factor surveillance. Diabetes Res Clin Pract 2008;80:159–68.

22. Mohan V, Shanthirani S, Deepa R, et al. Intra-urban differences in the prevalence of the metabolic syndrome in southern India—the Chennai Urban Population Study (CUPS No. 4). Diabet Med 2001;18:280–7.

23. Joseph A, Kutty VR, Soman CR. High risk for coronary heart disease in Thiruvananthapuram city: a study of serum lipids and other risk factors. Indian Heart J 2000;52: 29–35.

24. Kutty VR, Soman CR, Joseph A, et al. Type 2 diabetes in southern Kerala: variation in prevalence among geographic divisions within a region. Natl Med J India 2000;13: 287–92.

25. Iyer SR, Iyer RR, Upasani SV, et al. Diabetes mellitus in Dombivli—an urban population study. J Assoc Physicians India 2001;49:713–6.

26. Misra A, Pandey RM, Devi JR, et al. High prevalence of diabetes, obesity and dyslipidaemia in urban slum population in northern India. Int J Obes Relat Metab Disord 2001;25:1722–9.

27. Prabhakaran D, Shah P, Chaturvedi V, et al. Cardiovascular risk factor prevalence among men in a large industry of northern India. Natl Med J India 2005;18:59–65.

28. Gupta A, Gupta R, Sarna M, et al. Prevalence of diabetes, impaired fasting glucose and insulin resistance syndrome in an urban Indian population. Diabetes Res Clin Pract 2003;61:69–76.

29. Shah SK, Saikia M, Burman NN, et al. High prevalence of type 2 diabetes in urban population in north-eastern India. Int J Diab Dev Countries 1999;18:97–101.

30. Ramachandran A, Snehalatha C, Kapur A, et al. High prevalence of diabetes and impaired glucose tolerance in India: National Urban Diabetes Survey. Diabetologia 2001;44:1094–101.

31. Reddy KS, Prabhakaran D, Chaturvedi V, et al. Methods for establishing a surveillance system for cardiovascular diseases in Indian industrial populations. Bull World Health Organ 2006;84:461–9.

32. Manson JE, Nathan DM, Krolewski AS, et al. A prospective study of exercise and incidence of diabetes among US male physicians. JAMA 1992;268:63–7.

33. Manson JE, Rimm EB, Stampfer MJ, et al. Physical activity and incidence of non-insulin-dependent diabetes mellitus in women. Lancet 1991;338:774–8.

34. Kamath SK, Hussain EA, Amin D, et al. Cardiovascular disease risk factors in 2 distinct ethnic groups: Indian and Pakistani compared with American premenopausal women. Am J Clin Nutr 1999;69:621–31.

35. Hayes L, White M, Unwin N, et al. Patterns of physical activity and relationship with risk markers for cardiovascular disease and diabetes in Indian, Pakistani, Bangladeshi and European adults in a UK population. J Public Health Med 2002;24:170–8.

36. Mohan V, Gokulakrishnan K, Deepa R, et al. Association of physical inactivity with components of metabolic syndrome and coronary artery disease—the Chennai Urban Population Study (CUPS no. 15). Diabet Med 2005;22:1206–11.

37. Misra A, Sharma R, Gulati S, et al. Consensus dietary guidelines for healthy living and prevention of obesity, the metabolic syndrome, diabetes, and related disorders in Asian Indians. Diabetes Technol Ther 2011;13:683–94.

38. Misra A, Nigam P, Hills AP, et al. Consensus physical activity guidelines for Asian Indians. Diabetes Technol Ther 2012;14(1):83–98.

39. Chowdhury AM, Helman C, Greenhalgh T. Food beliefs and practices among British Bangladeshis with diabetes: implications for health education. Anthropol Med 2000; 7:219–26.

40. Macaden L, Clarke CL. Risk perception among older South Asian people in the UK with type 2 diabetes. Int J Older People Nurs 2006;1:177–81.

41. Samanta A, Campbell JE, Spaulding DL, et al. Eating habits in Asian diabetics. Diabet Med 1986;3:283–4.

42. Aslam M, Healy MA. Compliance and drug therapy in fasting Moslem patients. J Clin Hosp Pharm 1986;11:321–5.

43. Hawthorne K, Mello M, Tomlinson S. Cultural and religious influences in diabetes care in Great Britain. Diabet Med 1993;10:8–12.

44. Mather HM. Diabetes in elderly Asians. J R Soc Med 1994;87:615–6.

45. Hawthorne K. Asian diabetics attending a British hospital clinic: a pilot study to evaluate their care. Br J Gen Pract 1990;40:243–7.

46. Ashavaid TF, Todur SP, Dherai AJ. Health status of Indian population—current scenario. J Assoc Physicians India 2004;52:363–9.

47. Ashavaid TF, Kondkar AA, Todur SP, et al. Lipid, lipoprotein, apolipoprotein and lipoprotein(a) levels: reference intervals in a healthy Indian population. J Atheroscler Thromb 2005;12(5):251–9.

48. Steyn NP, Mann J, Bennett PH, et al. Diet, nutrition and the prevention of type 2 diabetes. Public Health Nutr 2004;7:147–65.

Cardiovascular Disease in India

Tester F. Ashavaid, PhD, CSci[a],*, Chandrashekhar K. Ponde, MD[b],
Swarup Shah, PhD[c], Monika Jawanjal, MBBS[b]

KEYWORDS

- Cardiovascular diseases • Young Indians • Risk factors • Biomarkers
- Genetic screening

KEY POINTS

- Cardiovascular disease (CVD) is one of the leading cause of mortality in India.
- It is estimated that 23.6 million CVD cases will be reported in subjects younger than 40 years of age by 2015, suggesting that young Indians are at higher cardiac risk.
- Evaluation of biomarkers in acute coronary syndrome (ACS) and at various stages of the disease such as inflammation, ischemia, and heart failure would indeed help to assess cardiac risk in Indian subjects.
- Identification of newer genetic markers through the candidate and/or genome-wide association approach would prove to be beneficial in developing a diagnostic assay for screening young asymptomatic Indian subjects.

INTRODUCTION

According to the projections by the World Health Organization (WHO), a substantial shift in the distribution of deaths from younger to older age groups and from communicable diseases to noncommunicable diseases (NCDs) will occur during the next 25 years. The proportion of deaths from cardiovascular disease (CVD) is greater in comparison to that from other NCDs (diabetes, cancer, stroke). According to the World Health Statistics 2008 report,[1] global deaths from CVD will rise from 17.1 million in 2004 to 23.4 million in 2030, thus projecting CVD as the leading cause of morbidity and mortality worldwide. This is true for developed as well as developing countries such as India, which are expected to face a phenomenal increase in the

The authors have nothing to disclose.
[a] Department of Laboratory Medicine, P.D. Hinduja National Hospital and Medical Research Center, Veer Savarkar Marg, Mahim, Mumbai 400016, Maharashtra, India; [b] Department of Cardiology, P.D. Hinduja National Hospital and Medical Research Centre, V. S. Marg, Mahim, Mumbai 400016, Maharashtra, India; [c] Department of Biochemistry and Research Laboratories, P.D. Hinduja National Hospital and Research Centre, V. S. Marg, Mahim, Mumbai 400016, Maharashtra, India
* Corresponding author.
E-mail address: dr_tashavaid@hindujahospital.com

burden of CVD in the near future. This risk in Indians is 3 to 4 times higher than in white Americans, 6 times higher than in Chinese, and 20 times higher than in Japanese.[2]

An estimate published in India's National Commission on Macroeconomics and Health report projects that cases of CVD would increase from 38 million in 2005 to 64.1 million in 2015, 95% of which would be due to coronary artery disease (CAD)/coronary heart disease (CHD) as compared to congenital heart disease, rheumatic heart disease, and stroke.[3] The same report also states that in 2015, of the 66.3 million persons with CVD, 23.6 million will be younger than 40 years of age, suggesting that the young Indian population is at a higher risk of developing CAD. A similar observation was found in a study on young Indian adults in whom the prevalence of dyslipidemia was higher in subjects aged 40 years or younger.[4] The likely cause of this epidemic lies in the country's epidemiologic transition. The health system in India has dramatically changed from what it was a few decades ago. This transition is characterized by liberalization of the economy, which has expanded opportunities for additional employment and generation of additional incomes, which in turn have helped to reduce poverty levels. However, such a developmental process has also caused adverse lifestyle changes (eg, drug and alcohol addictions, unhealthy diet, and physical inactivity), increased urbanization, and connectivity and enhanced access to information and services not available earlier.

According to the Global Burden of Diseases (GBD) study in India, in the year 1990 CAD caused 0.62 million deaths in men and 0.56 million deaths in women (total 1.18 million). By 2000, CAD had led to 1.59 million deaths. The reported prevalence of CAD in adults has risen 4-fold over the last 40 years (to a present level of around 10%), and even in rural areas the prevalence has doubled over the past 30 years (to a present level of around 4%). It is estimated that by 2020, CVD will be largest cause of morbidity and mortality in India. As per the WHO global report of 2005, it is estimated that India lost 9 billion dollars in national income from premature deaths due to heart diseases, stroke, and diabetes in 2005 and is likely to lose 237 billion dollars by 2015. Therefore CVD remains a growing public health burden in India.

PATHOGENESIS OF CVD

Atherosclerosis is the underlying cause of the majority of CVD cases. Human atherosclerosis involves two distinct pathologic processes: conventional atherogenesis at the early stage and atherothrombosis at advanced stages, which is responsible for acute manifestations of the disease.[5] Some of the clinical manifestations of atherosclerosis result from progressive narrowing by an atherosclerotic plaque; however, it is the development of a thrombus over a ruptured underlying plaque that causes the most acute and serious clinical manifestations of atherosclerotic vascular disease. Coronary thrombosis therefore is responsible for the vast majority of cases of unstable angina, acute coronary syndrome (ACS), and ischemic sudden death.

TRADITIONAL AND EMERGING RISK FACTORS/MARKERS FOR CVD

The development of CVD can be silent, often without any signs and symptoms. Many cases of CVD can be prevented by identifying modifiable risk factors. Various studies have so far identified several risk factors (modifiable and nonmodifiable) for CVD endpoints such as angina, myocardial infarction, and sudden ischemic death. The nonmodifiable risk factors for CVD include older age, gender, race, and family history of premature CVD; the modifiable risk factors include hypertension, diabetes mellitus, dyslipidemia (elevated total cholesterol levels, elevated low-density lipoprotein, decreased high-density lipoprotein), smoking/tobacco use, obesity, and physical inactivity.

So far most of the research associated with CVD has revolved around the aforementioned traditional risk factors. However, many adverse cardiac events, particularly premature CVD, could not be traced to these traditional risk factors because of the influence of unfamiliar and newer risk factors. Many CVD risk markers have also been identified such that the marker helps to identify people at high risk of CVD without actually causing it. Many emerging risk factors/markers for CVD such as chronic kidney disease, obstructive sleep apnea, low socioeconomic status; peripheral vascular disease, elevated C-reactive protein (CRP), elevated lipoprotein(a), and elevated homocysteine have been identified.

RISK ASSESSMENT OF CVD

With the increasing prevalence of CVD in the Indian population, assessment of cardiac risk has become of paramount importance. Various laboratory investigations have been developed that are aimed at identifying individuals at risk of CVD. The disease presents broadly in two different ways: ACS and chronic stable angina (CSA).

ACS

The term **acute coronary syndrome** refers to a group of conditions precipitated due to acute myocardial ischemia; these include ST-segment elevation myocardial infarction (STEMI), non-ST-segment elevation myocardial infarction (NSTEMI), and unstable angina (UA). Clinical outcomes in ACS depend upon accurate early diagnosis, optimal medical therapy, and real-time risk stratification, which can guide early revascularization. The therapeutic options, both medical and interventional, have been evolving at an extremely rapid pace. The 12-lead electrocardiogram (ECG) is the most readily available bedside investigation. However, the ECG has a sensitivity of only around 60% for a detection of acute MI, and as many as one third of patients with ACS present with symptoms other than chest pain. Imaging modality such as a bedside two-dimensional echocardiogram or at-rest perfusion scan may not be readily available in all centers, and therefore the role of biomarkers is of utmost importance.[6]

STEMI

STEMI is characterized by total occlusion of the infarct-related coronary artery with red thrombus. The plaques responsible for STEMI are generally more complex, irregular, and rich in thrombus, which is usually white containing platelets and fibrin. The thrombus in STEMI is totally occlusive and therefore generally leads to transmural infarction. The diagnosis of STEMI is based primarily on ECG showing more than 1 mm ST-segment elevation in at least two consecutive leads. Patients with STEMI then undergo rapid assessment for coronary reperfusion therapy, either pharmacologic (fibrinolysis) or mechanical (primary angioplasty) or a combination of both (pharmacoinvasive strategy). The most important concept here is to minimize time gap between initiation of therapy and establishment of reperfusion. Thus in the STEMI scenario the use of cardiac biomarkers for diagnosis has taken a back seat and they are used primarily for the assessment of reperfusion and estimation of infarct size.

NSTEMI

In NSTEMI or UA the underlying pathology is a nonocclusive white thrombus in the affected artery, with distal embolization of the white thrombus in the microcirculation superimposed with or without coronary spasm. The goal of the therapy is to prevent thrombosis, reduce microembolization and prevent reocclusion. The only difference between NSTEMI and UA is positive biomarkers in the first 24 hours in the former and their striking absence in the latter. In fact, the only distinction between NSTEMI and UA is that in NSTEMI the biomarkers are clearly elevated and in UA they remain within normal limits in serial sampling in 24 hours.[7]

Biomarkers in Initial Evaluation of ACS

Myocardial necrosis is accompanied by the release of structural proteins and other intracellular macromolecules into the cardiac interstitium as a consequence of compromise of the integrity of cellular membranes. The biomarkers for detection of early myocardial necrosis are myoglobin, creatine kinase MB_2 (CK-MB) isoform, copeptin, pregnancy associated plasma protein A, and platelet collagen receptor glycoprotein VI. However, these biomarkers are not routinely used either because they are not specific or not stable or their turnaround time is more than 30 minutes. The intermediate marker for detection of ACS of myocardial necrosis includes cardiac troponins I and T and CK-MB.

Cardiac troponins (troponin T and I)

Cardiac troponin is the preferred biomarker for the detection of myocardial injury based on its improved sensitivity. The troponins regulate the calcium-mediated contractile process in the heart muscle and include troponin C, which binds calcium; tropinin I (TnI), which binds to actin; and troponin T (TnT), which binds to tropomyosin. TnT usually increases up to about 20-fold above the reference range in patients with STEMI. The elevation is detectable in the serum at around 4 to 6 hours and persists for 7 to 10 days after MI. In contrast to CK, cardiac TnI and cardiac TnT have isoforms that are unique to cardiac myocytes and may be measured by assays employing monoclonal antibodies specific to epitopes of the cardiac form. The advantage of cardiac troponin over other biomarkers of necrosis has been firmly established in clinical studies.[8] The diagnosis of MI therefore must be associated with at least one of the following along with elevated TnT:

1. Significant ECG changes
2. Imaging evidence of new regional wall motion abnormalities
3. Perfusion defects.

The association between an increased concentration of cardiac troponin and a higher risk of recurrent cardiac events in patients with normal serum concentration of CK-MB and suspected ACS has confirmed the clinical relevance of detecting circulating troponin in patients previously classified with UA.[9]

When cardiac troponin is not available, the next best alternative is CK-MB and is measured by mass assay. Although total CK is a sensitive marker of myocardial damage, it has poor specificity owing to its high concentration in skeletal muscle. By virtue of its greater concentration in cardiac versus skeletal myocytes, the MB isoenzyme of CK offers an improvement in sensitivity and specificity compared with total CK. CK-MB is predominantly found in myocardium and starts elevating at around 6 hours after the onset of MI and remains elevated for 24 to 48 hours. Similar to cardiac troponins, serial testing of CK-MB has been recommended and the kinetics favor the marker to be used for detection of reinfarction.[8] Also, CK-MB constitutes 1% to 3% of the CK in skeletal muscle, and is present in minor quantities in intestine, diaphragm, uterus, and prostate. Therefore, the specificity of CK-MB may be impaired in the setting of major injury to these organs, especially skeletal muscle.

Biomarkers of Ischemia

In approximately one third of patients with ACS, the initial troponin concentrations are below the diagnostic range. Some present very early after the onset of pain and in some there is extensive ischemia without myocardial necrosis. Thus a biomarker that can reliably detect extensive ischemia in the absence of necrosis will always be helpful for the clinician.[10]

The following markers can be elevated with extensive ischemia with minimal necrosis:

1. Ischemia modified albumin (IMA)
2. Unbound free fatty acids (FFA$_u$s)
3. Heart-type fatty acid binding protein (H-FABP).

However, these three markers need to be established for day-to-day use and are not easily available in India.

Biomarkers of Inflammation

There is almost convincing evidence that inflammation is a central trigger for plaque rupture and subsequent thrombosis. Inflammation not only enters the picture in an acute event but is also responsible in the early stages of atherogenesis. Finally, inflammation plays a central role in rupturing the protective fibrous cap that forms the barrier between the thrombogenic contents of atheroma core and the circulatory platelets.[11]

Five inflammatory markers, described in the following subsections, are detectable in the majority of patients with ACS including even those without evidence of myocardial necrosis.

High-sensitivity CRP

The high-sensitivity CRP (hs-CRP) assay measures very low levels of CRP (<10 mg/L). hs-CRP certainly rises as a result of an inflammatory response to myocardial necrosis but has also been implicated to play a direct role in atherothrombosis. CRP is known to contribute directly in several adverse cascades in ACS.

In ACS, a cutoff point of more than 10 mg/L is validated in public studies.[12,13] There have been 25 clinical studies demonstrating the prognostic value of hs-CRP in patients with NSTEMI. Data in patients with STEMI are few. However, limitations to hs-CRP include not very well defined windows for sampling and the fact that as many as 30% of patients with NSTEMI ACS do not have elevated hs-CRP.

Myeloperoxidase

Myeloperoxidase (MPO) is a lysosomal enzyme and is usually released from neutrophilic granules, monocytes, and tissue macrophages. Neutrophils engulf the pathogens and then use MPO to produce a strongly antiseptic hypochlorite ion to destroy them. Unfortunately, MPO is linked with oxidation of low-density lipoprotein (LDL) and consumption of nitric oxide, thereby rendering the normal antithrombotic endothelial surface thrombogenic. MPO plays a central role in destabilization of the fibrous cap.[14]

Interleukin-6

In ACS the causative plaque is infiltrated by activated macrophages that produce cytokines to perpetuate an inflammatory process. Interleukin-6 (IL-6) is a cytokine with proinflammatory properties. It affects β-cell immunoglobulin production and

T-cell cytotoxic activity, increases platelet reactivity, increases gene expression of clotting factors, promotes endothelial passage of neutrophil, and induces synthesis of all acute-phase reactants by the liver. IL-6 has a relatively short plasma half-life of 4 hours and should be measured by enzyme-linked immunosorbent assay (ELISA).[15]

Interleukin-18

Interleukin-18 (IL-18) is a member of the cytokine family and is localized mainly in plaque macrophages. Animal studies have supported a proatherogenic effect of IL-18 on plaque progression.[16] IL-18 participates in all stages of plaque development:

1. IL-18 secretion promotes production of tumor necrosis factor-α (TNF-α) and IL-1β, creating a viscous positive feedback loop.
2. IL-18 affects T cells inside the plaque.
3. IL-18 weakens the fibrous cap.
4. Significantly higher levels of IL-18 are found in sera of patients with ACS.

Placenta growth factor

Placenta growth factor (PIGF) stimulates vascular smooth muscle cell growth, directs macrophages into atherosclerotic lesions, and upregulates production of human necrosis factor and stimulates pathologic angiogenesis. PIGF initiates the inflammatory process in the plaque, and in one study increased PIGF levels were associated with increased risk of recurrent instability after hospital discharge in patients with ACS.[17]

Biomarkers for Heart Failure

The biomarkers for heart failure are brain natriuretic peptide and N-terminal pro brain natriuretic peptide. Brain natriuretic peptide (BNP) was first isolated from porcine brain in 1998. BNP is released from cardiac myocytes in response to increased wall stress in the absence of necrosis. Pro BNP is then converted to biologically active BNP and biologically inactive N-terminal BNP (NT-BNP). BNP has shorter half-life 15 to 20 minutes and NT-proBNP has a longer half-life of 1 to 2 hours. BNP levels directly correlate to an increase in wall stress, left ventricular end diastolic pressure, and adverse ventricular remodeling either singly or in combination. Thus extensive ischemia can also release BNP in the absence of necrosis.[18]

After MI the plasma concentration of BNP rises rapidly and peaks at more than 24 hours, with peak values proportional to the size of the MI.[19] In patients who develop clinical heart failure later, a second peak occurs at more than 5 to 7 days, which reflects an increase in left ventricular end diastolic pressure (LVEDP) and adverse ventricular remodeling. In patients with acute MI, higher values of BNP and NT-proBNP both have been shown to be associated and predict a greater incidence of death and heart failure independent of other prognostic variables. It is noteworthy that BNP and NT-proBNP identify individuals without signs of heart failure who are at higher risk of death and heart failure, and this information is complementary to that offered through CK-MB and troponins.[20]

A cutoff limit of 80 ng/mL has been validated for BNP in patients with ACS using two different BNP assays. NT-proBNP has also been evaluated in clinical studies, and a cutoff value of less than 250 pg/mL is considered as lowest quartile (2nd, 250–670; 3rd, 670–1870; and 4th quartile, >1870). The higher the quartile the patient is in, the worse the prognosis. At least two samples, one within 24 hours of symptom onset and a second at approximately 5 days, are recommended.[21]

CSA

Chronic CAD is becoming a worldwide pandemic. Based on the Framinngham Heart study, the life time risk of developing symptomatic CAD is approximately 50% in men and 30% in women. The clinician's task in the management of these patients primarily is that of risk stratification on noninvasive testing. Recently there has been a focus on noninvasive detection of vulnerable plaques in this group of patients and use of biomarkers in risk stratification.

GENETIC MARKERS FOR CVD IN THE INDIAN POPULATION

Many of the current traditional and newer factors and/or markers for CVD identified so far are unable to fully predict the risk for CVD. It is a well established fact that Indians are more susceptible to heart diseases as compared to other populations, which may be the result of lifestyle and partly genetically inherited. The genetics of CVD is complex, and most of the gene and gene–environment interactions that influence risk of disease among Indian populations are largely unknown. Genetic studies that focus on identification of disease causing genes provide new insights into the pathogenesis of CVD. Therefore in an attempt to identify atherosclerotic genes, whole-genome scans for loci associated with hyperlipidemia, low concentration of high-density lipoprotein cholesterol (HDL-C), elevated lipoprotein(a) [Lp(a)], homocysteine, hypertension, and vascular disorders have been performed. Numerous mutations and/or polymorphisms have been identified across the entire length of the genome that are known to be associated with CVD. Thus, identification of genetic variants in candidate genes in the Indian population has been an important approach for identifying individuals at higher risk for CVD.

GENETIC VARIATIONS ASSOCIATED WITH DYSLIPIDEMIA

A large number of rare genetic variants are known to cause conditions such as dyslipidemia, leading directly to the development of coronary atherosclerosis.

LDL Receptor Genetic Variations

So far the best understood inborn error of metabolism determining elevated levels of plasma lipids and thus risk of CAD is the disorder familial hypercholesterolemia (FH). It is caused by mutations in the LDL receptor (*LDLR*) gene. There is little information on monogenic disorder of hypercholesterolemia in India. Neither the prevalence of FH nor the types of *LDLR* mutations causing FH among the Indian subjects are known. In a study conducted by Ashavaid and colleagues on patients with clinical features of FH, two novel single-nucleotide G insertion mutations in exon 3 (242insG) and in exon 4 (397insG)[22] were identified. These mutations are designated as FH Bombay–1 and FH Bombay–2 and are registered at the UMD-LDLR database, INSERM Necker-Enfants Institute, France (www.umd.necker.fr/disease.html). However, a screening study in a large number of clinically diagnosed FH patients for *LDLR* defects is needed to obtain genetic epidemiologic information on Indians.

Apolipoprotein B-100 Genetic Variation

Increased LDL concentrations in circulation may also result from inefficient clearance of LDL particles from defects in its ligand, apolipoprotein B-100 (apoB-100), which is classified as familial defective apoB-100 (FDB) genetic disorder. The prevalence of FDB in India is not yet known. The most studied Apo B-100 genetic variants are R3500W, R3531C, and signal peptide insertion/deletion (Sp Ins/Del) polymorphism.[23]

However, neither of the two variants (R3500W and R3531C) was identified in Indian patients with clinical features of possible type IIa hypercholesterolemia, suggesting that common mutations known to cause FDB are absent and possibly not associated with hypercholesterolemia among Indians.[24] In our study, the *Del* allele of the signal peptide I/D polymorphism was not found to be significantly associated with CAD in Indian subjects (Ashavaid and colleagues, unpublished data, 2012). However, the possibility of low rate or other unknown genetic variation at the *apoB* locus cannot be ruled out.

Apolipoprotein E Genetic Variations

Three common alleles (ε2, ε3, and ε4) of the *apoE* gene have been found to influence lipoprotein levels and thus increase the risk of CAD in the general population. The most common allele is ε3 (frequency 0.75), followed by ε4 (frequency 0.15) and ε2 (frequency 0.1). Based on the average impact of ε2 and ε4 on serum cholesterol, carriers of the ε4 allele have been estimated to have a risk of developing premature CAD 1.4 times higher than carriers of the ε2 allele. Substantial data on *apoE* polymorphism is lacking in India. In our previous study,[25] it was observed that the distribution of the allele frequencies in the normolipemic healthy population was 0.920 for ε3 and 0.040 for ε2 and ε4. In addition, the ε4 allele was significantly more prevalent in both the hypercholesterolemic ($P<.025$) and the CAD group ($P<.05$) as compared to the controls. It was further observed that the ε4 allele significantly contributes to the increase in total cholesterol by 7.5% in the hypercholesterolemic group ($P<.05$) and by 16.6% in the CAD group ($P<.05$) as compared to the ε3 allele. It can therefore be inferred that the apoE isoform could explain 7% to 16% of variation in total cholesterol levels, thus making a small but significant contribution to the risk of developing CAD among the Indian population. A larger study is required to strengthen this observation.

GENETIC VARIATIONS LEADING TO DECREASED HIGH-DENSITY LIPOPROTEIN CHOLESTEROL AND CAD

Decreased high-density lipoprotein cholesterol (HDL-C) is one of the common features observed in young Asian Indian. The Coronary Artery Disease among Indians (CADI) study showed that only 14% of Asian Indian men and 5% of women have optimal HDL-C levels. Various epidemiologic studies indicate that abnormalities in HDL-C metabolism play an important role in development of CAD in the Indian population.

Genes Involved in HDL-C Biosynthesis

The biosynthesis of HDL-C is complex and involves the synthesis and secretion of the major protein components of HDL-C followed by the largely extracellular acquisition of lipid (phospholipids and cholesterol) and the assembly and generation of mature HDL particle. The liver and intestine secretes the lipoprotein apolipoprotein A-1 (ApoA-1), a major constituent of HDL that causes specific efflux of free cholesterol and phospholipids from peripheral blood cells, particularly macrophages via ATP binding cassette A-1 (ABCA-1), thus forming nascent discoidal HDL. Maturation of HDL-C requires the esterification of cholesterol to form cholesterol esters and hydrophilic lipid core of HDL, a process mediated by the action of the enzyme lecithin cholesterol acyltransferase (LCAT). Thus genetic variation identified in *ABCA-1*, *APOA1*, and *LCAT* genes, which are involved in HDL-C biosynthesis, could lead to low circulating plasma HDL-C levels, causing attenuated antiatherogenic activity and thus favor accelerated atherosclerosis. So far, there have been no studies on complete genetic analysis of these genes involved in HDL-C biosynthesis in the Indian population. In our current case-control study, we identified a total of 40 genetic variants in three genes (ABCA, APOA1, and LCAT1), out of which four novel mutations were identified in ABCA1 along with one novel mutation in APOA1. Interestingly, we observed that three mutations including a novel mutation in ABCA1 gene was observed in 40% of subjects with low HDL-C (Sawant and colleagues, unpublished data, 2012); suggesting that these mutations might help to assess the CAD risk in young healthy asymptomatic individuals in the Indian population.

Cholesterol Ester Transfer Protein

Cholesterol ester transfer protein (CETP) activity is inversely associated with HDL-C levels. It increases LDL- and very low-density lipoprotein (VLDL)-cholesterol levels by transferring cholesteryl esters from HDL in exchange for triglycerides and thus is proatherogenic. The relation between the plasma concentration of CETP and HDL-C and atherosclerosis is complex. It has been suggested that this association might be population specific and highly influenced by environmental factors such as alcohol consumption and tobacco smoking. Several common polymorphisms have been reported in the CETP gene locus, of which TaqIB has been most studied. The allele carrying the cutting site for Taq1 enzyme is called B1 and the one in which it is missing is called B2. The B2 allele has been associated with increased levels of HDL-C and decreased CETP activity. In normolipemic healthy Indian subjects, B2 allele frequency was 0.49 and the HDL-C levels did not differ between the three genotypes in the normolipemic as well as the low HDL-C group.[26] However, B2 allele frequency in subjects with HDL-C less than 0.9065 mmol/L was found to be lower (0.4) as compared to the B1 allele (0.6). Thus, though significant association of Taq1 polymorphism of the CETP gene with low HDL-C levels was not observed, decreased B2 allele frequency, one of the features documented in the low HDL-C group, was observed in our study. Poduri and colleagues evaluated a panel of single-nucleotide polymorphisms (SNPs) known to influence lipid levels in Asian Indians. They observed that genetic predisposition to CAD was due to the cumulative effect of multiple genetic variants, possibly as a result of a synergistic association between them.[27]

Apolipoprotein CIII

Apolipoprotein CIII (ApoCIII), a major component of triglyceride-rich lipoprotein, chylomicrons, and VLDL, and a major component of HDL, is important in the regulation of plasma triglyceride concentrations. It is noncompetitive inhibitor of lipoprotein lipase (LPL) and thereby plays a role in reducing hydrolysis of triglyceride-rich lipoproteins. It has been reported that overexpression of the apoCIII gene results in hypertriglyceridemia with a positive linear relation between apoCIII, triglyceride concentration, and reduced HDL-C levels. Miller and colleagues[28] have reported a higher frequency of two promoter polymorphisms (C-482T and T-455C) in young Asian Indians than in Caucasians, especially in those with a family history of premature CAD and subjects with low HDL-C. However, we did not find significant association of these promoter variants with low HDL-C levels. The frequencies of −482T and −455C in our study were 0.47 and 0.55 respectively, similar to those reported by Miller and colleagues for Asian Indians. Thus in our population these promoter polymorphisms were shown to make a minor contribution in the polygenic context.

GENETIC VARIATION ASSOCIATED WITH OBESITY

Obesity is emerging as an important health problem in India, particularly in urban areas. Almost 30% to 65% of adult urban Indians are either overweight or obese or have abdominal obesity. The rising prevalence of overweight and obesity in India has a direct correlation with the increasing prevalence of obesity-related comorbidities: hypertension, the metabolic syndrome, dyslipidemia, type 2 diabetes mellitus, and CVD. Indians exhibit unique features of obesity; excess body fat, abdominal adiposity, increased subcutaneous and intra-abdominal fat, and deposition of fat in ectopic sites (liver and muscle). A recent genome-wide association studies (GWAS) in Asian Indians from the United Kingdom reported a strong association of variant (rs12970134) near the melanocortin-4 receptor (*MC4R*) gene with several obesity-related traits and increased risk to central obesity and insulin resistance.[29] This finding was further replicated in a Sikh population from North India. The study demonstrated that the genetic variation in the *MC4R* locus has a moderate contribution in the regional fat deposition and development of central obesity in Asian Indians.[30]

GENETIC VARIATIONS ASSOCIATED WITH HYPERTENSION

The renin–angiotensin system (RAS) plays a key role in the regulation of blood pressure. Angiotensin II, the main effector molecule of the system, has direct toxic effects on myocardial cells. In the past few years, therapeutic success has been achieved in reducing the risk of MI by using angiotensin I–converting enzyme (ACE) inhibitors and the risk of hypertension is reduced by using ACE and angiotensin II type I receptor (AGTR1) antagonists. Genes that encode components of the RAS are thought to play a role in determining genetic susceptibility to hypertension and CAD. Various mutations have been reported in these genes: 287-bp insertion/deletion (I/D) in the *ACE* gene, A/C 1166 polymorphism in the *AGTR1* gene, and *M235T* mutation in the *AGT* gene. However, none of these genetic variants showed any significant association with CAD or MI and hypertension in the Indian population.

GENETIC VARIATION ASSOCIATED WITH HOMOCYSTEINE METABOLISM

An elevated plasma level of the amino acid homocysteine (hcy) has been identified as an independent risk factor for coronary atherosclerosis. A plasma hcy concentration exceeding 15 mmol/L is now termed as hyperhomocysteinemia (Hhcy). Elevated plasma homocysteine levels have been reported in patients with premature CAD lacking the traditional risk factors. In Indians we have observed hyperhomocysteinemia to be 19.13% and 18.26% in patients with CAD and controls, respectively.[31] Although the majority of cases of HHcy are thought to be caused by an interplay between dietary and genetic factors, the genetic disorders are associated with the highest plasma levels of hcy, with inherited deficiency of several enzymes. The most common are methylene tetrahydrofolate reductase (MTHFR), cystathionine β-synthase (CBS), and methionine synthase (MS).

MTHFR Genetic Variation

The most extensively studied mutation in the *MTHFR* gene is the C677T genetic variant. In our previous study, the C/T heterozygous genotype was found in 48% of the Hhcy patients as compared to 12% of control. The difference was statistically significant (*P*<.05),[32] and hence heterozygosity for the thermolabile *MTHFR* mutation was found to be associated with Hhcy. There is another variant documented in the

MTHFR gene, A1298C. This genotype alone shows no effect on MTHFR activity but in combination with the C677T genotype it causes significant decrease in the MTHFR activity. Markan and colleagues observed that the co-occurrence of MTHFR 677C and 1298C mutant alleles is significantly associated with elevated homocysteine levels and also with increased risk of hypertension.[33]

CBS Genetic Variation

Homozygosity for defects in the enzyme CBS gives rise to the autosomal dominant recessive condition hereditary homocystinuria. Among various mutations reported so far in the CBS gene, 68-bp insertion, T833C and G919A variants are studied in CAD; 844ins68 variant is reported so far to be a neutral insertion. In our study, 3.47% of the controls were heterozygous for the CBS T833C mutation.[34]

MS Genetic Variation

MS is a vitamin B_{12}–dependent enzyme catalyzing the remethylation of homocysteine to methionine. Reduced activity increases the plasma homocysteine. A point mutation in the encoding region of MS (A2756G) that results in the substitution of an aspartic acid for a glycine residue (D919G) has been reported. Our previous study shows that the A/G heterozygous genotype was found in 44% of the Hhcy patients as compared to 16% of control. The difference between the Hhcy patient group and controls was statistically significant ($P<.0$) in our study.[32]

Nitric Oxide Synthase Genetic Variation

Endothelial function, of which decreased vasodilator activity of nitric oxide (NO) is a hallmark, and which is a component of early atherogenesis, including CAD, has been shown to be of prognostic significance. Hence, factors that influence NO availability are likely to be of considerable clinical importance. The synthesis of endothelial NO from L-arginine is regulated by the enzyme nitric oxide synthase (eNOS), and a number of polymorphisms in the eNOS gene sequence have been identified. The two polymorphisms in the eNOS gene that have been studied in association with CAD are Glu298Asp and T-786C. In vitro and animal models studies have demonstrated a relationship between HHcy, endothelial dysfunction, and accelerated atherosclerosis. In our previous study, association of Glu298Asp polymorphism of the eNOS gene was not significantly associated with the Hhcy.[32] The T-786C polymorphism in the 5′ flanking region of the eNOS gene was also not significantly associated with the presence of HHcy in our patients as well.[32]

GENETIC VARIATIONS ASSOCIATED WITH THROMBOSIS AND FIBRINOLYSIS

The main clinical manifestation of CAD involves the rupture of atherosclerotic plaque followed by the total occlusion of the coronary artery which leads to MI. Platelets play a critical role in normal blood hemostasis and thrombus formation in MI. Several genetic variations in genes involved in platelet activation and fibrinolysis have been reported to be associated with MI. Our recent study aimed to determine the frequency distribution and association of polymorphisms in these genes with CAD among Indian. A case-control genetic association study was performed for polymorphisms in platelet glycoprotein receptors (GPIIb/IIIa [HPA1a/1b], GPIb-IX-V [VNTR], and GPIa/IIa [C807T]), fibrinogen β-chain (BclI), α-chain (Aα312), tissue plasminogen activator (tPA) [I/D], and plasminogen activator inhibitor-I (PAI-1) [4G/5G] in 473 healthy controls and 446 patients with stable and unstable angina. The insertion allele frequency of the tPA I/D polymorphism was significantly higher in our patients ($P<.01$)

and no other polymorphisms varied significantly between patients and controls. Also, none of the polymorphisms seemed to affect the severity of the disease, the only exception being the mutant alleles of the β-chain of fibrinogen gene, which were significantly elevated in single-vessel disease. This is the first study to evaluate the role of gene polymorphisms in both the thrombotic and fibrinolytic pathway in the Indian population and suggests that tPA I/D polymorphism confers CAD risk in our population.[35]

Another genetic association study was conducted to evaluate the role of thrombomodulin genetic variant in the Indian population with cardiac risk. It was observed that the presence of *Ala455Val* variant significantly increases the CAD risk by 3-fold in subjects younger than 49 years and the risk is more apparent in presence of risk factors (Shah and colleagues, unpublished data, 2012). Thus it would indeed be worthwhile to further validate this finding to screen young asymptomatic subjects for future CAD risk. Various genome-wide association studies have shown strong association between a 58-bp region on chromosome 9p21 and CAD risk in European and East Asian ancestry. Bhanushali and colleagues evaluated an SNP rs10757278 at the *9p21* locus in a western Indian population and observed a stronger association of variant with CAD risk as compared to other populations.[36]

SUMMARY

Population variability, sample size, and selection of sample, in addition to the environmental risk factors, complex nature of the disease, and interaction of various genes overshadow the polymorphic influence of the single gene on the disease. In spite of that, the strong genetic effects observed in small subgroups of patients emphasize the role of these polymorphisms on the disease. Future genetic studies will promise to revolutionize the early diagnosis, treatment, and prevention of CVD. A unique advantage for the management of CVD is that a significant number of cases are potentially preventable. The early diagnosis by genetic testing will force lifestyle modifications in individuals with genetic risk factors, which alone or in combination with other therapeutic options may delay the onset of the disease or prevent MI and sudden death.

ACKNOWLEDGMENTS

We are extremely grateful to the National Health Education Society (NHES) of the P. D. Hinduja National Hospital and Medical Research Centre for their financial support.

REFERENCES

1. World Health Organization (WHO). A report on World Health Statistics by World Health Organization, 2007. Available at: http://www.who.int/whosis/whostat2007.pdf. Accessed April 19, 2012.
2. Enas EA, Garg A, Davidson MA, et al. Coronary heart disease and its risk factors in first-generation immigrant Asian Indians to the United States of America. Indian Heart J 1996;48(4):343–53.
3. National Commission on Macroeconomics and Health report, Ministry of Health and Family Welfare, Government of India, New Delhi, August 2005. Available at: http://www.who.int/macrohealth/action/Report%20of%20the%20National%20Commission.pdf. Accessed April 19, 2012.
4. Sawant AM, Shetty D, Mankeshwar R, et al. Prevalence of dyslipidemia in young adult Indian population. J Assoc Physicians India 2008;56:99–102.
5. Lusis AJ. Atherosclerosis. Nature 2000;407(6801):233–41.

6. Alpert JS, Thygesen K, Antman E, et al. Myocardial infarction redefined a consensus document of The Joint European Society of Cardiology/American College of Cardiology Committee for the redefinition of myocardial infarction. J Am Coll Cardiol 2000; 36:959–69.

7. Boden WE, Shah PK, Gupta V, et al. Contemporary approach to the diagnosis and management of non-ST-segment elevation acute coronary syndromes. Prog Cardiovase Dis 2008;50:311–51.

8. Morrow DA, Cannon CP, Jesse RL, et al. National Academy of Clinical Biochemistry Laboratory Medicine Practice Guidelines: clinical characteristics and utilization of biochemical markers in acute coronary syndromes. Clin Chem 2007;53:552–74.

9. Morrow DA. Troponins in patients with acute coronary syndromes: biologic, diagnostic, and therapeutic implications. Cardiovasc Toxicol 2001;1:105–10.

10. Jesse RL, Kukreja R. Rationale for the early clinical application of markers of ischemia in patients with suspected acute coronary syndromes. Cardiovasc Toxicol 2001;1: 125–33.

11. Morrow DA, Ridker PM. Inflammation in cardiovascular disease. In: Topol E, editor. Textbook of cardiovascular medicine updates. Cedar Knolls (NJ): Lippincott Williams & Wilkins; 1999. p. 1–12.

12. Blake GJ, Ridker PM. C-reactive protein and other inflammatory risk markers in acute coronary syndromes. J Am Coll Cardiol 2003;41:37S–42S.

13. Heeschen C, Hamm CW, Bruemmer J, et al. Predictive value of C-reactive protein and troponin T in patients with unstable angina: a comparative analysis. J Am Coll Cardiol 2000;35:1535–42.

14. Brennan, ML, Penn MS, Van Lente F, et al. Prognostic value of myeloperoxidase in patients with chest pain. N Engl J Med 2003;346:1595–604.

15. Barton BE. The biological effects of interleukin 6. Med Res Rev 1996;16:87–109.

16. Blankenberg S, Tiret L, Bickel C, et al. Interleukin-18 is a strong predictor of cardiovascular death in stable and unstable angina. Circulation 2002;106:24–30.

17. Heeschen D, Dimmeler S, Fichtlscherer S, et al. Prognostic value of placental growth factor in patients with acute chest pain. JAMA 2004;291:435–41.

18. de Lemos JA, Morrow DA. Brain natriuretic peptide measurement in acute coronary syndromes: ready for clinical application? Circulation 2002;106:2868–70.

19. Morita E, Yasue H, Yoshimura M, et al. Increased plasma levels of brain natriuretic peptide in patients with acute myocardial infarction. Circulation 1993;88:82–91.

20. James SK, Wallentin L, Armstrong PW, et al. N-terminal pro brain natriuretic peptide and other risk markers for the separate prediction of mortality and subsequent myocardial infarction in patients with unstable coronary disease: a GUSTO IV substudy. Circulation 2003;108:275–81.

21. Morrow DA, de Lemos JA, Sabatine MS, et al. Evaluation of B-type natriuretic peptide for risk assessment in unstable angina/non-ST elevation MI: BNP and prognosis in TACTICS-TIMI 18. J Am Coll Cardiol 2003;41:1264–72.

22. Ashavaid TF, Kondkar AA, Nair KG. Identification of two LDL receptor mutations causing familial hypercholesterolemia in Indian subjects. J Clin Lab Anal 2000;14(6): 293–8.

23. Chiodini BD, Barlera S, Franzosi MG, et al. APO B gene polymorphisms and coronary artery disease: a metaanalysis. Atherosclerosis 2003;167(2):355–66.

24. Kondkar AA, Nair KG, Ashavaid TF. Genetic analysis of Indian subjects with clinical features of possible type IIa hypercholesterolemia. J Clin Lab Anal 2007;21(6):375–81.

25. Ashavaid TF, Todur SP, Nair KG. Apolipoprotein E4 polymorphism as a risk factor for coronary heart disease among Indian subjects. Indian J Clin Biochem 2002;17:83–93.

26. Ashavaid TF, Shalia KK, Altaf AK, et al. Taq 1B polymorphism of cholesterol ester transfer protein and high density lipoprotein cholesterol in Indian population. AACC Mol Pathol Division Newsletter 2001;13:2–3.

27. Poduri A, Khullar M, Bahl A, et al. A combination of proatherogenic single-nucleotide polymorphisms is associated with increased risk of coronary artery disease and myocardial infarction in Asian Indians. DNA Cell Biol 2009;28(9):451–60.

28. Miller M, Rhyne J, Khatta M, et al. Prevalence of the APOC3 promoter polymorphisms T-455C and C-482T in Asian-Indians. Am J Cardiol 2001;87(2):220–1, A8.

29. Chambers JC, Elliott P, Zabaneh D, et al. Common genetic variation near MC4R is associated with waist circumference and insulin resistance. Nat Genet 2008;40(6): 716–8.

30. Been LF, Nath SK, Ralhan SK, et al. Replication of association between a common variant near melanocortin-4 receptor gene and obesity-related traits in Asian Sikhs. Obesity (MD) 2010;18(2):425–9.

31. Nair KG, Nair SR, Ashavaid TF, et al. Methylenetetrahydrafolate reductase gene mutation and hyperhomocysteinemia as a risk factor for coronary heart disease in the Indian population. J Assoc Phys Ind 2002;50:9–15.

32. Eghlim FF, Ashavaid TF, Nair KG. Genetic determinants of hyperhomocysteinemia in atherosclerosis. Indian J Clin Biochem 2006;21(2):4–11.

33. Markan S, Sachdeva M, Sehrawat BS, et al. MTHFR 677 CT/MTHFR 1298 CC genotypes are associated with increased risk of hypertension in Indians. Mol Cell Biochem 2007;302(1-2):125–31.

34. Tsai MY, Bignell M, Schwichtenberg K, et al. High prevalence of a mutation in the cystathionine beta-synthase gene. Am J Hum Genet 1996;59(6):1262–7.

35. Ashavaid TF, Todur SP, Kondkar AA, et al. Platelet polymorphisms: frequency distribution and association with coronary artery disease in an Indian population. Platelets 2011;22(2):85–91.

36. Bhanushali AA, Parmar N, Contractor A, et al. Variant on 9p21 is strongly associated with coronary artery disease but lacks association with myocardial infarction and disease severity in a population in Western India. Arch Med Res 2011;42(6):469–74.

Down Syndrome in India—Diagnosis, Screening, and Prenatal Diagnosis

Ishwar C. Verma, MBBS, FRCP*,
Meena Lall, PhD, Ratna Dua Puri, MD, DM

KEYWORDS

- Down syndrome • Cytogenetic studies • Folate metabolism
- Screening and prenatal diagnosis • Noninvasive prenatal diagnosis
- Future therapies

KEY POINTS

- Down syndrome (DS) is the most common genetic cause of mental retardation.
- Clinical manifestations are variable, and children have psychomotor impairment, multiple malformations, and medical conditions.
- Confirmation of the diagnosis is by karyotype analysis. The cytogenetic abnormality can be classified into pure trisomy 21, translocation, or mosaicism.
- Risk of recurrence depends on the primary cytogenetic abnormality in the proband.
- Prenatal screening is by biochemical and ultrasound markers in the first and second trimester. Definitive prenatal diagnosis is by analysis of fetal chromosomes in fetal chorionic villi, amniocytes, or cord blood.
- A noninvasive test for trisomy 21 in maternal blood has been developed by massively parallel shotgun sequencing.
- Therapeutic studies in Ts65Dn mice suggest an exciting prospect of improvement of learning ability and memory deficits.

INTRODUCTION

Down syndrome (DS) is the most common genetic cause of mental retardation around the world and is one of the best studied. John Langdon Down described the phenotype of the syndrome named after him in 1866. However, as is usual in medicine, the physical characteristics of Down syndrome had been described 20 years earlier by Esquirol and also Sequin. Lejeune and colleagues reported in 1959 that Down syndrome is caused by trisomy of chromosome 21, starting the chapter of cytogenetic disorders.[1] Chromosome 21 was sequenced in 2000 by Hattori and

The authors have nothing to disclose.
Center of Medical Genetics, Sir Ganga Ram Hospital, Rajender Nagar, New Delhi, India 110060
* Corresponding author.
E-mail address: icverma@yahoo.com

colleagues.[2] It is estimated that chromosome 21 encodes approximately160 "classical" protein-coding annotated genes, 5 microRNAs, and more than 350 genes of unassigned function.[3] The recent advances in genomics have led to a better understanding of the consequences of dosage imbalance attributable to trisomy 21. The recent evidence-based therapeutic approaches to ameliorate the harmful effects of trisomy 21 effects on brain structure and function in animal models are very encouraging and hold great promise for human application.[4]

EPIDEMIOLOGY

The incidence of trisomy 21 is influenced by maternal age and differs between populations.[5,6] Canfield and colleagues[7] estimated maternal age-adjusted prevalence of DS based on the surveillance of 22% of live births in the United States to be 1 in 732 live births. However, estimation of the frequency of DS depends on whether maternal age, gestational timing of diagnosis, and case loss caused by prenatal diagnosis and termination of pregnancy are taken into account.[8] Therefore, although the number of fetuses conceived with DS has increased in recent years as the mean age of pregnant women has increased in the United States, the number of terminated pregnancies with DS has also increased, so that the current prevalence is likely to have decreased to about 1 in 1000. On the other hand, extremely high frequencies have been recorded in the Middle Eastern countries, varying from 18 to 3.5 per 1000.[6] The reasons for this are that conceptions continue until women are in their late 40s, and abortion is not allowed. Murthy and coworkers[6] observed that 20% of the mothers in the United Arab Emirates (UAE) belonging to the younger age group of 17 to 25 years had a child with DS compared with 9.75% of the mothers in this age group belonging to non-UAE nations, suggesting the presence of some possible predisposing factor.

In India, meta-analysis of the earlier data on a study of 75,103 live births, with 82 cases of DS gave a frequency of 1 in 916.[9] In a 3-center study of 94,600 births that specifically investigated DS, 1 per 1150 births was affected.[9] In this study, the diagnosis of DS was confirmed by cytogenetic analysis. However, these data pertain to 1993 to 1997. The authors estimated the frequency of DS, based on the data provided by Baird and coworkers[10] from Vancouver and the maternal age distribution at birth in 2010 in Delhi,[11] to be 1 in 1200. The picture is muddied by widespread ultrasound studies during pregnancy, biochemical screening, amniotic fluid studies, and abortion of affected fetuses. However, in India, only 2% to 5 % of women at delivery are more than 35 years in age, which is much lower than that observed in the West or the Middle East.[11]

CLINICAL PRESENTATION

Children with DS have cognitive and psychomotor impairment, multiple malformations and medical conditions. The manifestations are varied, and all features may not be present in every affected child. The diagnosis is particularly difficult at birth, as the child often keeps the eyes closed, and the common diagnostic sign of upward slant of the palpebral fissures is not observed. However, presence of moderately severe hypotonia is more characteristic, and fewer cases would be missed if attention is paid to this sign. Additional features that are helpful in diagnosis at birth are increased skin at the nape of the neck, brachycephaly, flat midfacies with depressed bridge of nose, epicanthic folds, dysmorphic and small ears, protruding tongue, small fifth finger with clinodactyly, Simian crease, and deep vertical groove on the plantar surface of the foot between the first and second toes. The developmental retardation is difficult to judge in the neonatal period, although a poor Moro reflex is suggestive. Brushfield spots are not observed in Asian Indians and all those who have brown iris. Recall of the facial gestalt is usually enough for an experienced clinician to diagnosis DS. Some signs change with age; hypotonia, epicanthic fold, and upward slant of eyes all become less prominent as the child grows. Cognitive impairment can vary from mild to moderate to severe intellectual disability. About 5% of children with DS have mild mental retardation. Caution is necessary in labeling a child with DS who has 1 or 2 minor anomalies, like simian crease and clinodactyly, which can be present in normal individuals also. Kava and colleagues[12] reported the frequency of various physical signs in 524 patients with DS as follows: upward eye slant (83.9%), ear abnormalities (66.9%), epicanthic folds (56.9%), flat facies (50.9%), and hypotonia (76.3%).

ASSOSCIATED CONDITIONS
Mental Retardation

Mental retardation is a prominent symptom of DS. However, a great deal of heterogeneity is encountered in the expression of most symptoms and extent of abnormality. The measure of intelligence (IQ) in DS varies from 20 to 85. Its highest value may reach close to the lower range in normal individuals, but the lower values reveal a highly challenged condition. Developmental milestones of 134 noninstitutionalized DS patients in north India were studied by Menon and colleagues.[13] The mean ages for social smile, holding the head erect, sitting unsupported, standing unsupported, walking alone, and speaking at least 3 words to form a meaningful sentence were 6.3, 8.6, 15.7, 25.2, 32.0 and 42 months, respectively. However, the distribution of these milestones had a wide range. Bhattacharyya and coworkers[14] have shown a significant correlation between the minor physical anomalies and behavior phenotype of children with DS.

Congenital Heart Disease

It is important to exclude the presence of congenital heart disease in every case by echocardiography, as this is the major determinant of survival. It is present in 40% to 50% of the cases. The most common defects are atrioventricular canal malformation, ventricular septal defect, and atrial septal defect.[15] Kava and colleagues[12] reported heart disease in only 18.3% of cases, as echocardiography was not done in every case. However, in a recent follow-up of 378 children, the authors detected congenital heart disease in 37.8 % of subjects with DS (Nahar and colleagues unpublished data, 2012).

Thyroid Disease

Thyroid disease, or hypothyroidism, is present in 4% to 18% of the cases. This must be tested in every case. The prevalence of hypothyroidism increases with age, and it is advisable that thyroid function should be tested every year. There are rare reports of Graves disease.[16,17]

Hematologic Problems

Hematologic problems were present in 15 of 239 cases of DS between 1992 and 2003 in a study by Awasthi and coworkers.[18] These comprised 4 cases of transient myeloproliferative disorder (TMD), 3 cases of TMD/acute leukemia, 4 cases of acute leukemia, 2 of dual deficiency anemia, and 1 case each of myelofibrosis and idiopathic thrombocytopenia. TMD can be differentiated from acute leukemia only on follow-up. Transient aplastic anemia is a rare complication with only 7 reported cases to date.[19]

Other Medical Conditions

Other medical conditions associated with DS include visual problems (refractive errors, cataracts) in 60%, hearing defects in 75%, and otitis media in 50% of children. Twelve percent of cases have gastrointestinal atresia, and its presence during ultrasonography of the fetus strongly suggests the presence of DS. Obstructive sleep apnea occurs in 50% to 75% of the cases because of the presence of a small oropharynx with a relatively large tongue. Delayed dental eruption and hypodontia, seizures, celiac disease, and symptomatic atlanto-axial instability are also reported. Multiple reports from India highlight various complications encountered in these children, including rare manifestations like interstitial lung disease.[20]

Epilepsy

Epilepsy is reported in 1% to 13% of children with DS, the most common epileptic syndrome being infantile spasm/West syndrome.[21] Curiously, these patients have electroencephalographic (EEG) characteristics of idiopathic rather than symptomatic West syndrome. Lennox-Gastaut syndrome also exhibits some distinctive features in children with DS, including later onset and high incidence of reflex seizures. There is a high rate of EEG abnormalities in children with DS, even among children without epilepsy. However, no patterns specific to DS have been identified, and EEG does not correlate with outcome. Various cellular and molecular mechanisms contribute to epileptogenesis in DS and offer an interesting field of study.

Infections

Increased rate of infections is well known in DS. There are subtle abnormalities in both humoral and cellular arms of the immune response in children with DS compared with the control subjects.[22] In this study, there were no differences in the percentage of cases and controls who responded to inactivated influenza vaccine, but the response to polysaccharide pneumococcal vaccine was suboptimal in the cases.

Physical Growth

Physical growth of children with DS up to the age of 5 years in India was reported by Sachdev and colleagues.[23] The height curves of these children decreased to less than the 50th centile of normal children in the first 9 months of life and subsequently decreased to less than the 10th centile. The weight curves remained less than the 10th centile from the beginning. Head circumference curves decreased appreciably to less than the 10 centile at all ages, although the head continued to grow during the period of the study.

Lifespan

The lifespan of individuals with DS has greatly increased, and, in the West, approximately 85% live to about 60 years of age.[24] Mortality is maximum in the first 2 years of life because of congenital heart disease, recurrent infections, and rarely, leukemia. In India, longevity depends on the care that the family takes to look after the child, whether heart disease is present, and, if present, whether it is successfully operated. Adults with DS theoretically have a 50% chance of having a DS-affected child and 65% when both partners are affected. However, fertility in males is rare, although it has been reported.[25] Women are fertile, and have a 30% to 50% chance of having a child with DS. Individuals with mosaic DS have a 50% chance of an offspring with DS, but this is dependent on the percentage of trisomic cells in the gonads.

Table 1
Distribution of different types of cytogenetic abnormalities in DS in different studies

Report	No. of Subjects Studied	Trisomy (%)	Translocation (%)	Mosaic (%)
Meta-analysis of 18 studies[26] (1966–1987)	2410	91.64	4.12	4.12
Verma et al[26]	645	93.0	4.0	2.6
Mutton et al[27]	5737	95	4	1
Jyothy et al[28]	1001	87.92	7.69	4.39
Mokhtar et al[29]	146	96.6	2.7	0.7
Devlin & Morrison[30]	208	94.7	1.45	3.85
Kava et al[12]	1000	95	3.2	1.8
Ahmed et al[31]	295	95.6	3.7	0.7
Sheth et al[32]	382	84.8	8.9	3.9
OMIM entry 190685[33]		95	5	2–4% of free trisomy
Mandava et al[34]	1572	89.05	7.06	1.78
Authors' data, unpublished	830	94.8	3.6	1.20

CYTOGENETIC DIAGNOSIS

DS is easily confirmed by cytogenetic laboratory tests. The cytogenetic abnormality can be classified into pure trisomy 21, translocation, or mosaicism. Diagnostic testing involves taking 2 mL of heparinized sample of blood for lymphocyte culture with high resolution GTG banding. Chromosomes are counted in 20 metaphases and karyotyped. This detects the presence of an extra copy of chromosome 21 and classifies the syndrome as pure trisomy, mosaic, or translocation. If a rapid diagnosis is required, fluorescent in situ hybridization with probe for chromosome 21 may be used.

Pure trisomy consists of 3 complete copies of chromosome 21, caused by meiotic nondisjunction (NDJ) producing a gamete (ie, a sperm or egg cell) with an extra copy of chromosome 21. This gamete fertilizes with a normal gamete from the other parent to form an embryo with 47 chromosomes. This is the cause of DS in approximately 95% patients, with 88% caused by NDJ in the maternal gamete and 8% by NDJ in the paternal gamete. The trisomy of chromosome 21 is present in all cells in the body.

Mosaic DS is present when the subject has 2 cell lines, one with a normal set of chromosomes and the other with trisomy 21. This can occur in 1 of 2 ways: a NDJ event during an early cell division in a normal embryo leads to a fraction of the cells with trisomy 21 or an aneuploid embryo with trisomy 21 undergoes NDJ, and some of the cells in the embryo revert to the normal chromosomal arrangement. There is considerable variability in the percentage of trisomy 21 cells, both as a whole and among tissues. Mosaicism occurs in 1% to 2% of patients with DS.

Robertsonian translocations are present in 3% to 4% of the patients of DS and involve chromosome 21 and another acrocentric chromosome, number 14 being the most common type. Translocation DS does not show the maternal age effect and can be inherited from the father or the mother if they are carriers of this translocation.

The rates of the cytogenetic abnormalities in DS are similar in all ethnic groups, as shown in **Table 1**. However, 0.3% to 1.34 % of patients with DS have other chromosome rearrangements.[26] These abnormalities may consist of an additional sex chromosome, or ESAC (extra structurally abnormal chromosome) or rare transloca-tion (2:21).[35,36] The authors have observed a case with 18:21 translocation.

DOWN SYNDROME AND MATERNAL AGE

Maternal age as a risk factor was suspected even before the discovery of the chromosomal origin of DS. There is an exponential increase in the frequency of DS in mothers older than 35 years. This association has been shown to be universal. Verma and colleagues[37] reported that of 615 cases of DS in Delhi, 33% were born to mothers older than 35 years. A multicentric study from 1993 to 1997 showed that only 2.2% of women who delivered normal babies were in the age range 35 and older, whereas 8.9% of the 78 cases were in this age group (Verma and coworkers, unpublished data).

Even though high maternal age predisposes to DS, most cases are born to young couples. Therefore, much research has gone into establishing the parental origin of the extra chromosome in the patient and in unraveling the cause(s) of this anomaly. Analysis of parental origin as well as identification of the meiotic stage of NDJ, has been greatly improved by the use of chromosome 21–specific microsatellite mark-ers.[38] A meta-analysis of the data obtained from microsatellite-based analysis shows that greater than 85% cases of free trisomy 21 arise as a result of maternal aneupoidy and about 10% as a result of paternal aneupoidy.[39] The rest of the cases arise as a result of postzygotic mitosis. Further, in the majority of cases, NDJ occurs in the first meiotic division in ova (MI 65%; MII 23%), whereas in males, the error occurs more frequently in MII (MI 3%; MII 5%). The incidence of aneuploidy in human ova (~20%) is 10 to 20 times greater than in the sperm (1%–2%).[40]

Ghosh and colleagues[41] genotyped 212 unrelated Indian families with a DS child, using short tandem repeats. The maternal meiotic error was recorded as 88.06% of all cases, in contrast to 9.95% paternal and only 1.99% postzygotic mitotic errors. The estimated values of maternal meiotic I and meiotic II NDJ errors of chromosome 21 (Ch 21) were 78% and 22%, respectively. Within the paternal outcome group, about 47% and 53% accounted for NDJ at meiosis I and meiosis II, respectively. Malini and Ramachandra[42] reported that young mothers (18 to 29 years) born to their mothers at the age 30 years and older produced as high as 91.3% of children with DS in their study. The logistic regression of case-control study of DS children found that the odds ratio of age of grandmother was significant. The effect of age of mother and father was smaller than the effect of age of maternal grandmother.

DOWN SYNDROME AND FOLATE METABOLISM

Methylation is one of the mechanisms of suppression of transcriptional activity of the centromeric DNA. Inadequate methylation of centromeric DNA interferes with chro-mosomal segregation during cell division, leading to NDJ.[43] James and coworkers[44] were the first to demonstrate from their study on MTHFR C677T mutations in parents of children with DS that the frequency of T-allele–bearing mothers was significantly greater in the DS mothers than in the age-matched random controls. Hobbs and colleagues[45] confirmed that both MTHFR and MTRR mutations are risk factors in DS mothers. There are, however, reports that do not find an increased frequency of these single nucleotide polymorphisms in the DS mothers studied.[46] Analysis of 36 parents with DS children and 60 healthy couples from Tamil Nadu and Karnataka (South India) found that MTHFR 677CT polymorphism was associated with a risk for DS.[47] However, among 104 north Indian mothers of babies with DS and 109 control mothers, the prevalence of MTHFR C677T polymorphism was not significantly different in mothers of babies with DS compared with controls.[48] As part of the population-based, case-control National Down Syndrome Project involving 1011 mothers of infants with DS, Bean and colleagues[49] reported lack of maternal folic acid supplementation was more frequent among infants with DS and atrioventricular septal defects and atrial septal defects than among infants with DS and no heart defect. Based on the above studies, it would appear to be prudent to carry out periconceptional supplementation with folate-rich diet or tablets to reduce the number of new cases of DS or reduce the frequency of congenital heart disease in DS.

GENETIC COUNSELING AND MANAGEMENT
Breaking the News

In the majority of the cases, the parents are expecting the birth of a normal child. Appreciating and understating these expectations of the family, the disclosure of the news should be in a sensitive and caring manner. It is best done once the mother has recovered from the ordeal of childbirth and in the presence of the partner/family members, as the situation demands. The pediatrician should first discuss with the family his or her suspicion of DS in the neonate and order blood chromosomal analysis to confirm the diagnosis. FISH analysis can be ordered for an early report, but karyotype must be done to exclude a translocation state, as this has implications for counseling for future pregnancies and possibly other family members. If diagnosis was confirmed antenatally, the formal cytogenetic report must be seen by the physician. The information given should be correct, but it is not necessary to detail all complications associated with DS at the first contact. All children do not develop every complication. Physicians should use their experience to guide and support the family. Printed material on DS and access to other families and patient support groups can help the parents to deal with the unexpected news. Girisha and colleagues[50] studied the background information, concerns, and specific queries of families of children with DS. The majority of the parents were aware that their child has DS and will have mental retardation. However, most of the families were ignorant about the chromosomal nature of the disorder and prenatal screening and testing options.

Evaluation and Management

Details of evaluation and management at different age groups are available, and the reader should refer to the guidelines recently laid down by the American Academy of Pediatrics, and Weijerman and de Winter.[51,52]

Recurrence

The risk of another affected child to a couple who have a previous trisomy 21 child is related to the maternal age–related baseline risk. Women less than 30 years of age have an 8-fold increase from the age-related risk. In women older than 30 years, the risk is doubled. Practically, the risk of recurrence is low, approaching 1% by the mid 30s.[53] Recurrence risk after 2 previous conceptions with trisomy 21 is 10% to 20%, in view of a high possibility of the presence of gonadal mosaicism. Where the index child has a Robertsonian translocation, the karyotype of the parents to differentiate de novo and familial forms is crucial. For de novo translocations, the recurrence risk is less than 1%. In situations of familial Robertsonian translocation DS, of which rob (14q21q) is the most frequent, recurrence varies based on the sex of the carrier. The recurrence is about 1% if the male carries a translocation, and 10% to 15% for a female carrier. In a familial 21:21 translocation, the genetic risk is 100%, and all pregnancies continuing to term have an affected child.[53] In familial translocations, the family should be counseled about siblings at risk and the need to perform chromosomal analysis in them. Availability of prenatal diagnosis for DS in the next pregnancy should be discussed.

ANTENATAL SCREENING

The aim of a prenatal screening program is to refine a woman's risk of carrying a fetus with a chromosomal disease beyond her age-related risk. The risk of a woman to have a baby with DS increases in a gradual, linear fashion until age 30 years and thereafter increases exponentially. Maternal age was, therefore, the first screening test used, and amniocentesis was offered to women older than 35 years. However, this detected only 30% of all affected fetuses, and research for more sensitive markers with improved detection rates has now allowed screening of all pregnant women. In the 1980s, recognition of biochemical and ultrasound markers in the second trimester for trisomy 21 was introduced. The focus shifted to using screening markers in the first trimester in 1990s, greatly increasing the sensitivity and specificity of the screening tests. Screening tests are simple, relatively less-expensive tests, which can be offered to a population at large. They ascertain whether the fetus has a high or low risk of being affected. In a screening test, there is considerable distribution overlap between affected and nonaffected pregnancies. Therefore, a positive result in a screening test only places the patient in a high-risk group and does not in any way imply that the fetus is affected.[54]

Based on the results of these screening tests, definitive tests are offered to determine the actual fetal chromosomes. These are discussed below in the prenatal diagnostic studies section. As more and more women are delaying pregnancy until they are older, antenatal diagnosis of DS is gaining more relevance in current medical practice.

Pretest Counseling

This is a prerequisite to antenatal screening. This includes detailed explanation that the screening tests will only generate a risk of having a baby with DS. It does not confirm the presence or absence of DS or guarantee a normal baby. It should include a discussion of the diagnostic tests and the risks associated with them.

First Trimester Screen

This screening first began in 1992 with measurement of nuchal translucency on ultrasound scan and serum biochemistry combining free β-human chorionic gonadotropin (fβHCG) and pregnancy-associated plasma protein A (PAPP-A level), with the maternal age, to generate a risk for trisomy 21. The appropriate time for this is 10 to 13 weeks plus 6 days. Nuchal translucency (NT) is measured at a crown–rump length between 45 and 84 mm by a transabdominal or transvaginal scan. It is important to adhere to the standard ultrasound technique for correct measurement of the NT.[55,56]

Biochemical markers

Pregnancies with trisomy 21 are associated with increased fbHCG and low PAPP-A levels. For analysis, the measured marker concentration is converted to multiples of median of unaffected pregnancies at the same gestation. It is imperative to have normal medians of the population under analysis for improved sensitivity. In trisomy 21 pregnancies, the fbHCG is about twice as high, and the PAPP-A is reduced to half compared with euploid pregnancies. Other variables that affect the risk generated include maternal age, weight, racial origin, smoking, and method of conception and

Table 2
Comparative performance of different screening modalities for fetal chromosomal disease

Test	Sensitivity (%)	False-Positive Rate (%)
Maternal age (MA)	30	5
MA + Nuchal translucency	75–80	5
MA+ serum free βhCG & PAPP-A	60–70	5
MA+ NT+ serum free βhCG & PAPP-A (First trimester combined screening)	85–95	5
Combined test + nasal bone or tricuspid regurgitation or ductus venosus flow	93–96	2.5
MA+ serum AFP + free βhCG + uE3 + Inhibin A (quadruple test)	70–75	5
MA+ serum AFP + free βhCG + uE3 (triple test)	65–70	5

must be included in the analysis. New data are emerging on increase in detection rate and decrease in false-positive rate, with inclusion of alpha-fetoprotein (AFP) measurement in the first trimester.[57] Because there is no significant association between the biochemical and ultrasound markers in euploid and affected pregnancies, the 2 can be combined to generate more sensitive risk estimates (**Table 2**).[58]

Timing of ultrasound and serum screening in the first trimester:

1. OSCAR (One stop clinic for assessment of risk) combines counseling, risk assessment, and definitive testing in 1 patient visit. This is possible by current automated biochemical analyzers that provide random access and precise measurements of metabolites in a blood sample. The best time for OSCAR is 12 weeks when improved ultrasound detection of fetal malformations can be combined with the biochemical testing for aneuploidies. For a false-positive rate of 5%, this has a detection rate of 90%.
2. Two-visit screening refers to biochemical testing at 9 to 10 weeks of gestation, when the PAPP-A performance is best to differentiate the affected from the euploid fetus. Ultrasound scanning is done at the second visit at 12 weeks and then composite risk is estimated. This improves the detection rate to 93% to 94% but may be negated by poor patient compliance.

Additional markers in the first trimester

Absent nasal bone, tricuspid regurgitation, reversal of blood flow in the ductus venosus, and increased peak systolic velocity in the hepatic artery are some of the other signs checked for in the scan at 11 to 13 weeks. The absent nasal bone is observed in 60% of fetuses with trisomy 21 and 2.5% of euploid fetuses.[59] The sensitivity of the other markers for trisomy 21 is 55%, 60%, and 80% with a false-positive rate of 1.0%, 3.0%, and 5%, respectively.[56,60] Addition of these markers to the first trimester combined screening increases the detection rate to 93% to 96% for a false-positive rate of 2.5%.[56,61–63]

Identification of the above markers for DS has shifted the contingent screening to the first trimester. The first step with maternal age, NT, fbHCG, and PAPP-A stratifies the risk to high if more than 1 in 50 and low if less than 1 in 1000. The patients with the intermediate risk (1 in 51 to 1 in 1000) undergo the second-stage screening with nasal bone, ductus venosus, or tricuspid valve flows. This reclassifies as screen negative if less than 1 in 100 and screen positive if more than 1 in 100. The advantage of this lies in increased sensitivity, whereas only 15% to 20% of the total women screened require additional screening tests.

Second Trimester Biochemical Screening

Traditionally, at 15 to 22 weeks, the concentration of α-fetoprotein, unconjugated estriol, and human chorionic gonadotropin (HCG) in the "triple screen," and additionally inhibin A in the "quadruple screen" are measured and the composite risk for neural tube defect, trisomy 21, and trisomy 18 is estimated. To calculate the risk for DS, the results of the maternal serum screen are used to adjust a woman's age-related risk for DS. For a 5% false-positive rate, the sensitivity of the triple test is 70% and that of the quadruple test is 75%. Maternal variables as stated above, including pregnancy gestation dating by ultrasound scan, are important for improved accuracy of the screening test. In fetuses with DS, the AFP and estriol levels are decreased and the HCG and inhibin levels are higher. In trisomy 18, the levels of all the 3 markers are decreased. In twin pregnancies, the overall sensitivity of second trimester screening is lower, and only approximately 50% of affected fetuses may be identified.[54]

First Trimester Screening Followed by Second Trimester Screening

Integrated test combines the biochemical and ultrasound markers of the first trimester with the biochemical markers in the second trimester to generate a risk with a mid-trimester cutoff of 1 in 250. The final risk assessment is based on both screen tests considered together with nondisclosure of the first trimester results.

Sequential screening is a stepwise test, like the integrated test, but with disclosure of the first trimester screen result to the patient. A chorionic villus sampling (CVS) is recommended to all with a positive first trimester screen. Those with a negative screen are offered a triple/quadruple test.

Contingent screening combines the best of screening in the first and second trimester. It is similar to sequential screening but the results after the first trimester screen are divided into 3: screen negative, intermediate risk, and screen positive. A low first trimester screen offers early reassurance. It selects a subgroup of high-risk screen patients for early confirmatory testing and only measures the second trimester markers in a small subset with borderline/intermediate results on the first trimester screen.

The advantage of an additional second trimester screening after a woman has received the first trimester test is an improvement in the detection rate with a decrease in the false-positive rate. This improves the overall performance of the screening tests. The advantage of the sequential and contingent screening tests over the integrated test is that it allows a higher proportion of affected pregnancies to be identified in the first trimester. Overall, the contingent-based approach is the most efficient, with minimal additional screening in the second trimester, while maintaining a high detection rate and low false-positive rate.[64]

Screening in twin pregnancies requires special mention. The nuchal translucency of each twin is mentioned separately. In dichorionic twins, the biochemical markers of fbHCG and PAPP-A are twice that of singleton pregnancies, and those of monochorionic twins are slightly lower. Appropriate adjustments in the software are required for risk assessment. Biochemical screening is generally associated with detection rates at least 15% less than those for singleton fetuses.

GENETIC SONOGRAM

The systematic use of multiple sonographic markers to detect fetal aneuploidy at 18 to 22 weeks of gestation is referred to as the *genetic sonogram*. On ultrasound major structural malformations like cardiac defects, duodenal atresia, and other nonspecific markers termed *soft markers*. Of these, nuchal fold thickness is the most sensitive marker. Other ultrasonographic markers include short femur and humerus, ventriculomegaly, intrauterine growth retardation, renal pyelectasis, echogenic bowel, clinodactyly, and sandal gap. Because these markers may also be seen in normal fetuses, two approaches were popularized to assess their significance in counseling for confirmatory testing. Benacerraf and colleagues[65] had popularized the index scoring system, and Nyberg and coworkers[66] applied the likelihood ratio for each marker to an apriori risk of maternal age/biochemical screening. Gupta and colleagues[67] observed that after 20 weeks of gestation, the ratio of femoral/tibial length can be a marker of DS in utero.

Genetic services in India are undergoing a transition with increasing education, awareness, and availability of genetic tests. There is no uniform policy or national program on prenatal screening for DS. However, in the cities, these tests are being ordered by many obstetricians. Ultrasound screening for DS in both first and second trimesters is also performed in urban cities. The Society of Fetal Medicine, a national, scientific organization to promote fetal well being and care, is also involved in education of doctors and obstetricians for prenatal screening including counseling, interpretation of screening results, and appropriate ultrasound techniques for measurement of nuchal translucency and other markers of DS. In these centers, there is a slow but obvious shift of screening to the first trimester with the major limitation being late registration of pregnancies.

PRENATAL DIAGNOSTIC STUDIES

Prenatal diagnosis is offered to parents with increased risk of DS because of positive biochemical screening tests, high maternal age, or previous child with DS or when fetal ultrasound soft markers, such as increased nuchal fold thickness, cardiac defect, or duodenal atresia are suggestive of DS. Amniocentesis, chorionic villus sampling, or cordocentesis, followed by culture of cells from either of these samples and subsequent karyotyping, can confirm the diagnosis of DS in the fetus. Chorionic villus sampling is usually done between 10 and 14 weeks of gestation. This test carries a 1 in 100 risk of miscarriage. Amniocentesis can be done after 15 weeks of gestation. The test carries a 1 in 500 risk of miscarriage. Percutaneous umbilical blood sampling is done after 18 weeks of gestation. The risk for miscarriage is higher than amniocentesis or chorionic villus sampling. It is only done when results of other tests are unclear, if mosaicism is suggested on amniotic fluid studies, or if the woman presents late in pregnancy. Kabra and colleagues[68] analyzed 99 fetal blood samples for chromosomal abnormalities. The most common indications for the procedure were abnormalities detected on ultrasonography (47.7%) and previous child with DS. Analysis of the 67 successful cultures showed 4 (5.9%) karyotypic abnormalities. Mathur and coworkers[69] also studied 187 cases for prenatal karyotyping using cord blood. Karyotypic abnormalities were observed in 5.2% of the cases.

Novel methodologies for detection of chromosomal abnormalities have become available in recent years, and clinical utility in prenatal settings is being explored.[70] These include FISH, quantitative fluorescence polymerase chain reaction (QF-PCR), multiplex ligation-dependent probe amplification (MLA), Bacs-on-beads microarrays, microarrays, and non-invasive prenatal diagnosis. These are briefly discussed below.

Amniotic cell cultures, FISH studies, QF-PCR, and MLPA studies are being carried out in many laboratories in India. Bacs-on-beads technology will be available soon.

Amniotic Fluid Cultures

Since 1970, amniotic fluid cultures with subsequent complete karyotyping are used as the gold standard for prenatal diagnosis of chromosomal abnormalities. Amniocytes are cultured in monolayers and harvested at the exponential phase of the culture to analyze the chromosomes in the mitotic cells. This method can detect aneuploidies and structural chromosomal abnormalities at metaphase/prometaphase in 12 to 14 days. The culture technique requires technical expertise and is time consuming. The long waiting period can cause emotional stress to the parents; therefore, rapid aneuploidy detection tests such as FISH, QF-PCR, or MLPA should always be done as well.

Fluorescence in Situ Hybridization

FISH is a targeted approach by which fluorescently labeled, region-specific probes of 5 common aneuploidies of chromosomes 13, 18, 21, X, and Y are hybridized on fetal cells followed by washes of the excess probe and enumeration of the fluorescent signals. The number of fluorescent signals per cell indicates the number of copies of the targeted chromosomes. Three signals of chromosome 21 will detect trisomy 21. To exclude mosaicism, 100 to 200 cells are enumerated. A big advantage is that interphase cells can be used to detect or rule out trisomy 21 and other targeted aneuploidies within 24 to 48 hours. The technique is highly sensitive and specific for detection of targeted aneuploidies. It can detect triploidy and mosaicism. Cultures are not required. The test is rapid but can miss other unexpected chromosomal abnormalities in the fetus. Therefore, most centers use FISH as an adjunct test along with amniotic fluid cultures for karyotyping. In the presence of abnormal ultrasound studies, targeted FISH for certain microdeletions can be carried out.

Quantitative Fluorescence Polymerase Chain Reaction

QF-PCR consists of selective amplification of polymorphic DNA markers (specific for chromosomes 13,18, 21, X, and Y regions) on genomic DNA, after binding of fluorescent-labeled primers, which are unique for that region. Computer-based measurement of the intensity of the fluorescent signal quantifies the copy number of the target sequence of each chromosome. Results can be obtained from uncultured CVS or amniocytes to detect or rule out trisomy 21 and other targeted aneuploidies within 24 hours. QF-PCR is as reliable as FISH and karyotype for the targeted aneuploidies. The sensitivity of QF-PCR is 95.65% and specificity is 99.97%. It can be automated; therefore, it is more useful if a large number of samples have to be analyzed. These analyses suggest that QF-PCR alone is appropriate for patients with uncomplicated pregnancies who are referred solely for an increased risk of a common trisomy. QF-PCR can replace conventional cytogenetic analysis whenever prenatal testing is performed solely because of an increased risk of aneuploidy in chromosomes 13, 18, 21, X, or Y. As with all tests, pretest counseling should include a discussion of the benefits and limitations of the test. Both conventional cytogenetics and QF-PCR should be performed in all cases of prenatal diagnosis referred for a fetal ultrasound abnormality (including an increased nuchal translucency measurement >3.5 mm) or a familial chromosomal rearrangement. Cytogenetic follow-up of QF-PCR findings of trisomy 13 and 21 is recommended to rule out inherited Robertsonian translocations.

Multiplex Ligation-Dependent Probe Amplification

MLPA allows detection of copy number changes of specific DNA sequences. MLPA uses 2-part probes of unique length that, when hybridized to adjacent target sequences on genomic DNA, can be joined together by enzyme DNA ligase. This then allows all target sites to be amplified using a single primer pair that is complimentary to the 2 free ends common to all probes. Using a series of normalization calculations, copy number can be determined for each target sequence and, therefore, each chromosome. Results can be obtained on uncultured CVS or amniocytes to detect or rule out trisomy 21 and other targeted aneuploidies within 24 hours. The sensitivity of 100% and specificity of 99% for nonmosaic-targeted aneuploidies has been reported.

BACs-on-Beads

BACs-on-beads technology is comparable to FISH in a liquid format. It utilizes DNA probes generated from selected PCR-amplified bacterial artificial chromosomes (BACs), which are fluorescently coded and immobilized on Luminex beads. Five independent BACs on beads probes of chromosome 13, 18, 21, X, and Y can be used for aneuploidy detection. BACs of 9-12 microdeletion syndromes are included to extend the sensitivity for diagnosis of chromosomal abnormalities in a cost-effective manner. DNA extracted from uncultured fetal cells is used to detect or rule out trisomy 21 and other targeted aneuploidies, along with 9-12 microdeletion syndromes. It is a rapid test, a form of multiplex FISH, which can be automated. Disadvantages include the inability to detect triploidy, and sensitivity for detection of mosaicism is low. Shaffer and colleagues[71] report prenatal BACs-on-beads as a robust technology for the investigation of fetuses with normal karyotype with or without sonographic abnormalities.

Non-Invasive Tests for Detection of Trisomy 21 from Maternal Blood

Circulating cell-free DNA fragments are isolated from maternal plasma and quantified with an assay that determines the fetal contribution (fetal fraction), using massively parallel shotgun sequencing (MPSS). This technique sequences millions of DNA fragments to determine their specific chromosomal origin. If the fetus has a third chromosome 21, the percentage of chromosome 21 fragments is higher than expected. When applied to high-risk pregnancies for Down syndrome, a detection rate of at least 98% can be achieved at a false-positive rate of 2% or lower. This method substantially reduces the need for invasive diagnostic procedures and procedure-related losses. MPSS testing does not address other chromosome abnormalities or events such as twin pregnancies. Recently, a number of investigators have shown that in high-risk populations, massively parallel sequencing can detect a large proportion of DS with a low false-positive rate.[72–74] However, this test is not fully diagnostic and therefore constitutes an advanced screening test. Accordingly, confirmation of MPSS-positive results through invasive testing would still be required. It is also important to recognize that for women who are screen-positive using current screening protocols, DS represents only about half of the fetal chromosomal abnormalities identified through amniocentesis and CVS.[75,76]

THERAPY OF DOWN SYNDROME

Recent advances in our understanding of the genetics of DS indicate that the trisomy of only a fraction of these genes may result in the development of DS-associated conditions. Ts65Dn mice are trisomic for at least 104 of the genes on human chromosome 21 and exhibit many of the features of DS, including specific deficits in learning and memory. Fernandez and colleagues[77] showed increased inhibition of inputs in hippocampus of Ts-65Dn mice. They treated these mice with the noncompetitive GABAA antagonists, picrotoxin, and PTZ (pentylenetetrazole) for 10 days. The mice showed improved performance in novel object recognition and the T-maze tasks. Improvement persisted for several months after treatment. Costa and coworkers[78] showed that NMDA receptor function is perturbed by the integrated effects of increased expression of several chromosome 21 genes, including *RCAN1, APP, TIAM1, ITSN1,* and *DYRK1A.* They treated Ts65Dn mice with uncompetitive NMDA receptor antagonist, memantine. Memantine is US Food and Drug Administration approved for Alzheimer's disease, and a pilot study in humans has been started. Most promising have been the studies by Salehi and colleagues,[79] which showed that in the brain of the Ts65Dn mouse neurons in a particular brain stem nucleus— the locus coeruleus—degenerate. They noted that the amount of norepinephrine in the hippocampus of the Ts65Dn mice was reduced compared with the amounts present in control (euploid) mice, but it remained responsive to norepinephrine. When they treated the Ts65Dn mice with a combination of drugs that restored norepinephrine concentrations in the hippocampus, learning and memory deficits in the mice were alleviated. This observation suggests the exciting prospect that the delivery of norepinephrine to the central nervous system of people with DS may improve their learning ability and memory. These studies give hope that new therapies for DS are on the horizon.[80]

REFERENCES

1. Megarbane A, Ravel A, Mircher C, et al. The 50th anniversary of the discovery of trisomy 21: The past, present, and future of research and treatment of Down syndrome. Genet Med 2009;11(9):611–6.
2. Hattori M, Fujiyama A, Taylor TD, et al. Chromosome 21 mapping and sequencing consortium. Nature 2000;405:311–9.
3. Gardiner K, Herault Y, Lott IT, et al. Down syndrome: from understanding the neurobiology to therapy. J Neuroscience, 2010;30(45):14943–5.
4. Antonarakis SE, Lyle R, Dermitzakis ET, et al. Chromosome 21 and Down syndrome: from genomics to pathophysiology. Nat Rev Genet 2004;5:725–38.
5. Wiseman FK, Alford KA, Tybulewicz VL,et al. Down syndrome—recent progress and future prospects. Hum Mol Genet 2009;18 (R1):R75–83.
6. Murthy SK, Malhotra AK, Mani S, et al. Incidence of Down Syndrome in Dubai, UAE. Med Princ Pract 2007;16:25–8.
7. Canfield MA, Honein MA, Yuskiv N, et al. National estimates and race/ethnic-specific variation of selected birth defects in the United States, 1999–2001. Birth Defects Res A Clin Mol Teratol 2006;76:747–56.
8. Roizen NJ, Patterson D. Down's syndrome. Lancet 2003;361:1281–9.
9. Verma IC, Bijarnia S. The burden of genetic disorders in India and a framework for community control. Community Genetics 2002;5(3):192–6.
10. Baird PA, Sadovnick AD. Maternal age-specific rates for Down syndrome: changes over time. Am J Med Genet 1988;29:917–27.
11. Annual Report on Registration of Births & Deaths in Delhi. 2010. Directorate of Economics and Statistics, & Office of the Chief Registrar (Births and Deaths), Civil Lines, Vikas Bhavan II, New Delhi.
12. Kava MP, Tullu MS, Muranjan MN, et al. Down syndrome: clinical profile from India. Arch Med Res 2004;35(1):31–5.

13. Menon PS, Sachdev HP, Verma IC, et al. Developmental milestones of Down's syndrome patients in north India. Indian J Med Res 1981;73:369–73.
14. Bhattacharyya R, Sanyal D, Roy K, et al. Correlation between physical anomaly and behavioral abnormalities in Down syndrome. J Pediatr Neurosci 2010;5(2):105–10.
15. Bhatia S, Verma IC, Shrivastava S. Congenital heart disease in Down syndrome: an echocardiographic study. Indian Pediatrics 1992;29(9):1113–6.
16. Nebesio TD, Eugster EA. Unusual thyroid constellation in Down syndrome: congenital hypothyroidism, Graves' disease, and hemiagenesis in the same child. J Pediatr Endocrinol Metab 2009;22(3):263–8.
17. Bhat MH, Saba S, Ahmed I, et al. Graves' disease in a Down's syndrome patient. J Pediatr Endocrinol Metab 2010;23(11):1181–3.
18. Awasthi A, Das R, Varma N, et al. Hematological disorders in Down syndrome: ten-year experience at a tertiary care centre in North India. Pediatr Hematol Oncol 2005;22(6):507–2.
19. Gathwala G, Dalal P, Dalal JS, et al. Transient aplastic anemia in Down's syndrome—a rare association. Eur J Med Genet 2011;54(3):341–2.
20. Sinha R, Thangaswamy CR, Muthiah T, et al. Prolonged postoperative desaturation in a child with Down syndrome and atrial septal defect. Indian J Anaesth 2011;55(6):608–10.
21. Arya R, Kabra M, Gulati S. Epilepsy in children with Down syndrome. Epileptic disorders: international epilepsy journal with videotape. 2011;13(1):1–7.
22. Joshi AY, Abraham RS, Snyder MR, et al. Immune evaluation and vaccine responses in Down syndrome: evidence of immunodeficiency? Vaccine 2011;29(31):5040–6.
23. Sachdev HS, Menon PS, Verma IC, et al. Physical growth of children with Down syndrome in India. Indian Journal Pediatr 1981;48(390):85–9.
24. Glasson N, Sullivan EJ, Hussain SG, et al. The changing survival profile of people with Down's syndrome: implications for genetic counselling. Clinical Genet 2002;62(5):390–3.
25. Pradhan M, Dalal A, Khan F, et al. Fertility in men with Down syndrome: a case report. Fertil Steril 2006;86(6):1765,e1–3.
26. Verma IC, Mathew S, Elango E, et al. Cytogenetic studies in Down syndrome. Indian Pediatrics 1991;28:991–6.
27. Mutton D, Alberman E, Hook EB. Cytogenetic and epidemiological findings in Down syndrome, England and Wales 1989 to 1993. National Down Syndrome Cytogenetic Register and the Association of Clinical Cytogeneticists. J Med Genet 1996;33:387–94.
28. Jyothy A, Kumar KS, Rao GN, et al. Cytogenetic studies of 1001 Down syndrome cases from Andhra Pradesh, India. Indian J Med Res 2000;111:133–7.
29. Mokhtar MM, Abdel-Aziz AM, Nazmy NA, et al. Cytogenetic profile of Down syndrome in Alexandria, Egypt. Eastern Med Health J 2003;9:37–44.
30. Devlin L, Morrison PJ. Mosaic Down's syndrome prevalence in a complete population study. Arch Dis Child 2004;89:1177–8.
31. Ahmed I, Ghafoor T, Samore NA, et al. Down syndrome: clinical and cytogenetic analysis. J Coll Physicians Surg Pak 2005;15(7):426–9.
32. Sheth F, Rao S, Desai M, et al. Cytogenetic analysis of Down syndrome in Gujarat. Indian Pediatr 2007;44:774–7.
33. Available at: http://omim.org/entry/190685. Acessed May 20, 2012.
34. Mandava S, Koppaka N, Bhatia V, et al. Cytogenetic analysis of 1572 cases of Down syndrome: a report of double aneuploidy and novel findings 47,XY, t(14;21)(q13;q22.3)mat,+21 and 45,XX,t(14;21) in an Indian population. Genet Test Mol Biomarkers 2010;14(4):499–504.

35. Kotwaliwale SV, Dicholkar VV, Motashaw ND. Maternal transmission of translocation 2;21 associated with Down's syndrome. Journal Med Genet 1991;28(6):415–6.

36. Balwan WK, Kumar P, Raina TR, et al. Double trisomy with 48, XXX+21 karyotype in a Down's syndrome child from Jammu and Kashmir, India. J Genet 2008;87(3): 257–9.

37. Verma IC, Gupta AK, Devanagondi BS. Down syndrome: maternal age in 615 cases in india and its implications in genetic counseling. Indian pediatrics. 1975;12(12): 1239–45.

38. Dagna-Bricarelli F, Pierluigi M, Perroni L, et al. High efficiency in the attribution of parental origin of nondisjunction in trisomy 21 by both cytogenetic and molecular polymorphisms. Hum Genet 1988;79:124–7.

39. Jacobs PA, Hassold TJ. The origin of numerical chromosomal abnormalities. In Adv Hum Genet 1995;33:101–33.

40. Raman R. Down syndrome in India. In: Kumar D, editor. Genetic disorders of the Indian subcontinent. Dordrecht: Kluwer Academic Publishers; 2004. p.171–84.

41. Ghosh S, Bhaumik P, Ghosh P, et al. Chromosome 21 non-disjunction and Down syndrome birth in an Indian cohort: analysis of incidence and aetiology from family linkage data. Genet Res 2010;92(3):189–97.

42. Malini SS, Ramachandra NB. Influence of advanced age of maternal grandmothers on Down syndrome. BMC Med Genet 2006;7:4.

43. Leyton C, Mergudich D, de la Torre D, et al. Impaired chromosome segregation in plant anaphase after moderate hypomethylation of DNA. Cell Prolif 1995;28:481–96.

44. James SJ, Pogribna M, Pogribny IP, et al. Abnormal folate metabolism and mutation in the methylenetetrahydrofolate reductase (MTHFR) gene may be maternal risk factors for Down syndrome. Am J Clin Nutr 1999;70:495–501.

45. Hobbs CA, Sherman SL, Yi P, et al. Polymorphisms in genes involved in folate metabolism as maternal risk factors for Down syndrome. Am J Hum Genet 2000;67: 623–30.

46. Petersen M, Grigoriadou M, Mikkelsen M. A common mutation in the methylenetetrahydrofolate reductase gene is not a risk factor for Down syndrome. Am J Hum Genet 2000;67(Suppl 2):141.

47. Cyril C, Rai P, Chandra N, et al. MTHFR Gene variants C677T, A1298C and association with Down syndrome: a Case-control study from South India. Indian J Hum Genet 2009;15(2):60–4.

48. Kohli U, Arora S, Kabra M, et al. Prevalence of MTHFR C677T polymorphism in north Indian mothers having babies with Trisomy 21 Down syndrome. Down's syndrome, research and practice. Journal of the Sarah Duffen Centre/University of Portsmouth 2008;12(2):133–7.

49. Bean LJ, Allen EG, Tinker SW, et al. Lack of maternal folic acid supplementation is associated with heart defects in Down syndrome: a report from the National Down Syndrome Project. Birth defects research Part A, Clinical and Molecular Teratology 2011;91(10):885–93.

50. Girisha KM, Sharda SV, Phadke SR. Issues in counseling for Down syndrome. Indian Pediatr 2007;44(2):131–3.

51. Bull MJ. Committee on Genetics. Health supervision for children with Down syndrome. Pediatrics 2011;128(2):393–406.

52. Weijerman ME, de Winter JP. Clinical practice. The care of children with Down syndrome. Eur J Pediatr 2010;169(12):1445–52.

53. Gardner RJM, Sutherland GR. Down syndrome. Other Full aneuploides, and Polyploidy, In: Chromosome abnormalities and genetic counseling. Oxford Monographs on Medical Genetics. No 46. 3rd edition. New York: Oxford University Press; 2004. p. 249–63.

54. Driscoll DA, Gross SJ; Professional Practice Guidelines Committee. Screening for fetal aneuploidy and neural tube defects. Genet Med 2009;11(11):818–21.
55. Malone FD, Canick JA, Ball RH, et al. First-trimester or second-trimester screening, or both, for Down's syndrome for the first trimester and second trimester evaluation of risk (FASTER) research consortium. N Engl J Med 2005;353:2001–11.
56. Pandya PP, Goldberg H, Walton B, et al. The implementation of first-trimester scanning at 10–13 weeks' gestation and the measurement of fetal nuchal translucency thickness in two maternity units. Ultrasound Obstet Gynecol 1995;5(1):20–5.
57. Bredaki FE, Wright D, Matos P, et al. First-trimester screening for trisomy 21 using alpha-fetoprotein. Fetal Diagn Ther 2011;30:215–8.
58. Nicolaides KH. Screening for fetal aneuploides at 11–13 weeks. Prenat Diag 2011; 31:7–15.
59. Cicero S, Curcio P, Papageorghiou A, et al. Absence of nasal bone infetuses with trisomy 21 at 11–14 weeks of gestation: an observational study. Lancet 2001;358: 1665–7.
60. Nicolaides KH. Turning the pyramis of prenatal care. Fetal Diagn Ther 2011;29: 183–96.
61. Kagan KO, Cicero S, Staboulidou I, et al. Fetal nasal bone in screening for trisomies 21, 18 and 13 and Turner syndrome at 11–13 weeks of gestation. Ultrasound Obstet Gynecol 2009;33:259–64.
62. Maiz N, Valencia C, Kagan KO, et al. Ductus venosus Doppler in screening for trisomies 21, 18 and 13 and Turner syndrome at 11–13 weeks of gestation. Ultrasound Obstet Gynecol 2009;33:512–7.
63. Kagan KO, Valencia C, Livanos P, et al. Tricuspid regurgitation in screening for trisomies 21, 18 and 13 and Turner syndrome at 11 + 0–13 + 6 weeks of gestation. Ultrasound Obstet Gynecol 2009;33:18–22.
64. Guanciali-Franchi P, Iezzi I, Palka C, et al. Comparison of combined, stepwise sequential, contingent, and integrated screening in 7292 high-risk pregnant women. Prenat Diagn 2011;31(11):1077–81.
65. Benacerraf BR, Neuberg D, Bromley B, et al. Sonographic scoring index for prenatal detection of chromosomal abnormalities. J Ultrasound Med 1992;11:449–58.
66. Nyberg DA, Luthy DA,Williams MA, et al. Genetic sonogram: computerized assessment of risk for Down syndrome based on obstetric US findings during the second trimester (abstr). Radiology 1996;201(P):160.
67. Gupta R, Thomas RD, Sreenivas V, et al. Ultrasonographic femur-tibial length ratio: a marker of Down syndrome from the late second trimester. Am J Perinatol 2001;18(4): 217–24.
68. Kabra M, Saxena R, Chinnappan D, et al. Karyotyping of at risk fetuses by cordocentesis in advanced gestation. Indian J Med Res 1996;104:288–91.
69. Mathur R, Dubey S, Hamilton S, et al. Rapid prenatal karyotyping using foetal blood obtained by cordocentesis. Nat Med J India 2002;15(2):75–7.
70. Hahn S, Jackson LG, Zimmermann BG. Prenatal diagnosis of fetal aneuploidies: post-genomic developments. Genome Med 2010;2(8):50.
71. Shaffer LG, Coppinger J, Morton SA, et al. The development of a rapid assay for prenatal testing of common aneuploidies and microdeletion syndromes. Prenat Diagn 2011;31(8):778–87.
72. Chiu RW, Akolekar R, Zheng YW, et al. Non-invasive prenatal assessment of trisomy 21 by multiplexed maternal plasma DNA sequencing: large scale validation study. BMJ 2011;342:c7401.

73. Palomaki GE, Kloza EM, Lambert-Messerlian GM, et al. DNA sequencing of maternal plasma to detect Down syndrome: an international clinical validation study. Genet Med 2011;13:913–20.

74. Papageorgiou EA, Karagrigoriou A, Tsaliki E, et al. Fetal-specific DNA methylation ratio permits noninvasive prenatal diagnosis of trisomy 21. Nat Med 2011;17:510–3.

75. ISPD Rapid Response Statement. Prenatal detection of Down syndrome using massively parallel sequencing (MPS): a rapid response statement from a committee on behalf of the Board of the International Society for Prenatal Diagnosis, 24 October 2011. Available at www.ispdhome.org. Accessed April 1, 2012.

76. Benn P, Cuckle H, Pergament E. Non-invasive prenatal diagnosis for Down syndrome: the paradigm will shift, but slowly. Ultrasound Obstet Gynecol 2012;39:127–30.

77. Fernandez F, Morishita W, Zuniga E, et al. Pharmacotherapy for cognitive impairment in a mouse model of Down syndrome. Nat Neurosci 2007;10:411–3.

78. Costa C, Scott-McKean JJ, Stasko MR. Acute injections of the NMDA receptor antagonist memantine rescue performance deficits of the Ts65Dn mouse model of Down syndrome on a fear conditioning test. Neuropsychopharmacology 2007;33: 1624–32.

79. Salehi M, Faizi D, Colas J, et al. Restoration of norepinephrine-modulated contextual memory in a mouse model of Down syndrome. Sci Transl Med 2009;1:7ra17.

80. Wiseman FK. Cognitive enhancement therapy for a model of Downs syndrome. Sci Transl Med 2009;1:1.

Hemoglobinopathies in India—Clinical and Laboratory Aspects

Ishwar C. Verma, MBBS, FRCP[a],*, Renu Saxena, PhD[b],
Sudha Kohli, PhD[b]

KEYWORDS

- β-thalassemia • α-thalassemia • Epidemiology • Molecular mutations
- Molecular methods • Prenatal diagnosis

KEY POINTS

- β-thalassemia is the most common autosomal recessive genetic disorder in India with a mean carrier frequency of 3.3%, and 7500 to 12,000 children with β-thalassemia major are born every year.
- Subjects with thalassemia trait, also known as carriers, have low mean corpuscular volume, low mean corpuscular hemoglobin, and increased hemoglobin A2 (>4%).
- Patients with β-thalassemia major have severe anemia and require blood transfusions by 1 year of age, whereas β-thalassemia intermedia patients have mild to moderate anemia and in most cases require no or infrequent blood transfusions.
- Genotype/phenotype correlation is helpful for the prediction of the phenotype, and deciding treatment options for β-thalassemia patients.
- Genetic analyses include determining the type of β-globin gene mutation, co-inheritance of α-globin gene deletions/duplications, and Xmn1 polymorphism in γ gene.
- Success of a β-thalassemia control program depends on prospective carrier screening followed by genetic counseling and prenatal diagnosis.

INTRODUCTION

The hemoglobinopathies comprise inherited disorders of the structure or synthesis of hemoglobin. They are the commonest single gene disorders in the world. It is estimated that about 450,000 infants with hemoglobinopathies are born in the world. Almost 85.9% of these hemoglobinopathies are sickle cell disease (SCD). Births of children with β-thalassemia alone or combined with hemoglobin (Hb) E are about 44, 000 (9.7%) per year, whereas infants affected with Hb Barts and HbH disease are

---

The authors have nothing to disclose.
[a] Center of Medical Genetics, Sir Ganga Ram Hospital, Rajender Nagar, New Delhi 110060, India;
[b] Division of Molecular Genetics, Center of Medical Genetics, Sir Ganga Ram Hospital, Rajender Nagar, New Delhi 110060, India
* Corresponding author.
E-mail address: dr_icverma@yahoo.com

Clin Lab Med 32 (2012) 249–262
http://dx.doi.org/10.1016/j.cll.2012.04.011
0272-2712/12/$ – see front matter © 2012 Elsevier Inc. All rights reserved.

about 20,000 (4.4%). Approximately 80% of the annual births of babies with these disorders occur in low- or middle-income countries. These disorders originated in populations in tropical Africa, Asia, and the Mediterranean region and have spread via migration throughout the world. They are, therefore, of concern in all countries. In North and South America and Western Europe, the birth prevalence of hemoglobinopathies is related to the proportion of the population that originated from Africa and Southeast Asia.

EPIDEMIOLOGY

The prevalence of the β-thalassemia trait in India in different regions varies from 1% to 17% with a mean prevalence of about 3.3%. A multicentric study sponsored by the Indian Council of Medical Research conducted among school children age 11 to 18 years in Delhi, Bombay, and Calcutta showed a β-thalassemia carrier rate of 5.5%, 2.6%, and 10.2%, respectively.[1] Recently, Mohanty and colleagues[2] screened 29,898 college students and 26,916 pregnant women living in 6 cities in India with a high prevalence of hemoglobinopathies—Mumbai (Maharashtra), Vadodora (Gujarat), Dibrugarh (Assam), Kolkata (West Bengal), Ludhiana (Punjab), and Bangalore (Karnataka). The prevalence of the β-thalassemia trait varied from 1.5% to 3.4% among college students and 1.3% to 4.2% among pregnant women. A high frequency of carriers is reported among certain communities: Punjabis who have migrated from West Pakistan, especially Aroras, Lohanas, Sindhis, Bengalis, Gujaratis, Bhanushalis, Gujarati Khojas, Jains, Vellalas, Mandls, Pillais, Khatirs. and Baidyas.[3] Based on the above carrier frequencies, it is estimated that there are almost 36 to 39 million carriers of β-thalassemia in India, and about 7500 to 12,000 babies with β-thalassemia major are born each year.[4] Micromapping studies at the district level in 2 States, Maharashtra and Gujarat in western India, showed that the prevalence of β-thalassemia trait varied from 0% to 9.5%. Based on these frequencies, the authors estimated that there would be around 1000 births of babies with β-thalassemia major each year in these 2 States alone.[5] A recent study of 35,413 individuals in rural areas of West Bengal[6] found the frequency of β-thalassemia trait to be 10.38%, HbE trait 4.30%, and sickle cell trait 1.12%. These micromapping studies suggest that the earlier figures of the number of births with thalassemia major are likely to be an underestimate.

HbS is prevalent in central India with the carrier rate varying from 1 to 40%. The tribal communities with sustained high frequencies of the sickle cell trait include the Irula/Kurumba/Paniyan in Tamil Nadu (up to 40%); the Gonds in Andra Pradesh, Madhya Pradesh, Chhatisgarh, Maharashtra, Orissa, and Uttar Pradesh (up to 34%); the Bhils in Madhya Pradesh, Chhatisgarh, Maharashtra, Gujarat, and Rajasthan (up to 31%); and the Kolarian in Maharastra and Gujarat (up to 18%).[7] With a trait frequency of 20% in a population, it can be estimated that 1% of births would have homozygous SCD (10,000 cases of SCD per million births). Given a frequency of 10%, 625 affected infants would be born in 1 million births. It is not possible to derive the precise figure for birth of infants with SCD in India because the number of people in different tribes is not available. Patra and coworkers[8] recently screened 359,823 subjects among 2087 villages in Raipur District, Chhattisgarh State, India. The sickle cell trait occurred in 33,467 people (9.30%) and SS phenotype in 747 subjects (0.21%). The gene frequencies were not in Hardy-Weinberg equilibrium, which is likely to be because of a deficiency of the SS phenotype failing to enter the sampled population from either sickness or early death. These figures suggest that the disease in India is at least as prevalent as it is in Equatorial Africa, and that the oft-quoted figure of 5000 to 6000 babies with SCD born each year is an underestimate.[7]

Considering the lifelong care needed for patients with a genetic condition, this would represent a huge burden on the health care services.

Hemoglobin E is widespread in the northeastern States in Assam, Mizoram, Manipur, Arunachal Pradesh, and Tripura, the prevalence of HbE trait being highest (64%) among the Bodo-Kacharis in Assam and going up to 30% to 40% in some other populations in this region. In eastern India, the prevalence of HbE trait varies from 3% to 10% in West Bengal. Both HbE and HbS when co-inherited with β-thalassemia result in a disorder of variable clinical severity.[9]

Prevalence of α-thalassemia was investigated by Nadkarni and colleagues[10] in 1235 blood samples from different regions of India. Deletion of a single α gene was observed in 10.5% and 2 α-gene deletions in 2.31%, whereas α-gene triplication was present in 1.1% of cases. All the samples showed the presence of the rightward deletion ($-\alpha^{3.7}$) except 1 sample, which showed the leftward deletion ($-\alpha^{4.2}$). Among the different ethnic groups, the Punjabis showed the highest prevalence of α-thalassemia (26.3%), followed by Sindhis (23.5%). In the other caste groups, the prevalence of α-thalassemia varied from 7.2% to 16.8%. Garewal and coworkers[11] have also reported a high incidence of α-thalassemia (10%) in the Punjabi population. These studies show that the most common hemoglobinopathy in India is α-thalassemia, but it does not cause any serious problem, as the milder form α-thal-2 ($-\alpha/\alpha\alpha$) of α-thalassemia is predominant. However, knowing the α-genotype is useful for genetic counseling in subjects who have reduced red cell indices coupled with a raised red blood cell count and normal HbA2 levels.

CLINICAL PRESENTATION

Three classes of β-thalassemia are recognized clinically: β-thalassemia major, intermedia, and minor. These are differentiated clinically by the degree of anemia, with thalassemia major and minor having the most and least severe anemia, respectively. The clinical presentation of children with β-thalassemia major in India is no different than that in other parts of the world. Anemia is severe and commonly presents after 6 months of birth. Other clinical manifestations include listlessness, poor appetite and growth, flat facial profile, and hepatosplenomegaly. The children often require blood transfusions by 1 year of age. In India, growth and pubertal failure as well cardiac problems arise as a result of inadequate chelation therapy. Only about 20 adults with thalassemia major are known in India who have married and have had children.

Patients with β-thalassemia intermedia have mild to moderate anemia, and, in most cases, require no or infrequent blood transfusions. There is no consensus on the clinical definition of thalassemia intermedia. A severity scoring system has been described to determine its grade. Common clinical features include moderate degree of anemia and splenic enlargement with risk of iron overload in part caused by increased intestinal absorption.

Thalassemia minor is also known as the "thalassemia trait," and such individuals are generally asymptomatic. Hemoglobin levels tend to be slightly lower than those in the general population, especially during stress of fever or pregnancy. The red cells are microcytic, and there is low mean corpuscular volume (MCV) and low mean corpuscular hemoglobin (MCH). Characteristically, HbA2 is increased to greater than 4.0%. Patients with thalassemia trait commonly do not need iron therapy. However, in India, very often iron deficiency coexists with thalassemia trait. This is especially important during pregnancy, as giving iron therapy raises the hemoglobin level. It is known that iron deficiency may lower the HbA2 level but not to the extent that HbA2 falls into the normal range. When HbA2 is in the intermediate range (3%–4%), it becomes difficult to decide whether the patient is a carrier of β-thalassemia. Rangan and coworkers[12] sequenced the β-globin gene in a number of such patients and observed that 8 (32%) of the 25 cases with HbA2 levels ranging from 3.5% to 3.9% had mutations in the β-globin gene - IVS-I-5 (G>C) in 3, 619 bp deletion in 2, codons 41/42 (-TTCT) in 1 case, and CAP +1 (A>C) mutation in 2 cases. In patients with HbA2 between 3% and 3.5%, there were no carriers of β-thalassemia.

HbE/β-thalassemia is the most common form of severe thalassemia observed in West Bengal and Northeastern states in India. It has variable clinical features, as is observed in the rest of the world. Nadkarni and coworkers[13] showed that the variability was not caused by the character of β thal mutation but the coinheritance of α and γ gene abnormalities. In a multicountry study of cases of thalassemia intermedia, the XmnI Gγ polymorphism -158 (C>T) was positive (T) in the majority of β⁺-thal/HbE compound heterozygote patients (88.6%) and β⁰-thal/HbE patients (84.8%), suggesting that it is associated with a milder phenotype.[14]

Carriers (heterozygotes) of α thalassemia are clinically asymptomatic, although it may give rise to mild to moderate microcytic hypochromic anemia. HbH disease has been reported from India, but it is rare. Of 105 with unexplained anemia, Dastidar and coworkers[15] observed 17 cases to have HbH disease. The predominant features were mild to moderate anemia (2.6–13.3 g/dL) with variable amounts of HbH (0.8%–40%). The patients usually have splenomegaly, jaundice may be present in variable degree, and children may have growth retardation. Older patients often have some degree of iron overload. The severity of the clinical features is clearly related to the molecular mutations. Patients with nondeletional types of HbH disease are more severely affected than those with the common deletional types. Hb Bart's hydrops fetalis syndrome has the most severe deficiency in α-globin expression. The clinical features are those of a pale edematous infant with signs of cardiac failure, prolonged intrauterine anemia, pronounced hepatosplenomegaly, and gross enlargement of the placenta. These infants almost always either die in utero (23–38 weeks) or shortly after birth. Hb Barts hydrops has not been reported in the Indian subcontinent.

LABORATORY DIAGNOSIS

The hematologic profile in thalassemia major, intermedia, and minor is similar to that observed globally. Laboratory abnormalities in thalassemia major include microcytic anemia with abnormally shaped and nucleated red blood cells, and abnormally raised fetal hemoglobin. The diagnosis often is difficult on hematologic criteria in the first year because of the high fetal hemoglobin in early life. Molecular diagnosis is more useful. In thalassemia minor, the hemoglobin is reduced and the red cell count is relatively high, whereas the MCV and MCH are reduced. The crucial investigation is estimation of HbA2, which is increased (>4.0%). There are many electrophoretic and chromatographic approaches for estimation of HbA2 and HbF, but cation exchange high performance liquid chromatography (CE-HPLC) systems have become the method of choice for these investigations.[16] Kar and Sharma[17] pointed out that one should be vigilant not to mistake the presence of a bilirubin peak (caused by liver failure), for Hb Bart's or HbH on HbHPLC. Correlation with the clinical context and biochemical parameters, coupled with repeating the run after washing the sample, can resolve this problem.

CE-HPLC also helps in the presumptive identification of many abnormal hemoglobin variants. For Example, HPLC analysis of samples in India disclosed the following Hb variants: HbS, HbE, HbD, Hb Q-India, Hb-Lepore, δβ-thalassemia/HPFH, HbD-Iran, HbJ-Meerut, HbH, and Hb Lepore disease.[18,19] It has also proved useful for second trimester prenatal diagnosis of thalassemia by fetal blood analysis in cases in which mutations remain unidentified or in which patients present late in pregnancy.

Rao and coworkers[20] evaluated the reliability of this technique to measure low concentrations of adult hemoglobin (HbA) in fetal blood to enable differentiation between affected and unaffected fetuses at risk for β-thalassemia (n = 85). The HbA for 27 affected fetuses was 0%, whereas 2 showed an HbA value of 0.5%. The mean HbA for 61 unaffected fetuses was 4.8% $\pm$ 2.08%. AX-HPLC was found to be a simple and rapid procedure with high sensitivity, and there was a good correlation between the HbA values obtained by AX-HPLC and the diagnosis by carboxymethyl cellulose chromatography. Wadia and colleagues[21] evaluated the usefulness of analysis of fetal blood on the Biorad Variant Hemoglobin Testing System using the β-thalassemia short program in comparison with the conventional globin biosynthesis in 58 pregnancies. The β/α biosynthesis ratios in 13 homozygous fetuses ranged from 0 to 0.03, and the adult hemoglobin (HbA) levels by automated chromatography varied from 0% to 0.4%. The normal or heterozygous fetuses had β/α ratios of greater than 0.04 and HbA levels ranging from 2.1% to 10.6%. Rao and coworkers[22] evaluated 112 cord blood samples and found that 74 were informative for analyzing HbA levels by CE-HPLC between 18 and 22 weeks of gestation.

Rao and colleagues[18] observed a significant decrease in the level of HbA2 associated with iron deficiency anemia (P = .004) and increase in megaloblastic anemia ($P<.001$) among subjects with normal HPLC pattern. Madan and colleagues[23] also observed a significant decrease in HbA2 levels in the presence of anemia during pregnancy but not to the extent that it would lead to errors in detection of β-thalassemia carriers. Colah and coworkers[24] designed a kit for collecting capillary blood in remote areas for population studies for hemoglobinopathies. The stability of the sample was maintained for 12 to 15 days up to 37°C. HbE was stable for 3 days up to at 37°C and HbD and HbQ for 3 days up to 42°C.

The hematologic profile of SCD in India differs from that in Jamaica and the United States by having a lower hemoglobin, MCV, MCH, and MCH concentration levels. The differences could be attributed to severe iron deficiency anemia and associated α-thalassemia. The lower MCH and MCV levels are likely to diminish the amount of intravascular sickling and reduced complications. Similar findings were reported earlier in sickle heterozygotes from Eastern India. The high reticulocyte level seen in many of African patients is also not observed in Indian sickle homozygous patients.

MOLECULAR DIAGNOSIS

During the first year of life, the diagnosis of thalassemia is difficult on hematologic studies. The presence of other factors such as α- and γ-thalassemia or iron deficiency may distort the hematologic findings and lead to misdiagnosis. Molecular techniques help to resolve the diagnostic problem. Thalassemia International Federation recommends that at first diagnosis molecular studies should be done to determine the mutations in the β-globin gene as well the status of the α- and γ-globin genes, as these are useful for prognosis and response to therapy.

There is striking heterogeneity in the molecular basis of β-thalassemia, as almost 200 different mutations in the β-globin gene have been reported so far. However, population studies indicate that probably only 20 β-thalassemia alleles account for greater than 80% of the β-thalassemia mutations in the whole world. This is caused by the phenomenon of geographical clustering, in which each population has few very common mutations together with a varying number of rare ones. For molecular diagnosis of β-thalassemia in a country, it is essential first to characterize the spectrum of mutations present so that common mutations are identified. In India, about 64 mutations have been characterized by studies done at different centers.[25] Seven mutations (IVS 1-5 [G>C], 619 bp deletion, IVS 1-1 [G>T], codon 8/9 [+G], codons 41/42 [-CTTT], codon 15 [G>A], codon 30 [G>C]) are common, accounting for 85% to 95% of mutant alleles. However, regional differences in their frequencies have been noted.[26] This knowledge on the distribution of mutations in different regions and in people of different ethnic backgrounds has facilitated molecular diagnosis using techniques like allele-specific oligonucleotide hybridization, dot-blot analysis, reverse dot-blot analysis (RDB), allele-specific priming or amplification refractory mutation system (ARMS), restriction enzyme analysis, gap-polymerase chain reaction (PCR) (for common deletions), and DNA sequencing. PCR-based approaches to screen unknown mutations can be done by denaturing gradient gel electrophoresis, single-strand conformation polymorphism, and heteroduplex analysis followed by sequencing of the altered fragment. Nowadays, considering the small size of the β-globin gene (1.2 kb) and the easy availability of sequencers, most investigators proceed to sequence, once testing for the common 7 mutations is negative. Every laboratory has its own strategy of identifying the mutations. For example, the RDB procedure for detection of 6 common Indian β-thalassemia mutations along with 2 abnormal hemoglobins (HbE and HbS) is followed by some investigators. In the authors' laboratory, the 5 common mutations are first tested by ARMS method. This technique is rapid and cost effective and provided reliable results. If the common mutations are negative, sequencing is carried out. Some large deletions involving the β-globin, such as in δβ-thalassemia and hereditary persistence of fetal hemoglobin (HPFH) can be identified by gap-PCR.

MOLECULAR TECHNIQUES

The most popular technique for mutation detection is the ARMS technique. This was applied for molecular diagnosis for thalassemia by Old and colleagues[27] It has proved to be a good technique and easy to learn. However, its disadvantage is that separate primers are required to analyze each mutation. Primers are designed that generate specific amplification products, one with the mutant allele and the other with the normal sequence. The nucleotide at the 3' end of the primer is complementary to the base in the respective target sequence at the site of the mutation. In addition, a deliberate mismatch to the target sequence is included at the 3rd or the 4th base from the 3'end. The deliberate mismatch enhances the specificity of the primer. ARMS technique is used to characterize the 4 mutations common in India, whereas the control fragment is generated from the 3' end of the β-globin gene by primers that span the breakpoints of the 619 bp deletion.

Reverse Dot Blot (RDB) analysis is another very popular technique. The DNA region of interest is specifically amplified by PCR with biotinylated primers and are denatured and allowed to hybridize with DNA probes specific for the mutant and normal sequences, immobilized onto a membrane. Hybridization is detected by adding streptavidin-alkaline phosphatase conjugate, which binds to biotin, and on further addition of the chromogenic substances, 4-nitro blue tetrazolium chloride and 5-bromo-4-chloro-3-indolyl phosphate it gives a blue precipitate. A normal individual (N/N) will give positive results with each wild-type sequence but not with any mutant probe. Heterozygotes (M/N) show a reaction with a single mutation dot in addition to the normal dots, whereas homozygotes (M/M) will give a positive dot with that mutant probe but not with its corresponding normal sequence. Two mutant dots will be seen if the individual carries 2 different mutations together with positive spots for the remaining normal probes.

Restriction enzyme analysis can be used for detecting mutations that create or abolish restriction enzyme sites. Genomic DNA containing the mutation, the "target," is amplified by PCR, and the product is then digested by the diagnostic restriction enzyme and the resulting DNA fragments separated on a agarose gel electrophoresis. Incomplete or partial digests can be a problem for some restriction enzymes leading to false-negative or positives. Thus, positive and negative controls should always be included. Restriction enzyme analysis can be applied for some of the mutations, eg, HbS, codon6 (-A), codon5 (-CT), and IVS1-5 (G>A). For the mutations HbS, codon6 (-A), and codon5 (-CT), that destroy cutting site for the restriction enzyme DdeI, genotyping by ARMS or sequencing is essential.

Gap-PCR can be used for diagnosis of large deletions involving the β-globin gene (eg, Hb Lepore, some δβ-thal deletions, and HPFH1/2/3 deletion mutations). The gap PCR is the simplest of amplification techniques, using 2 primers complementary to the sense and antisense strand of DNA regions flanking the deletion. Amplified product is obtained only from the allele harboring a deletion, as the primers are too far apart to amplify successfully the normal DNA sequence. The type of deletion can be inferred by the size of the product because each deletion, if present, gives rise to an amplified product of characteristic size.

Automated DNA sequencing is replacing the other techniques for diagnosis of mutations in the β-globin gene, once the common mutations are not detected in a given sample. It is a multistage procedure requiring PCR amplification, cycle sequencing, and precipitation before the sequence can be determined. After this, the sequence must be analyzed and checked for any changes. This method is based on the introduction of chain terminating dideoxynucleotide triphosphates (ddNTPs) to stop the growing chain. 2'3' ddNTPs differ from conventional dNTPs in that they lack a hydroxyl residue at the 3' position of deoxyribose. They can be incorporated by sequenase into a growing DNA chain through their 5' triphosphate group. However, the absence of a 3' hydroxyl residue prevents formation of a phosphodiester bond with the succeeding dNTP. Further extension of the growing DNA chain is therefore stopped. In automated sequencing, all the dNTPs are tagged fluorescently with different fluorochromes and are incorporated into the growing chain. A single reaction is put up, and the reaction products containing different size of fragment length terminated at the incorporation of ddNTPs are then separated by capillary electrophoresis. The sequencing analysis software interprets the result calling the bases from the fluorescent intensity at each data point. The only pitfalls of using sequencing as a routine diagnostic technique are the cost and the time of analysis, which is more as increased compared with standard PCR assays.

DISTRIBUTION OF MUTATIONS IN INDIA

The distribution of mutations in the β-globin gene in various parts of India has been reported by a number of investigators. Sinha and colleagues[28] have recently summarized the regional distribution of 8,505 alleles with 64 β-globin gene mutations. Nationally, IVSI-5 (G>C), 619-bp del, IVSI-1 (G>T), codon 41/42 (-TCCT) and codon 8/9 (-G) comprised the 5 most common disease mutations and accounted for 82.5% of all mutations. Codon 15 (G>A), codon 30 (G>C), cap site +1 (A>C), codon 5 (-CT), and codon 16 (-C) accounted for an additional 11.0% of all mutant alleles. The Western region (Maharashtra, Gujarat, and Rajasthan) has a higher prevalence of the 619-bp deletion (14.2%) and IVSI-1 (G>T) (8.7%), and with codon 15 (G>A) as the fourth commonest mutation (7.6%). In the northern region (Uttar Pradesh, Punjab, Haryana, Himachal Pradesh, Uttarakhand and Jammu, and Kashmir), IVSI-5 (G>C) accounted for 44.8% of β-thalassemia alleles. The 5 most common mutations closely match the national pattern, with codon 16 (-C) and -88 (C>T) in the list of 10 common mutations along with codon 15 (G>A), codon 30 (G>C), and cap site +1 (A>C). The 4 southern States (Andhra Pradesh, Karnataka, Tamil Nadu, and Kerala) have a predominantly Dravidian population, ethnically and culturally quite distinct from the largely Indo-European populations of the north. IVSI-5(G>C) has a prevalence of 67.9%, the 619-bp deletion is present in only 1.8% of cases, whereas the second commonest allele (8.8%) is codon 15 (G>A). Poly A site (T>C) is the third most common allele (4.7%). The east region exhibited the highest prevalence of IVSI-5 (G>C) at 71.4%, with codon 30 (G>C) and codon 15 (G>A) the second and third most common alleles, accounting for 5.8% and 5.4% of the total, respectively.

PHENOTYPE-GENOTYPE CORRELATION

Understanding the relationship between genotype and phenotype is helpful in clinical practice for the prediction of the phenotype, in genetic counseling, in decisions regarding prenatal diagnosis, and for planning the appropriate treatment of β-thalassemia patients. Most patients with thalassemia major present with a severe transfusion-dependent anemia from the first year of life. This phenotype is caused by homozygosity or compound heterozygosity of β^0 mutations. However, some patients with these mutations show a mild clinical picture of survival without or with less-intensive requirement of regular transfusions. This condition, defined as *thalassemia intermedia*, is extremely heterogeneous and encompasses a wide spectrum of phenotypes. It is important to recognize patients with thalassemia intermedia, as their management and prognosis differs from cases of thalassemia major. The intermediate phenotype may be caused by the combination of β^0 mutation with milder β^+ mutations, interaction of β-globin gene with other globin genes, or polymorphisms of other nonglobin genes. In India, such interactions have been examined by many investigators. A multicentric study on the interaction of β, α, and γ genes in causing thalassemia intermedia found that the presence of α-thalassemia mutation is the main ameliorating factor in the presence of β^+ mutations,[14] whereas the γ gene polymorphism was the main ameliorating factor in β^0 mutations.

Type of β Globin Gene Mutation

The most clinically important mechanism consistently resulting in thalassemia intermedia is the coinheritance of homozygosity or compound heterozygosity for mild β-thalassemia alleles, leading to a consistent residual output of β chains from the affected β-globin locus. From India, a number of mild and silent mutations have been reported, which include mild β^{++} promoter region mutation- capsite +1 (A>C), poly A (T>C), -28 (A>G), and -88 (C>T). However, the IVS1-5 G>C mutation, which has been reported as a β^+ mutation worldwide has been found to behave as a β^0 severe mutation in the Indian population.[14]

α-Globin Genes

Mild β-thalassemia may be caused by the co-inheritance of homozygous β-thalassemia and an α-thalassemia determinant that, by reducing the α chain output, decreases the α/non-α chain imbalance. A single α-globin gene deletion is sufficient to improve the clinical phenotype of homozygous β^+ mutations, whereas in β^0 mutations, the deletion of 2 α-globin genes, or the presence of an inactivating mutation of the major α2-globin gene is necessary.

Xmn1 Polymorphism in γ-Globin Gene

Co-inheritance of a genetic determinant that leads to production of high HbF would, by reducing the extent of the β/non-β chain imbalance, result in a milder phenotype, eg, point mutations at G-gamma promoter region -158C>T (XMN1 polymorphism)

(Xmn1-HBG2 or rs7482144). HbF levels are reported to be significantly higher in Xmn1-(G)γ +/+ and Xmn1-(G)γ +/- β-thalassemia intermedia patients.[29]

BCL11A Gene Polymorphism

Coinheritance of genetic determinants capable of sustaining a continuous production of HbF in adult life and mapping outside the β-globin cluster has been shown to determine a mild phenotype. Two HPFH have been mapped on chromosome 2p16 and chromosome 6q23. The locus on chromosome 2p16 has been located by genomewide association study on the BCL11A gene, and the single nucleotide polymorphism rs11886868 in its intron 2 was found strongly associated with HbF levels. The BCL11A variants were shown to influence HbF levels also in nonanemic whites from a European twin study.[30] The same C variant was significantly higher in β^0-thalassemia homozygotes for the codon 39 nonsense mutation with a mild phenotype (thalassemia intermedia) compared with those with the same β-globin genotype, but with a severe phenotype, compensating for the imbalance of Hb production through the augmentation of HbF levels. Furthermore, the BCL11A variant C allele by increasing HbF levels was associated with a mild phenotype also in SCD. The BCL11A gene encodes a zinc-finger transcription factor, which regulates the globin switching during ontogeny by interacting with specific sequence in the β-globin cluster and repressing the HbF. According to these results, the identification of BCL11A polymorphism in young homozygous β-thalassemia and sickle cell anemia patients may serve as a prognostic marker for severity of the disease. Furthermore, targeted down-regulation of BCL11A in patients could elevate HbF levels, thereby ameliorating the severity of these inherited anemias.

HBS1L-MYB Region

Another HPFH locus was mapped many years ago on chromosome 6q23 by linkage analysis in a large Indian family with segregating β-thalassemia and confirmed more recently by twin studies. Further studies found that this variant maps in the HBS1L-MYB region. Specifically, the G allele of SNP rs9389268 is associated with high HbF levels. HBS1L is a putative member of the "GTPase superfamily," whereas MYB has a crucial role in normal erythropoiesis. The HBS1L-MYB intergenic polymorphisms contain regulatory sequences controlling MYB expression.[31] However, further studies are necessary to elucidate the precise biological role of these 2 genes in the modulation of HbF.

PRENATAL DIAGNOSIS

Prenatal diagnosis has been offered to high-risk families since late 1989 in Delhi. Initially, samples for prenatal diagnosis were sent to laboratories abroad. However, the ARMS/restriction fragment length polymorphism (RFLP) analysis using restriction enzymes method to detect the mutations was set up in Delhi, and by 1996 prenatal diagnosis was performed in 415 cases in the All India Institute of Medical Sciences, New Delhi.[32] In rapid succession it was established in Christian Medical College in Vellore [33] and in Mumbai at the National Institute of Immunohaematology and Wadia Hospital for Children.[34,35] Mahadik and colleagues[34] in Mumbai established the status of fetus in 494 of 787 fetuses by ARMS and the rest by GCS. Bandyopadhyay and coworkers[36] reported prenatal diagnosis in 63 couples by ARMS and RFLP studies in Kolkata. National Institute of Immuno-Hematology, Mumbai published their experience of providing prenatal diagnosis in 2,221 pregnancies at risk for β-thalassemia.[35] To date, the authors' laboratory in Delhi has carried out

2,355 prenatal diagnoses for thalassemia by ARMS and sequencing (Saxena and colleagues, unpublished data, 2012). RFLP within the β-globin gene cluster was used as secondary method to confirm the results diagnosis when an affected or normal child is available (in case of a "normal" child one has to be sure that the child is normal or carrier, as this would lead to misdiagnosis). This method is also useful in cases in which either 1 or both the maternal and paternal mutations are not known. The common RFLP markers linked to the β-globin gene studied are Hind II/ε, Xmn I/Gγ, HindIIIGγ, Hind III/Aγ, HindII/5'$\beta\Psi$, Hind II/3' $\beta\Psi$, Ava II/β, Hinf I/β, and (Bam HI/β) by previously described methods.

Fetal DNA for analysis can be obtained from either chorionic villus samples (CVS) or amniocytes. Because the risk of recurrence is 25%, fetal DNA is preferably obtained after 10 weeks of gestation by CVS to provide a prenatal diagnosis in the first trimester of pregnancy. The risk of miscarriage associated with chorionic villus sampling is about 1%. CVS provide a good yield of DNA. The villi are visualized under the microscope and carefully separated from the maternal tissue (decidua) to reduce the chance of maternal cell contamination. If the sample is too small, the CVS sample may need to be cultured. At the authors' laboratory, CVS sample is preferred over amniotic fluid. Even for those patients reporting late in pregnancy, chorionic villus biopsy can be carried or fetal blood collected for analysis. However, in certain centers, because of the lack of expertise in CVS sampling, amniocentesis is being done. In such cases, about 25 mL of amniotic fluid should be collected, and it is good practice to set up a backup culture of amniotic fluid cells. The results from amniotic fluid analysis have to be interpreted with caution, as there could be unseen maternal cell contamination, which can only be detected by molecular methods. In the presence of visible blood cells in the amniotic fluid sample, there is significant risk of maternal ell contamination.

Misdiagnosis may occur for several reasons: errors in the laboratory such as sample exchange, failure of molecular technique, maternal cell contamination, and mis-paternity. The most common cause for misdiagnosis is maternal cell contamination, and specific tests to exclude this should be done in all cases. The authors prefer analysis of DNA of the mother and the father along with the fetal tissue as a double check in place of only checking against the mother's sample. The biological father's sample is required to determine the paternal mutation. In each amplification reaction, a control fragment should be included to confirm that the technique is working. Meticulous laboratory practices should be followed to prevent errors as well as contamination of samples from the environment. It is necessary to separate the post-PCR processing area from pre-PCR work area. Positive and negative control samples for the parental mutations should always be set up. The risk of misdiagnosis because of failure of molecular technique is limited if one performs 2 alternate methods.

In recent years, there has been a changing pattern of referral for prenatal diagnosis. Earlier parents having an affected child would approach for prenatal diagnosis in a future pregnancy. Now many couples receive the diagnosis as carriers in their first pregnancy. This is a good sign that suggests there is increasing awareness of the disease among patients as well as professionals. Indeed, in developing countries, the obstetricians have an important role to play in controlling the disease, by ensuring that they check the carrier status for thalassemia in every pregnant woman at first encounter. Sadly, this good practice is not followed by many obstetricians so that we encounter cases being referred for prenatal diagnosis after 20 weeks of gestation.

The important steps for undertaking prenatal diagnosis can be listed as (1) Be certain that both parents are carriers, especially if there is no affected child. Even in families with an affected child who is on blood transfusions, it is better to establish that the parents are carriers by hematologic studies. Sometimes one of the parents turns out to have HbE or SCD, or the disorder may not be thalassemia all. Electronic cell count should invariably be done to support the results of HbA2 by HPLC. Estimation of HbA2 by electrophoresis is not always reliable and requires that the laboratories concerned participate in quality control programs. (2) When one of the partners is a carrier, particular care should be taken that the other partner is not a carrier. This is because they may carry mild or "silent" mutations of β-globin gene. In those with borderline values of red cell indices or HbA2, it is better to sequence the β-globin gene. (3) Know which combination of alleles is significant. For example, the combinations of the following alleles lead to clinical manifestations and require prenatal diagnosis: β-Thal/β-Thal (thalassemia major), β-Thal/HbS (sickle/β-thalassemia), β-Thal/HbE (E/β-thalassemia), HbS/HbS (sickle cell anemia), HbS/HbDPb/HbC (SCD/Symptomatic). On the other hand, the following combinations do not require prenatal diagnosis because these do not lead to any clinical problem: β-Thal/Hb D Punjab/Hb D Iran, β-Thal/Hb C/HbQ, homozygous HbE, HbD Punjab/HbD Iran.

SPECIMEN/TESTING GUIDELINES

For establishing a prenatal diagnostic service in developing countries the following strategy is recommended, based on the experience of the authors: (1) The fetal sampling technique should be performed by a limited number of obstetricians who should gain experience by performing CVS in cases undergoing medical termination of pregnancy. (2) Expertise in separating chorionic villus tissue from decidual (maternal) tissue must be learned from a person experienced in this technique. (3) The mutations causing β-thalassemia in a given region should be identified in at least 100 children with thalassemia major or their parents (200 mutant chromosomes). (4) Any of the nonisotopic PCR-based mutation detection methods such as reverse dot blot or ARMS technique should be set up. Primers for the common and rare mutations, as well as for normal sequences at that site, should be procured.

FUTURE OF THALASSEMIA CARE

Thalassemia is the most common single gene disorder in India. There are almost 40 million carriers of β-thalassemia and almost 12,000 infants born every year with thalassemia major in India. This is a huge burden for a resource-poor country. Fortunately, a number of centers exist that have trained physicians to manage the patients with thalassemia and trained scientists to carry out mutation studies for diagnosis, prognosis, and prenatal diagnosis. The need for prevention of thalassemia is obvious because of the high frequency of the condition, the great expense and difficulties in providing optimal treatment for patients, and the innumerable fatalities from untreated β-thalassemia. Prevention would not only be a good public health practice, as envisioned in the Alma Ata declaration, but it would also be cost effective, as the ratio of the cost of treatment to prevention is 4:1. It would help tremendously in reducing the burden of the disease for patients, families, and the health services. The strongest argument for prevention is that it would ensure the best possible care for the affected by curbing the increase in their number. The authors have recently summarized the experience in India for strategies to control this disorder in India.[37] Carrier screening during pregnancy and prenatal diagnosis should receive the highest priority to reduce drastically the birth of affected children. The Government of India is keen to initiate a control program for thalassemia, but the size of the country and the huge population is a deterrent. Hopefully, these will be set up in the states that have a high prevalence of carriers of β-thalassemia in the next 5-year national plan starting in 2012. There is a need to increase the number of centers in India able to perform prenatal diagnosis and provide this facility at a subsidized cost, or free for the poor, and introduce quality control programs. An important challenge is to develop preimplantation genetic diagnosis, as many couples are distressed by having affected children in consecutive pregnancies. Investment in noninvasive techniques for prenatal diagnosis would be worthwhile, as this would help provide prenatal diagnosis in peripheral areas also. The facilities for voluntary cord stem cell storage should be established in the government sector, as currently most of these exist in the private sector at a huge cost. Centers for bone marrow transplantation need to be expanded and facility subsidized. The patient organizations for thalassemia are strong and well organized and have played a key role for creating awareness in the population as well as the professionals.

REFERENCES

1. Sood SK, Madan N, Colah R, et al. Collaborative study on thalassemia. Report of ICMR Task Force study on thalassemia. New Delhi: Indian Council of Medical Research; 1993.
2. Mohanty D, Colah R, Gorakshakar. 124. Jai Vigyan S & T Mission Project on community control of thalassemia syndromes—Awareness, screening, genetic counseling and prevention. New Delhi: Indian Council of Medical Research; 2008.
3. Verma IC, Choudhry VP, Jain PK. Prevention of thalassemia: 96. A necessity in India. Indian J Pediatr 1992;59:649–54.
4. Verma IC. Burden of genetic disorders in India. Indian J Pediatr 2000;67(12):893–8.
5. Colah R, Gorakshakar A, Phanasgaonkar S, et al. Epidemiology of beta-thalassaemia in Western India: Mapping the frequencies and mutations in sub-regions of Maharashtra and Gujarat. Br J Haematol 2010;149:739–47.
6. Dolai TK, Dutta S, Bhattacharyya M, et al. Prevalence of Hemoglobinopathies in rural Bengal, India. Hemoglobin 2012;36:57–63.
7. Serjeant GR. The case for dedicated sickle cell centres. Indian J Hum Genet 2006; 12:148–51.
8. Patra PK, Chauhan VS, Khodiar PK, et al. Screening for the sickle cell gene in Chhattisgarh state, India: an approach to a major public health problem. J Community Genet 2011;2:147–51.
9. De M, Halder A, Podder S, et al. Anemia and hemoglobinopathies in tribal population of eastern and north eastern India. Hematology 2006;11:371–3.
10. Nadkarni AH, Gorakshakar AC, Mohanty D, et al. Alpha genotyping in a heterogeneous Indian population. Am J Hematol 1996;53:149–50.
11. Garewal G, Fearon CW, Warren TC, et al. The molecular basis of beta β-thalassaemia in Punjabi and Maharashtran Indians includes a multilocus aetiology involving triplicated alpha-globin loci. Br J Haematol 1994;86:372–6.
12. Rangan A, Sharma P, Dadu T, et al. β-Thalassemia mutations in subjects with borderline HbA(2) values: a pilot study in North India. Clin Chem Lab Med 2011;49: 2069–72.
13. Nadkarni A, Ghosh K, Gorakshakar A, et al. Variable clinical severity of Hb E beta-thalassemia among Indians. J Assoc Physicians India 1999;47:966–8.
14. Verma IC, Kleanthous M, Saxena R, et al. Multicenter study of the molecular basis of thalassemia intermedia in different ethnic populations. Hemoglobin 2007;31:439–52.

15. Dastidar R, Gajra B, De M. Molecular and hematological characterization of hemo-globin H disease in the Bengali population of Kolkata, India. Genet Test Mol Biomark-ers 2011;15:93–6.
16. Colah RB, Surve R, Sawant P, et al. HPLC studies in hemoglobinopathies. Indian J Pediatr 2007;74(7):657–62.
17. Kar R, Sharma CB. Bilirubin peak can be mistaken as Hb Bart's or Hb H on High-performance liquid chromatography. Hemoglobin 2011;35:171–4.
18. Rao S, Kar R, Gupta SK, et al. Spectrum of haemoglobinopathies diagnosed by cation exchange-HPLC & modulating effects of nutritional deficiency anaemias from north India. Indian J Med Res 2010;132:513–9.
19. Sachdev R, Dam AR, Tyagi G. Detection of Hb variants and hemoglobinopathies in Indian population using HPLC: report of 2600 cases. Indian J Pathol Microbiol 2010;53:57–62.
20. Rao VB, Natrajan PG, Lulla CP, et al. Rapid mid-trimester prenatal diagnosis of beta-thalassaemia and other haemoglobinopathies using a non-radioactive anion exchange HPLC technique—an Indian experience. Prenat Diagn 1997; 17:725–31.
21. Wadia MR, Phanasgaokar SP, Nadkarni AH, et al. Usefulness of automated chroma-tography for rapid fetal blood analysis for second trimester prenatal diagnosis of beta-thalassemia. Prenat Diagn 2002;22:153–7.
22. Rao S, Saxena R, Deka D, et al. Use of HbA estimation by CE-HPLC for prenatal diagnosis of beta-thalassemia; experience from a tertiary care centre in north India: a brief report. Hematology 2009;14:122–4.
23. Madan N, Sikka M, Sharma S, et al. Phenotypic expression of hemoglobin A2 in β-thalassemia trait with iron deficiency. Ann Hematol 1998;77:93–6.
24. Colah RB, Wadia M, D'Souza E, et al. Evaluation of a capillary blood collection system for screening for hemoglobinopathies in remote areas. Int J Lab Hematol 2010; 32:57–63.
25. Colah R, Gorakshakar A, Nadkarni A, et al. Regional heterogeneity of β-thalassemia mutations in the multi ethnic Indian population. Blood Cells Mol Dis 2009;42:241–6.
26. Verma IC, Saxena R, Thomas E, et al. Regional distribution of β-thalassemia muta-tions in India. Hum Genet 1997;100:109–13.
27. Old JM, Varawalla NY, Weatherall DJ. Rapid detection and prenatal diagnosis of β-thalassaemia: studies in Indian and Cypriot populations in the UK. Lancet 1990; 336:834–7.
28. Sinha S, Black ML, Agarwal S, et al. Profiling β-thalassaemia mutations in India at state and regional levels: implications for genetic education, screening and counseling programmes. Hugo J 2009;3:51–62.
29. Oberoi S, Das R, Panigrahi I, et al. Xmn1-(G) γ polymorphism and clinical predictors of severity of disease in β-thalassemia intermedia. Pediatr Blood Cancer 2011;57: 1025–8.
30. Lettre G, Sankaran VG, Bezerra MA, et al. DNA polymorphisms at the BCL11A, HBS1L-MYB, and beta-globin loci associate with fetal hemoglobin levels and pain crises in sickle cell disease. Proc Natl Acad Sci U S A 2008;105:11869–74.
31. Wahlberg K, Jiang J, Rooks H, et al. The HBS1L-MYB intergenic interval associated with elevated HbF levels shows characteristics of a distal regulatory region in erythroid cells. Blood 2009;114:1254–62.
32. Saxena R, Jain PK, Thomas E, et al. Prenatal diagnosis of β-thalassaemia: experience in a developing country. Prenatal Diagnosis 1998;18:1–7.
33. Muralitharan S, Srivastava A, Shaji RV, et al. Prenatal diagnosis of beta-thalassaemia mutations using the reverse dot blot technique. Natl Med J India 1996;9:70–1.

34. Thakur (Mahadik) C, Vaz F, Banerjee M, et al. Prenatal diagnosis of β-thalassaemia and other haemoglobinopathies in India. Prenatal Diagnosis 2000;20:194–201.
35. Colah RB, Gorakshakar AC, Nadkarni AH. Invasive & non-invasive approaches for prenatal diagnosis of haemoglobinopathies: experiences from India. Indian J Med Res 2011;134:552–60.
36. Bandyopadhyay A, Bandyopadhyay S, Basak J, et al. Profile of β-thalassemia in eastern India and its prenatal diagnosis. Prenat Diagn 2004;24:992–6.
37. Verma IC, Saxena R, Kohli S. Past, present & future scenario of thalassaemic care & control in India. Indian J Med Res 2011;134:507–21.

Inborn Errors of Metabolism and Their Status in India

Alpa J. Dherai, PhD

KEYWORDS

- Inborn errors of metabolism • Characteristics • Diagnosis
- Therapeutic management • Newborn screening • Inborn errors of metabolism in India

KEY POINTS

- Inborn errors of metabolism (IEM) have a characteristic clinical presentation overlapping with infection and intoxication.
- Diagnostic modalities for IEM vary from biochemical to molecular methods including next-generation sequencing.
- Therapeutic options including substrate restriction, enzyme replacement, chaperone administration, and organ transplant are promising for management of patients with IEM.
- Prenatal diagnosis and newborn screening help to reduce the societal burden as well as the morbidity due to IEM.
- IEM occur in India, and the need of the time is to have large diagnostic and screening programs to dilute the gene pool.

For if it be true that in every phenomenon of Nature there is something of the marvellous, surely that factor is nowhere more in evidence than in the workings of the metabolic processes of living things.

Archibald Garrod[1]

The dynamic pathways of *metabolism* represent a continuous stepwise movement through intermediary products, each having only a transient existence, but failure of a single step due to a defective gene as an inborn event affects this flow causing accumulation of a substrate or deficiency of a product leading to an inborn error of metabolism (IEM). The concept of inborn errors of metabolism was introduced by Archibald Garrod in the early 20th century through his documentation of four conditions, namely albinism, alkaptonuria, cystinuria, and benign pentosuria that were

Disclosure: The author has nothing to disclose.
Department of Laboratory Medicine, P.D. Hinduja National Hospital and Medical Research Center, Veer Savarkar Marg, Mahim, Mumbai 400016, Maharashtra, India
E-mail address: alpadherai@gmail.com

due to enzyme deficiencies inherited in an autosomal recessive manner.[2] Subsequently Folling described phenylketonuria (PKU) in 1934, and since then advances in medicine and diagnostic techniques have unveiled more than 500 IEM.[3]

Currently, IEM are recognized as a heterogeneous group of disorders resulting from abnormalities of synthesis, transport, and turnover of dietary and cellular components involving great complexity of the underlying pathophysiology and biochemical workup with complicated therapeutic and management options. Although IEM are individually rare, their conjunct frequency is as high as approximately 1 per 1000 births, accounting for about 20% of deaths from genetic diseases and about 38% accounting for hereditary neurologic or storage disorders.[3]

CHARACTERISTICS OF IEM

The clinical presentation of IEM is highly variable ranging from very mild to lethal forms with features overlapping those of infection and intoxication. There is also a substantial overlap within the group of an IEM, thus making laboratory evaluation crucial for confirmation of diagnosis. An infant with IEM would be normal at birth and become symptomatic later in life. The severity of the disease would be evident from the time of presentation, for example the earlier the presentation the more severe would be the disease. A high genotype-phenotype variation is also observed due to the mutational variability in these disorders with even individuals having the same mutation exhibiting a spectrum of clinical manifestations. Because many IEM are inherited as autosomal recessive traits, a history of consanguinity in the parents or an unexplained neonatal death in the family could raise suspicion of an inherited metabolic disease in a sick infant.

GENERAL CLASSIFICATION OF IEM BASED ON PATHOPHYSIOLOGY

The defects of metabolic pathways cause disease either by accumulation of a toxic metabolite or depletion of a metabolic byproduct required to maintain normal cellular function. Deficient enzyme activity may arise from mutations in the gene coding for the protein with loss of activity, abnormal processing of messenger RNA, or even mistaken intracellular localization of the protein. Metabolic defects may also result from defects of structural or transport proteins because of the aforesaid reasons. Based on pathophysiology with respect to the molecular type or the metabolite involved, IEM are classified into three groups.[4]

Disorders of Intermediary Metabolism

Disorders of intermediary metabolism lead to an acute or progressive intoxication due to accumulation of toxic compounds proximal to the metabolic block. The acute presentation may be due to dietary intake of a particular compound and may even be precipitated by a minor viral infection or fever. The disorders include aminoacidopathies, organic acidemias, congenital urea cycle defects, and sugar intolerances (galactosemia, hereditary fructose intolerance [HFI], etc). The symptoms may appear chiefly in the neonatal period or as late-onset. The clinical presentation may either be a disease-free interval followed by clinical signs of intoxication that could be acute (vomiting, lethargy, coma, liver failure, thromboembolic complications, etc) or chronic (progressive developmental delay, ectopia lentis, cardiomyopathy, etc).

Disorders Involving Energy Metabolism

Energy metabolism disorders are inborn errors of intermediary metabolism, with symptoms at least partly due to a deficiency in energy production or utilization resulting from a defect in the liver, myocardium, muscle, or brain. Clinically, they present with failure to thrive, hypoglycemia, hyperlactacidemia, severe generalized hypotonia, myopathy, cardiomyopathy, cardiac failure, circulatory collapse, sudden infant death syndrome, or malformation. They include defects in glycogenesis, gluconeogenesis, congenital lactic acidemias (pyruvate carboxylase and pyruvate dehydrogenase deficiency), fatty acid oxidation (FAO) defects, Krebs cycle defects, and mitochondrial respiratory chain disorders.

The previous two categories involve small molecules of intermediary and energy metabolisms and hence together can be termed as *small molecule disorders*.

Complex Molecule Disorders

Complex molecule disorders include diseases that disturb synthesis or the catabolism of complex molecules. The symptoms are permanent, progressive, independent of intercurrent events, and are not related to dietary intake. All lysosomal disorders, peroxisomal disorders, disorders of intracellular trafficking and processing such as α1-antitrypsin deficiency, congenital defects of glycosylation (CDG), and inborn errors of cholesterol synthesis come under this category.[4]

CLINICAL MANIFESTATION OF IEM

IEM essentially manifest in the pediatric age group in the early neonatal period, infancy, or later in childhood. The presentation is often multisystemic or with single organ involvement, and they majorly fall into categories like neurologic, hepatic, cardiac, storage syndrome, and dysmorphism.[4] Metabolic acidosis is a characteristic finding in several disorders.

Neurologic Syndrome

Neurologic presentations account for one-third of IEM and fall under five different categories viz, chronic encephalopathy, acute encephalopathy, movement disorders, myopathy, and psychiatric disorders (details are given in **Table 1**).[5]

Hepatic Syndrome

Liver involvement is a presenting feature of a number of inherited metabolic diseases, and the manifestations are difficult to distinguish from many acquired conditions such as infections, intoxications, developmental abnormalities, and neoplasia. The hepatic syndrome usually presents with features such as jaundice, hepatomegaly, hypoglycemia, and hepatocellular dysfunction.[5]

Jaundice

Jaundice presents either with unconjugated or conjugated hyperbilirubinemia. Unconjugated hyperbilirubinemia is characteristic of disorders presenting with increased bilirubin production and is usually caused by hemolysis. It is generally not accompanied by any clinical or biochemical evidence of hepatocellular dysfunction and includes disorders of erythrocyte energy metabolism (pyruvate kinase deficiency) and disorders of bilirubin metabolism (Crigler-Najjar syndrome). Conjugated hyperbilirubinemia presents with hepatocellular dysfunction and includes disorders such as galactosemia, hepatorenal tyrosinemia, and HFI.[5]

Hepatomegaly

Hepatomegaly is generally persistent and nontender with either isolated or associated splenomegaly. It can either be an intrinsic liver disease with minimal evidence of

Table 1 Neurologic presentations of IEM	
Presentation	Features
Chronic encephalopathy	Global developmental delay/psychomotor retardation that is usually progressive and associated with other neurologic dysfunctions such as tone disorders, impairment of special senses, seizures, pyramidal tract signs, evidence of extrapyramidal deficits, or cranial nerve deficits.
Acute encephalopathy	Occurs usually spontaneously and is rapidly progressive with no focal neurologic deficits in an otherwise healthy infant or child.
Movement disorders	Present with neurologic signs with other parts of the nervous system and include progressive ataxia (observed in late onset variants of organelle disease), intermittent ataxia (common manifestation of metabolic decompensation in small molecule disorders), choreoathetosis (Lesch-Nyhan syndrome, glutaric aciduria, and so forth), and parkinsonism.
Myopathy	Commonly disorders of energy metabolism and can present as progressive muscle weakness (Pompe disease, glycogen storage disease type III), exercise intolerance with cramps and myoglobinuria (McArdle disease, carnitine palmityl transferase II deficiency), and myopathy as a manifestation of multisystem disease (mitochondrial myopathies).
Psychiatric disorders	Usually present with hyperactivity, impulsiveness, short attention span (mucopolysaccharidosis type II and III), irritability (Krabbe disease), behavioral and personality changes, social withdrawal, episodes of social withdrawal (X-linked adrenoleukodystrophy, adult-onset metachromatic leukodystrophy), hallucinations (late-onset GM2 gangliosidosis, hyperornithinemia-hyperammonemia-homocitrullinuria [HHH] syndrome, etc).

hepatocellular dysfunction or an expansion of reticuloendothelial system (RES). Hepatocellular dysfunction is observed in glycogen storage disease, cholesterol ester storage disease, Niemann-Pick disease type C, and so forth, whereas expansion of RES is seen in lysosomal storage disorders (LSDs) such as mucopolysaccharidosis, mucolipidosis, sphingolipidosis, and so forth.[5]

Hypoglycemia

Hypoglycemia may occur as a result of primary or secondary defects in glucose production (ketotic hypoglycemia) or overutilization due to defects in fatty acid or ketone oxidation (nonketotic hypoglycemia). Ketotic hypoglycemia may be caused by defects in glycogen mobilization (glycogen storage diseases, GSDs), defects in gluconeogenesis (GSD type I and others such as fructose 1,6-diphosphatase deficiency, pyruvate carboxylase deficiency, HFI, galactosemia, hepatorenal tyrosinemia, etc). Nonketotic hypoglycemia may either be due to hyperinsulinism or FAO defects.[5]

Hepatocellular dysfunction

Hepatocellular dysfunction is also a common finding in several acquired disorders and hence is challenging to isolate from primary metabolic disorders. The presentation is in all age groups. The onset may be in the first few months of life as observed in galactosemia, hepatorenal tyrosinemia, long-chain 3-hydroxyacyl-coenzyme A (CoA) dehydrogenase (LCHAD) deficiency, α1-antitrypsin deficiency, HFI, GSD type IV, Wolman disease, peroxisomal disorders, mitochondrial depletion syndrome, and so forth The onset in later infancy or childhood is observed in GSD type III, Gaucher disease type III, Niemann-Pick disease type C, carnitine palmitoyltransferase I (CPT I) deficiency, and so forth, whereas onset in adolescence is observed in Wilson disease, cholesterol ester storage disease, and adult onset as in Niemann-Pick disease type B.[5]

Cardiac Syndrome

Cardiac involvement is a common serious complication although not a presenting symptom of several IEM. The clinical presentation may be cardiomyopathy as observed in disorders of glycogen metabolism and glycolysis, disorders of fatty acid oxidation, organic acidurias, aminoacidopathies, mitochondrial cardiomyopathies, and storage disorders. Arrhythmias are common relatively nonspecific complications and are observed in Kearns-Sayre syndrome, Fabry disease, Carnitine acyl translocase, propionic acidemia, and so forth, whereas coronary artery disease is observed in familial hypercholesterolemia.[5]

Storage Syndrome and Dysmorphism

The dysmorphic features associated with IEM are generally disturbances of shape rather than fusion, cellular migration abnormalities, or abnormalities of number such as polydactyly. However there are some exceptions such as cellular migration in Zellweger syndrome, glutaric acidurias (GA) type II, and pyruvate dehydrogenase (PDH) deficiency, whereas fusion abnormalities (polydactyly) may be observed in Smith-Lemli-Opitz (SLO) syndrome.[5] Microscopic and ultrastructural abnormalities are often prominent, and the dysmorphism progresses with age. These disorders predominantly involve defects of organelle metabolism, biosynthetic processes, or receptor defects.

Organelle disorders

Organelle Disorders include LSDs such as mucopolysaccharidosis (MPS), sphingolipidosis, glycoproteinoses, and combined defects such as I-cell disease, multiple sulfatase disease, and so forth; peroxisomal disorders such as Zellweger syndrome, rhizomelic chondrodysplasia punctata, adult Refsum disease, and so forth; and mitochondrial disorders like GA type II, 3-hydroxyisobutyric acidurias, PDH deficiency, and mitochondrial electron transport chain defects.

Biosynthetic pathway defects

Biosynthetic pathway defects include cholesterol synthesis (SLO syndrome), glycosylation defects (CDG syndrome), collagen synthesis, albinism, and so forth.

Receptor defects

Receptor defects include familial hypercholesterolemia, pseudohypoparathyroidism, and other hormone receptor defects.[5]

Metabolic Acidosis

Metabolic acidosis is a common presenting or coincident feature of many inherited metabolic diseases wherein the acidosis may be persistent but mild or with an acute episode of severe, even life-threatening acidosis. It could either be due to an abnormal bicarbonate loss or an accumulation of an acid. It is usually assessed by calculating the anion gap. In case of an abnormal bicarbonate loss either due to renal tubular dysfunction or gastrointestinal losses from diarrhea, the anion gap is usually normal, in spite of decreased HCO_3^- due to an increase in plasma Cl^-. Thus a history of diarrhea discriminates hyperchloremic metabolic acidosis due to gastrointestinal bicarbonate loss or renal tubular dysfunction. The IEM due to renal tubular dysfunction/acidosis (RTA) include galactosemia, HFI, hepatorenal tyrosinemia, cystinosis, GSD type I, congenital lactic acidosis, Wilson disease, vitamin D dependency, osteoporosis with RTA, Lowe syndrome, and so forth. Metabolic acidosis resulting from accumulation of organic acids caused by IEM is usually persistent with an increased anion gap. It is important to identify the increased anion by estimating specific ions such as lactate, 3-hydroxybutyrate, acetoacetate, and urinary organic acid analysis. Metabolic acidosis either involves primary lactic acidosis (PDH deficiency, pyruvate carboxylase deficiency and mitochondrial electron transport chain defects) or secondary lactic acidosis due to disorders of gluconeogenesis (GSD type I, HFI, phosphoenolpyruvate carboxykinase deficiency, and fructose-1,6-phosphatase deficiency), FAO defects, defects of biotin metabolism (biotinidase and holocarboxylase deficiencies), and defects of organic acid metabolism (methylmalonic acidemia, propionic acidemia, etc).[5]

IEM present in both neonatal period as well as in late infancy or childhood. In late infancy or childhood the presentation may be chronic progressive or with an acute episode. The symptoms are usually multisystemic[4] (**Table 2**).

PRELIMINARY LABORATORY ASSESSMENT IN IEM

The diagnosis is usually a multitier evaluation and begins with basic laboratory investigations (preliminary evaluation) followed by targeted biochemical and molecular evaluation. In an acute episode in a neonate, infant, or a child, the basic laboratory investigations as follows[3,4] have to be initiated as early as possible.

- Complete blood count. (Neutropenia or thrombocytopenia may be associated with organic acidurias such as methylmalonic acidemia, propionic acidemia, etc.)
- Blood gases and plasma electrolytes. (Acidosis and increased/normal anion gap associated with several organic acidemias.)
- Ammonia (urea cycle defects, organic acidemia).
- Amino acid quantification from plasma/cerebrospinal fluid (CSF)/urine (aminoacidopathy, CSF: plasma glycine >.06 in nonketotic hyperglycinemia, plasma and CSF glycine low in 3-phosphogyecerate dehydrogenase deficiency; plasma glycine markedly elevated in patients with organic acidemias).
- Lactate (lactic acidosis, respiratory chain defects, maple syrup urine disease [MSUD], etc).
- Calcium, magnesium, liver function tests, including albumin and prothrombin and partial thromboplastin time.
- Carnitine, plasma or serum total, and free (unesterified) urine levels. (Deficiency may develop in carnitine transport defects, disorders of fatty acid oxidation and branched chain amino acid metabolism, and valproic acid treatment.)
- Acylcarnitine profile (normal plasma acyl/free carnitine ratio: <.25).
- Ceruloplasmin. (Decreased in Wilson and Menkes disease, aceruloplasminemia.)
- Galactosemia screening test.

| Table 2 | | |
| Presentation of IEM | | |
Characteristic	Neonate or Acute Episode in Late Onset	Chronic Progressive Presentation in Infants and Children
Indicators	Deterioration after a period of apparent normalcy, parental consanguinity, neonatal death in the family, rapid progressive encephalopathy, seizures, metabolic acidosis, persistent vomiting, peculiar odor, etc.	Delayed onset acute presentations are preceded by premonitory symptoms involving several organs/systems that are usually ignored or misinterpreted in early stages.
Neurologic symptoms	Present with seizures that are usually inconsistent and occur later except in case of pyridoxine dependent seizures, refractory seizures, and convulsions.	Symptoms are very frequent and encompass progressive psychomotor retardation, seizures, a number of neurologic abnormalities in both the central and peripheral nervous system, and sensorineural defects.
Muscle disorder presentation	Severe hypotonia with lethargy, coma, seizures, and other neurologic symptoms, or an isolated hypotonia may be observed in hyperlactacidemias, respiratory chain distress, urea cycle defects, trifunctional enzyme deficiency etc. Both seizures and hypotonia are a common presentation in nonketotic hyperglycinemia, sulfite oxidase deficiency, peroxisomal disorders etc.	Several disorders such as late onset form of urea cycle disorder and many organic acidurias present with severe hypotonia, muscular weakness, and poor muscle mass. Severe neonatal generalized hypotonia and progressive myopathy associated with a nonobstructive idiopathic cardiomyopathy can be specific revealing symptoms of a number of inherited energy deficiencies.
Gastrointestinal symptoms	Hepatic symptoms associated with hypoglycemia and seizures are observed in glycogenesis type I and III; gluconeogenesis defects or severe hyperinsulinism, liver failure syndromes (jaundice, hemorrhagic syndrome, hepatocellular necrosis) are characteristic in HFI; galactosemia, tyrosinemia type 1, and cholestatic jaundice with failure to thrive are obtained in α1-antitrypsin deficiency, Byler disease, peroxisomal disorders, Niemann-Pick type C disease, CDG syndrome, cholesterol biosynthesis defects, IEM of bile acid metabolism etc.	Symptoms such as anorexia, failure to thrive, osteopenia, chronic vomiting etc overlapping with other acquired diseases of pediatrics.

- Urine ketones, reducing substances, ketoacids (dinitrophenylhydrazine test).
- Urine organic acids (gas chromatography mass spectrometry).

It is recommended to preserve 2 to 5 mL plasma and 10 to 20 mL urine in −20°C for further analysis.

Based on the preliminary laboratory results of the previously described investigations the patients often fall into one of the following categories.[5]

Encephalopathy without Metabolic Acidosis

Encephalopathy without metabolic acidosis is observed in MSUD, urea cycle disorders, nonketotic hyperglycinemia, pyridoxine-dependent seizures, Zellweger syndrome, molybdenum cofactor defect (sulfite oxidase, xanthine oxidase deficiency), and so forth.

Encephalopathy with Metabolic Acidosis

Encephalopathy with metabolic acidosis is usually associated with the anion gap greater than 25 mmol/L. The increased anion gap may be due to the unmeasured anions. These anions can be identified by urinary organic acid analysis. The presentation is a characteristic finding in organic acidurias, congenital lactic acidosis (defects in pyruvate metabolism or mitochondrial electron transport defects), or dicarboxylic acidurias (FAO defects).

Neonatal Hepatic Syndrome

The presentation of neonatal hepatic syndrome is dominated by jaundice (disorders of bilirubin metabolism, galactosemia, α1-antitrypsin deficiency, etc), severe hepatocellular dysfunction (hepatorenal tyrosinemia; HFI; GSD type IV; FAO defects such as medium-chain acyl-CoA dehydrogenase [MCAD], long-chain acyl-CoA dehydrogenase [LCAD], LCHAD, CPT II, etc; disorders of mitochondrial depletion syndrome; Niemann-Pick disease, etc).

Hypoglycemia

Hypoglycemia is a frequent nonspecific complication of almost any severe illness in newborns. In several IEM associated with hypoglycemia, low blood glucose is a trivial problem as compared with metabolic acidosis and hyperammonemia or severe hepatocellular dysfunction; however, in primary disorders of gluconeogenesis, hypoglycemia may be the only sign of presentation.

Nonimmune Fetal Hydrops

Nonimmune fetal hydrops is an associated finding in several conditions including the genetic conditions of IEM seen in hemoglobin disorders such as G6PD deficiency, pyruvate kinase deficiency, glycerophosphate isomerase deficiency, and LSDs like GM1 gangliosidosis, Gaucher disease, Niemann-Pick diseases, sialidosis, galactosialidosis, I-cell disease, sialic acid storage disorder, Morquio disease, Sly disease, and so forth.

Based on the previously described results the patients have to be categorized, and further diagnostic tests as mentioned in **Table 3**[4,6] have to be initiated.

LABORATORY DIAGNOSIS OF IEM

The diagnosis of IEM is complex and composed of both analytical and molecular methods. Among analytical methods, metabolite estimation using chromatographic and mass spectrometry methods and enzyme assays using artificial chromogenic,

Table 3
Categorization of IEM based on basic laboratory results

Ketones	Lactate	Acidosis	Glucose	Ammonia	Diagnosis	Secondary Tests
+/++	n/++	++	n/+	n/+,++	Organic acidurias (MMA, PA, IVA)	Organic acids, carnitine, and acyl carnitines
+	n	–	n	n	MSUD	Plasma and urine amino acids quantification
–	n/+	–/+	n	+/++++	Urea cycle disorders, HHH syndrome, fatty acid oxidation defects (GAII, CPT II, VLCAD, LCHAD, CAT)	Plasma and urine amino acids quantification, orotic acid estimation, liver or intestine enzyme studies
–	n/+	–	n	n	NKH, SO, XO, pyridoxine dependency, peroxisomal disorders, trifunctional enzyme deficiency etc	Amino acid (NKH, SO), VLCFA, phytanic acid, acyl carnitine, profile
n/++	+++	variable	variable	variable	Congenital lactic acidosis (PC, PDH, Krebs cycle, Respiratory chain disorders, PDH), MCD	Plasma redox state ratios (L/P, 3OHB/AA), organic acids, enzyme assays
++/–	+/++	variable	Low	n	Disorders of gluconeogenesis or glycogen storage	Fasting test, loading test, enzyme studies, liver, lymphoblasts, fibroblasts
–	n	–	n	n	α1-antitrypsin, IEM of bile acid metabolism, peroxisomal disorders, CDG, LCHAD, Niemann-Pick type C	Protein electrophoresis, organic acid, VLCFA, glycosylated transferrin, fibroblast studies

Abbreviations: CAT, carnitine acylcarnitine translocase; GAII, GA type II; GCMS, gas chromatography mass spectrometry; IVA, isovaleric acidemia; MCD, multiple carboxylase deficiency; MMA, methyl malonic acid; MSUD, maple syrup urine disease; n, normal; NKH, nonketotic hyperglycinemia; PA, propionic acidemia; PC, pyruvate carboxylase; PDH, pyruvate dehydrogenase; SO, sulfite oxidase; VLCAD, very-long-chain acyl-CoA dehydrogenase; VLCFA, very-long-chain fatty acids; XO, xanthine oxidase.

fluorogenic substrates, immunometric methods, radio immunoassays, and so forth form the key functional areas of a biochemical genetics laboratory.

IEM chiefly being monogenic disorders following an autosomal recessive inheritance, molecular genetic methods such as targeted mutation analysis or candidate gene sequencing are used for diagnosis. Gene sequencing can detect point mutations and small insertions/deletions but is not capable of detecting

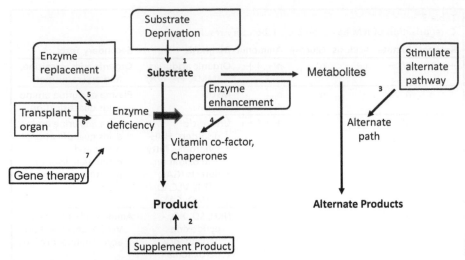

Fig. 1. Therapeutic management of IEM.

large duplications and rearrangements. In such cases other novel methods such as targeted comprehensive genomic hybridization (array comparative genomic hybridization methods),[7] microarray gene expression profiling,[8] parallel next generation sequencing,[9] and whole genome exome sequencing[10] are being used. Molecular analyses assist in prenatal diagnosis and for carrier detection in affected families. They also serve as a diagnostic modality in disorders wherein metabolite and enzyme assays do not confirm the diagnosis or also in institution of therapy; for example, pharmacologic chaperone therapy (PCT). Chaperones are small molecules that assist folding of mutated enzymes and improve their stability and lysosomal trafficking. PCT can only be initiated in patients carrying chaperone-responsive mutations.[11]

THERAPEUTIC MANAGEMENT OF IEM

Therapeutic management of an acute episode of IEM is common to almost all IEM. It aims at reducing the burden of toxic metabolites, ensuring adequate fluid and cofactor infusion and settling of coexisting conditions such as infection, electrolyte and acid-base balance, and so forth. Targeted long-term therapeutic interventions are usually disease-specific and are initiated once a definitive diagnosis is obtained. The therapeutic options focus on the following (**Fig. 1**).

Substrate deprivation: In case of small molecule disease, dietary restriction of the substrates such as phenylalanine in PKU, lysine and tryptophan in GA type I, and so forth are being administered, whereas in storage disorders such as LSDs, small molecules that inhibit synthesis of complex storage substances are used. For example, iminosugar N-butyl-deoxynojirimycin is the first such molecule used that inhibits ceramide-specific glucosyltransferase, thus preventing the formation of glucocerebroside in Gaucher disease.[12]

Enzyme enhancement: Providing a vitamin cofactor to activate residual enzyme activity such as vitamin B_{12} in methylmalnonic acidemia, and so forth. Treating with chaperones (low-molecular-weight molecules) help to unfold the proteins and hence enhances the residual activity of the lysosomal enzymes.[11]

Stimulation of alternate pathway: Supplementing the product or stimulation of an alternate metabolic pathway (sodium benzoate in urea cycle disorders, carnitine in organic acidemias, glycine in isovaleric acidemia, penicillamine in Wilson disease, and so forth).

Enzyme replacement therapy: Supplying the enzyme itself (enzyme replacement therapy for lysosomal disorders such as Gaucher disease, Pompe disease, Fabry disease, MPS I, etc).

Organ transplantation: Transplant of body organs such as liver in Wilson disease, hemochromatosis, tyrosinemia, urea cycle defects and hypercholesterolemia, MSUD,[13] hematopoietic stem cell transplant, and so forth.[14]

Gene therapy: It is in early stage and has been tried in mouse model.[15]

Treatment of IEM is complex and requires a multidisciplinary team effort of a pediatrician, geneticist, neuropediatrician, intensivist, and clinical pathologist in addition to other professionals such as a nutritionist, nurse, and physiotherapist.

PRENATAL DIAGNOSIS

Prenatal diagnosis will play a vital role in checking the incidence of IEM. Establishing a diagnosis in an index patient even from a postmortem sample is necessary to offer prenatal diagnosis in the subsequent pregnancies. The reliability of prenatal diagnosis depends on the quality of primary sample and sensitivity of the analytical method used. Advancements in prenatal sampling techniques and analytical methods have complemented each other in developing confident prenatal diagnosis for IEM. Several approaches such as chorionic villi sampling, amniocentesis, fetal blood, fetal liver biopsy, and so forth are attempted depending on the sample requirement. The analysis method of choice can again be aimed at biochemical or DNA targets depending on the diagnosis status of the index patient and extent of prior molecular diagnostic workup in the family.

NEWBORN SCREENING

The pathologic variations in IEM, particularly the CNS, are irreversible and hence an early diagnosis would help to initiate timely treatment and arrest further damage. Newborn screening (NBS) aims to screen the babies for possible IEM in the presymptomatic state. The foundation of NBS was laid by Dr Guthire in the early 1960s by using bacterial inhibition test for phenylketonuria. Since then several hematologic and endocrine disorders have been included in the panel. The inclusion criteria for NBS programs follow principles proposed by Wilson and Jungner; however, several modifications mainly driven by the advent of new screening techniques such as tandem mass spectrometry (MSMS) have been implemented. NBS can be a targeted screen for a particular disorder or a broad-spectrum analysis using multiplexed panel on MSMS.[16] The availability of enzyme replacement therapy for LSDs such as Gaucher, Pompe, Fabry, Hurler-Scheie, and so forth has substantially increased the need for newborn screening of LSDs[17] (**Table 4**).

The NBS panels are generally identified based on large epidemiologic studies available from a given geographic area. At present national NBS programs differ widely and are a part of standard care in many developed countries. The American College of Clinical Genetics recommends use of a panel of 29 core and 25 secondary conditions;[18] New Zealand screens for 28 disorders;[19] Germany for only 12;[20] United Kingdom for PKU, congenital hypothyroidism (CH), cystic fibrosis (CF), sickle cell disease, and medium-chain acyl-CoA dehydrogenase deficiency (MCADD);[21] and France screens PKU, CH, congenital adrenal hyperplasia (CAH), CF, and sickle cell

Table 4	
Disorders screened in NBS panels	
Mode of Screen	**Disorder**
Targeted tests	CH Galactosemia, CF, CAH, Biotinidase deficiency, G6PD deficiency. PKU
Multiplex testing using MSMS	**Amino acid disorders:** Argininemia, argininosuccinic aciduria (ASA lyase), carbamoylphosphate synthetase deficiency 1, citrullinemia (CIT-I or ASA synthetase), citrin deficiency[a], homocystinuria[b], hypermethioninemia, HHH syndrome, hyperornithinemia with gyral atrophy 1, MSUD[b], PKU and pterin disorders, tyrosinemia[a] **Organic acid disorders:** 2-methylbutyryl-CoA dehydrogenase deficiency, 3-hydroxy-3-methylglutaryl-CoA lyase deficiency, 3-methylcrotonyl-CoA carboxylase deficiency, 3-methylglutaconic aciduria type I deficiency, beta ketothiolase deficiency, biotinidase[b], cobalamin C disease, GA type I. holocarboxylase deficiency, beta-ketothiolase deficiency, cobalamin C disease, isobutyryl-CoA dehydrogenase[c], isovaleric acidemia, methylmalonic acidemias, propionic acidemia **Fatty acid oxidation disorders:** Carnitine: acyl carnitine translocase deficiency, CPT I deficiency, CPT II deficiency, Carnitine uptake defect LCHAD/trifunctional protein deficiency, MCAD deficiency, multiple acyl-CoA dehydrogenase deficiency, short-chain acyl-CoA dehydrogenase deficiency Short-chain hydroxy acyl-CoA dehydrogenase deficiency[c] VLCAD deficiency
MSMS for LSDs	Gaucher disease, Fabry disease, Krabbe disease, Hurler/Scheie disease, Pompe disease, Hunter disease, Niemann-Pick A/B

[a] Possibility of missing the cases.
[b] Milder forms may be missed.
[c] Clinical significance is uncertain.

disease.[22] In several other countries from the Asia Pacific region like China, Japan, Australia, Hong Kong, India, Singapore, and so forth newborn screening programs have been varying in the initiation time and also in the program design.[23]

INCIDENCE OF IEM

The availability of NBS and diagnostic methods have eased the estimation of incidence of IEM. The disorders, although individually rare, together form a group of disorders. The incidence of several disorders in the US population may be comparable with the international population;[24] however, a few ethnic groups may have a prevalence of a particular disorder.[25,26]

IEM IN INDIA

India has a relatively high birth rate of approximately 25 million babies born per year. There is also prevalence of consanguineous marriage across the country, which may suggest possibility of a high occurrence of IEM in India although comprehensive published reports are not available.

Unlike the developed countries, NBS in India has been limited to small-scale funded projects rather than a nationwide mandatory program. NBS is currently available in India as a voluntary or paid for service facility by private service providers. Neonatal screening for amino acids (N = 98,256) in Karnataka showed most common occurrence of disorders like homocystinuria (HCY), hyperglycinemia, MSUD, and PKU along with transient tyrosinaemia.[27] An extended screening program from Hyderabad showed CH (1:1700) to be the most common IEM followed by CAH (1: 2575).[28] A recent study on tandem mass spectrometry profile of around 4896 newborn babies from Andhra Pradesh showed out of range values for 47 babies.[29] As a first coordinated nationwide screening effort, Indian Council of Medical Research (ICMR) has taken an initiative to constitute a task force and has funded a multicenter project to assess feasibility of newborn screening for CH and CAH.

There have been case reports, independent small scale studies, and few multicentric efforts reporting occurrence of several IEM among Indians. A multicentric study published in 1991 by ICMR collaborating centers has reported metabolic defects as basis of mental retardation in 65 out of a total 1314 patients studied (ie, 5%).[30] In a subsequent study from north India, around 2.5% of the total 2560 patients evaluated for a suspected metabolic disorder were diagnosed as having an amino acid disorder.[31] Organic acid analysis by gas chromatography mass spectrometry (GCMS) has been only recently available in India, and hence occurrence of organic acidurias is underdiagnosed. A few reports available are collaborative work carried out with referral laboratories. One such hospital-based retrospective study has obtained organic acidurias in 27% of the 366 cases diagnosed with IEM over a period of 20 years. Among the organic acidemias, methylmalonic acidemia was the most common disorder followed by propionic acidemia. Hyperlacticacidemias (including respiratory chain disorders) were diagnosed in 12% and fatty acid oxidation defects in 8.3% of the cases.[32] A tertiary care public hospital in Mumbai had diagnosed around 1016 cases of inherited disorders over a period of 25 years, of which 20% had amino acid disorders, with albinism being the most common followed by alkaptonuria, urea cycle defects, and others; 5.7% had organic acidemia wherein GA type I was the most common followed by methylmalonic acidemia, propionic acidemia, fatty acid oxidation defects, and so forth; 4.3% had either mitochondrial or respiratory chain defects; 18.6% had mucopolysaccharidosis; 0.7% mucolipidosis; and 24.5% were cases of other LSDs.[33] An acyl carnitine profile in a high-risk group of around 3550 patients from southern India revealed evidence of an amino acid, organic acid, or fatty acid disorder in 3.2% of the patients, of which 54% had aminoacidopathies, 41.6% had organic acidemias, and 4.4 % had fatty acid oxidation defects.[34]

From eastern India there has been a report[35] on clinical and biochemical profile of around 49 patients diagnosed with Wilson disease over a period of 10 years. The study has reported an earlier age of onset of neurologic signs and symptoms with an initial deterioration in 50% of cases wherein the response to treatment was poor.

Among the LSDs, a small study from western India conducted on 150 suspected patients confirmed an enzyme defect in 21 patients (14%). GM2 gangliosidosis was the most prevalent (N = 10) followed by mucopolysaccharidosis (N = 7) and metachromatic leukodystrophy (N = 2).[36] A retrospective analysis of cerebral glycolipidosis (N = 41) diagnosed in a tertiary care center from southern India has reported metachromatic leukodystrophy in 20 patients, Tay-Sachs in 12, Sandhoff in 8, and multiple sulfatase deficiency in 1 patient.[37]

A few studies on molecular characterization of inherited disorders have also been carried out. Shukla and colleagues[38] assessed molecular profiling of arylsulfatase A gene in 20 patients of metachromatic leukodystrophy and ABCD1 gene in 3 patients with X-linked adrenoleukodystrophy.[39] The workers identified 9 pathogenic mutations of which 5 were novel mutations in ASA gene[38] and 3 novel mutations in the ABCD1 gene.[39] Among the small molecule diseases mutation profiling of phenylalanine hydroxylase gene in 7 Indian families with phenylalaninemia revealed 4 novel mutations,[40] whereas that in oculocutaneous albinism[41] mutation analysis of OCA2, TYRP1, SLC45A2, and SLC24A5 genes in 24 affected patients exhibited mutation in OCA2 and SLC5A2 genes, and no mutations were obtained on TYRP1 and SLC24A5 genes. Novel mutations have also been reported TYR[42] gene in Indian population.

Enzyme replacement therapy for LSDs is being administered in India to several patients under a humanitarian program. A report on enzyme replacement therapy administered in 25 Gaucher patients followed for a period of 6 months has shown remarkable improvement in organomegaly, hematologic parameters, and gain in height and weight of the patients.[43]

The present review does not include Indian data on small reports, case studies, and so forth on clinical presentation, molecular analysis, and management of individual inherited disorders.

SUMMARY

IEM are a group of more than 500 individually rare genetic disorders that collectively have an incidence of 1 in 1000 births. Timely diagnosis helps in early initiation of therapy preventing irreversible damage, genetic counseling, and prenatal diagnosis in subsequent pregnancies. But with overlapping clinical presentations and features similar to those of infection and intoxication, diagnosis and management of IEM become intricate. Advancements in biochemical and genetic diagnosis have enhanced precision in timely diagnosis of IEM. Newer therapeutic options like enzyme replacement, enzyme enhancement, organ transplantation, formulated food, and so forth are promising remedies in combating these diseases. Newborn screening aimed at presymptomatic identification of metabolic disorders guides diagnosis and therapy to counter irreversible damage to CNS.

A comprehensive report on incidence of IEM is lacking from India, although several independent groups and reports of multicenter studies focused on a few disorders have indicated presence of many IEM in Indian population. A relatively high birth rate and prevalence of consanguinity increase the suspicion of high incidence of IEM among Indians. Increase in general awareness, availability of NBS, and IEM diagnosis facilities are drawing the attention of clinicians to screen for IEM in a sick child. A nationwide NBS program or large-scale multicenter studies are warranted to access the incidence of IEM in the general population and to sensitize the clinical community about IEM. Leveraging on the advancements in biochemistry and genetic techniques would also benefit the development of novel diagnostic and prenatal screening modalities, which in turn will help in identifying at-risk families, providing genetic counseling, and ultimately diluting the genetic pool of IEM from the society.

ACKNOWLEDGMENTS

The author duly acknowledges the help extended by Tony Jose in compilation of the article.

REFERENCES

1. Garrod AE. Inborn Errors of Metabolism, The Croonian Lectures delivered before the Royal College of Physicians of London. London; 1908. p. 5–7.
2. Garrod AE. The incidence of alkaptonuria: a study in chemical individuality. Lancet 1902;2:1616–20.

3. Pastores GM. Inborn errors of metabolism of the nervous system. In: Bradley WJ, editor. Neurology in clinical practice. 5th edition. Philadelphia: Elsevier; 2008. p. 1761–83.

4. Saudubray JM, Ogier de Baulny H, Charpentier C. Clinical approach to inherited metabolic diseases. In: Fernandes J, Saudubray J-M, van den Berghe G, editors. Inborn metabolic diseases. Diagnosis and treatment. New York: Springer-Verlag; 2000. p. 3–41.

5. Clarke JT. Chapters 2–8. In: A clinical guide to inherited metabolic diseases. Cambridge (UK); University Press; 1996. p. 19–204.

6. Zschocke J, Hoffmann GF. General clinical situations. In: Zschocke J, Hoffmann GF, editors. Vademecum metabolicum: diagnosis and treatment of inborn errors of metabolism. 3rd revised edition. Stuttgart (Germany): Milupa Metabolics GmbH; 2011. p. 3–29.

7. Landsverk ML, Wang J, Schmitt ES, et al. Utilization of targeted array comparative genomic hybridization, MitoMet, in prenatal diagnosis of metabolic disorders. Mol Genet Metab 2011;103:148–52.

8. Hernandez MA, Schulz R, Chaplin T, et al. The diagnosis of inherited metabolic diseases by microarray gene expression profiling. Orphanet J Rare Dis 2010;5:34.

9. Vasta V, Ng SB, Turner EH, et al. Next generation sequence analysis for mitochondrial disorders. Genome Med 2009;1:100.

10. Jones MA, Ng BG, Bhide S, et al DDOST mutations identified by whole-exome sequencing are implicated in congenital disorders of glycosylation. Am J Hum Genet 2012;90:363–8.

11. Parenti G. Treating lysosomal storage diseases with pharmacological chaperones: from concept to clinics. EMBO Mol Med 2009;1:268–79.

12. Pastores GM. Miglustat: substrate reduction therapy for lysosomal storage disorders associated with primary central nervous system involvement. Recent Pat CNS Drug Discov 2006;1:77–82.

13. Moini M, Mistry P, Schilsky ML. Liver transplantation for inherited metabolic disorders of the liver. Curr Opin Organ Transplant 2010;15(3):269–76.

14. Vormoor J, Marquardt T. Hematopoietic cell transplantation in inborn errors of metabolism. Curr Opin Organ Transplant 2004;9:43–8.

15. Neri M, Ricca A, di Girolamo I, et al. Neural stem cell gene therapy ameliorates pathology and function in a mouse model of globoid cell leukodystrophy. Stem Cells 2011;Oct 29(10):1559–71.

16. Pitt JJ. Newborn screening. Clin Biochem Rev 2010;3:57–68.

17. Bennett MJ, Dietzen DJ, Rhead WJ, et al. Future directions in expanded newborn screening for metabolic diseases by tandem mass spectrometry. In: Bennett MJ, editor. Follow up testing for metabolic diseases identified by expanded newborn screening using tandem mass spectrometry. Washington, DC: National Academy of Clinical Biochemistry; 2007. p. 47–9.

18. American College of Medical Genetics in Newborn Screening Expert Group. Newborn screening: toward a uniform screening panel and system- executive summary. Pediatrics 2006;117:S296–307.

19. Newborn screening program, New Zealand. Available at: http://www.nsu.govt.nz/current-nsu-programmes/911.aspx. Accessed March 4, 2012.

20. Gemeinsamer Bundesausschuss der Arzte und Krankenkassen. Beschluss über eine änderung der richtlinen des bundesausschusses der ärzte und krankenkassen über die früherkennung von krankheiten bei kindern bis zur vollendung des 6. Lebensjahres (Kinder-Richtlinien) zur Einführung deserweiterten Neugeborenen-Screenings, 2005.

Available at: http://www.g-ba.de/informationen/beschluesse/zur-richtlinie/15/#170. Accessed May 18, 2011.

21. UK Newborn Screening Programme Center. NHS Newborn Bloodspot Screening Programme. Available at: http://newbornbloodspot.screening.nhs.uk. Accessed March 4, 2012.

22. Associatin Francaise pour le Dpeistage eta la Prevention des Handicaps de l'Enfant. Available at: http://www.afdphe.fr. Accessed March 4, 2012.

23. Padilla CD, Therrell BL. Newborn screening in the Asia Pacific region. J Inherit Metab Dis 2007;30:490–506.

24. Raghuveer T, Garg U. Inborn errors of metabolism in infancy and early childhood: an update. Am Fam Physician 2006;73(11):1981–90.

25. Yoon HR, Lee KR, Kang S, et al. Screening of newborns and high-risk group of children for inborn metabolic disorders using tandem mass spectrometry in South Korea: a three-year report. Clin Chim Acta 2005;354(1-2):167–80.

26. Applegarth DA, Toone JR, Lowry RB. Incidence of inborn errors of metabolism in British Columbia. Pediatrics 2000;105(1):1969–96.

27. Devi AR, Rao NA, Bittles AH. Neonatal screening for amino acid disorders in Karnataka, South India. Clin Genet 1988;34:60–3.

28. Devi AR, Naushad SM. Newborn screening in India. Indian J Pediatr 2004;71: 157–60.

29. Sahai I, Zytkowicz T, Rao Kotthuri S, et al. Neonatal screening for inborn errors of metabolism using tandem mass spectrometry: experience of the pilot study in Andhra Pradesh, India. Indian J Pediatr 2011;78(8):953–60.

30. Multicentric study on genetic causes of mental retardation in India. ICMR Collaborating Centres and Central Co-ordinating Unit. Indian J Med Res 1991;94: 161–9.

31. Kaur M, Das GP, Verma IC. Inborn errors of amino acid metabolism in North India. J Inherit Metab Dis 1994;17:1–14.

32. Muranjan M, Kondurkar P. Clinical features of organic acidemias: experience at a tertiary care center in Mumbai. Indian Pediatr 2001;38:518–24.

33. Kumta NB. Inborn errors of metabolism and Indian Perspective. Indian J Pediatr 2005;72(4):325–32.

34. Nagaraja D, Mamatha SN, De T, et al. Screening for inborn errors of metabolism using automated electrospray tandem mass spectrometry: study in high-risk Indian population. Clin Biochem 2010;43:581–8.

35. Sinha S, Jha DK, Sinha KK. Wilson's disease in Eastern India. J Assoc Physicians India 2001;49:881–4.

36. Sheth J, Patel P, Sheth F, et al. Lysosomal storage disorders. Indian Pediatr 2004; 41:260–6.

37. Nalini A, Christopher R. Cerebral glycolipidoses: clinical characteristics of 41 pediatric patients. J Child Neurol 2004;19(6):447–52.

38. Shukla P, Vasisht S, Srivastava R, et al. Molecular and structural analysis of metachromatic leukodystrophy patients in Indian population. J Neurol Sci 2011; 301(1-2):38–45.

39. Shukla P, Gupta N, Kabra M, et al. Three novel variants in X-linked adrenoleukodystrophy. Child Neurol 2009;24(7):857–60.

40. Bashyam MD, Chaudhary AK, Reddy EC, et al. Phenylalanine hydroxylase gene mutations in phenylketonuria patients from India: identification of novel mutations that affect PAH RNA. Mol Genet Metab 2010;100(1):96–9 [Erratum: Mol Genet Metab 2010;100(4):390].

41. Sengupta M, Mondal M, Jaiswal P, et al. Comprehensive analysis of the molecular basis of oculocutaneous albinism in Indian patients lacking a mutation in the tyrosinase gene. Br J Dermatol 2010;163(3):487–94.

42. Saxena R, Verma IC. Novel human pathological mutations. Gene symbol: TYR. Disease: Albinism, oculocutaneous 1. Hum Genet 2010;127(4):488.

43. Nagral A, Mewawalla P, Jagadeesh S. et al. Recombinant macrophage targeted enzyme replacement therapy for Gaucher disease in India. Indian Pediatr 2011; 48(10):779–84.

Clinical Laboratory Accreditation in India

Anil Handoo, MD, Swaroop Krishan Sood, MD, FISHBT*

KEYWORDS

- Clinical Laboratory Accreditation • Laboratory Quality Management
- Quality Assurance ISO 9001 Certification • ISO 15189 Accreditation • NABL India

KEY POINTS

- Test results from clinical laboratories must ensure accuracy, as these are crucial in several areas of health care. It is necessary that the laboratory implements quality assurance to achieve this goal. The implementation of quality should be audited by independent bodies, referred to as *accreditation bodies*.
- Accreditation is a third-party attestation by an authoritative body, which certifies that the applicant laboratory meets quality requirements of accreditation body and has demonstrated its competence to carry out specific tasks. Although in most of the countries, accreditation is mandatory, in India it is voluntary.
- The quality requirements are described in standards developed by many accreditation organizations. The internationally acceptable standard for clinical laboratories is ISO 15189, which is based on ISO/IEC standard 17025.
- The accreditation body in India is the National Accreditation Board for Testing and Calibration Laboratories, which has signed Mutual Recognition Agreement with the regional cooperation the Asia Pacific Laboratory Accreditation Cooperation and with the apex cooperation the International Laboratory Accreditation Cooperation.

INTRODUCTION

A medical/clinical laboratory is planned to provide results of tests performed on human specimens within a period that it is relevant for the purpose for which these are analyzed. The clinical laboratories receive specimens:

- From patients to reach a diagnosis, exclude disease, determine prognosis, monitor progress, and define targeted therapy
- From healthy subjects to exclude disease before employment and issuing visas and insurance

The authors have nothing to disclose.
Quality Management Department, BLK Super Speciality Hospital, Pusa Road, New Delhi 110005, India
* Corresponding author.
E-mail address: swaroopksood@hotmail.com

Clin Lab Med 32 (2012) 281–292
http://dx.doi.org/10.1016/j.cll.2012.04.009
0272-2712/12/$ – see front matter © 2012 Elsevier Inc. All rights reserved.

labmed.theclinics.com

- For regular health check of employees
- From populations for disease surveillance and national planning
- From patients or healthy subjects for clinical trials.

For all these purposes, it is important to ensure accuracy and precision and maintain turnaround time. These are accomplished by implementing quality assurance programs, which are described in detail in several text books of laboratory medicine[1,2] and can also be downloaded from the Internet.[3,4] This involves defining mission, vision, and objectives of the organization, planning, documenting, and establishing management requirements and achieving technical competence. The laboratory must ensure the following:

- Develop, document, implement, and monitor standard operating procedures (SOPs) for all key activities
- Appoint qualified, trained, and experienced staff
- Procure validated equipment and maintain its regular calibration
- Establish healthy environment and safety procedures
- Introduce correct sampling practices
- Use only validated analytical procedures
- Implement internal quality control
- Participate in external quality assessment schemes where available.

These elements have been defined in the standards laid down by the accreditation bodies (ABs), which conduct audits of the applicant laboratory to check implementation of defined requirements and the competence of the laboratory to provide reliable and accurate results. The test results generated by the accredited laboratory are accepted by the countries that are signatory to the Mutual Recognition Arrangement (MRA) for that standard.

LABORATORY ACCREDITATION STANDARDS AND LABORATORY ACCREDITATION BODIES

ISO/IEC 17025 "General requirements for the competence of testing and calibration laboratories"[5] and ISO 15189 "Medical laboratories—Particular requirements for quality and competence"[6,7] are the international standards by which clinical laboratories are accredited. The international standard ISO/IEC 17025 was developed by International Organization for Standardization (ISO) and is designed for testing and calibration laboratories. It started as Guide ISO/IEC 25, which later was upgraded to standard ISO/IEC 17025. The standard was essentially developed for industrial laboratories, such as biological, chemical, electrical, electronics, mechanical, photometry, and thermal. Later it was applied to clinical laboratories as well. It was realized that there were interpretation problems; hence, a closely related new standard ISO 15189 was developed specifically for clinical laboratories using language in harmony with the medical testing environment with the objective of giving quality service to patients and health care providers.[6] The process for preparation of these is through preparing a draft, circulating it among MRA partners, and reaching a consensus. Practically all standards have incorporated management requirements described in ISO 9001.

OTHER ACCREDITATION STANDARDS FOR CLINICAL LABORATORIES
Clinical Pathology Accreditation Standard

This standard is the national guideline for accreditation of medical laboratories in United Kingdom.[8] United Kingdom Assessment Scheme (UKAS) is the national accreditation body recognized by the European Cooperation for accreditation.

Clinical Pathology Accreditation and UKAS have recently formed a partnership to cooperate on the development of accreditation policy within the United Kingdom.[8]

College of American Pathologists Standard

The College of American Pathologists (CAP) started accreditation of clinical laboratories in 1961.[9] The CAP accreditation is voluntary. However, CAP-accredited laboratories do not need inspection by licensing authorities in most states of United States. Implementation of Clinical Laboratory Improvement Amendments in 1988 in the United States was a great impetus to accreditation. Drug industry supports clinical trials. The companies insisted that the laboratory tests must be performed in a CAP-accredited laboratory. For the last few years, however, these companies accept results of tests performed in laboratories accredited against ISO 15189. CAP accreditation is still more common than other accreditations. Internationally, however, accreditation against ISO 15189 is the most common and gaining ground.

Accreditation Bodies

Accreditation bodies exist practically in each field of human activity from education, food, hotels, environment, and laboratories. Laboratory accreditation is given to calibration and to testing laboratories. The ISO/IEC 17025 and ISO 15189 standards are being used around the globe by many accreditation bodies including International Laboratory Accreditation Cooperation (ILAC).

ACCREDITATION: WHAT, WHO, HOW, WHY, WHEN, WHERE
What

Accreditation is a third-party attestation related to a conformity assessment body conveying formal demonstration of its competence to carry out specific conformity tasks (ISO/IEC 17000:2004).[10] The competence of the laboratory is assessed for the tests in its scope and the laboratory's compliance with stated quality management system (QMS). It, thus, endorses the QMS of the audited laboratory.

Accreditation should not be confused with licensing. The latter requires compliance with minimal criteria, does not involve a compliance or implementation audit, and, more importantly, does not assure technical quality. In fact, in some instances, licensing may require accreditation.[11–13]

The laboratory accreditation certifies validity of technical procedures, competence of the laboratory to carry out the scope of tests, and compliance with stated QMS. It, therefore, endorses the quality management system of the audited laboratory.[14,15] It may seem that accreditation is akin to licensing. However, they are not the same. Licensing requires compliance with minimal criteria, does not involve a compliance or implementation audit, and, more importantly, does not assure technical quality. In fact, in some instances, licensing may require accreditation (**Table 1**).

Who

The ILAC first started as a conference in 1977 with the aim of developing international cooperation for facilitating trade by promotion of the acceptance of accredited test and calibration results. In 1996, ILAC became a formal cooperation with a charter to establish a network of mutual recognition agreements (later modified to arrangements) among accreditation bodies that would fulfil this aim. The ILAC arrangement is the culmination of 22 years of intensive work. The ILAC network consists of 135 bodies representing 88 different economies. Worldwide there are almost 35,000 laboratories accredited by an ILAC signatory (**Box 1**). There are more than 6000 accredited inspection bodies.

Table 1
Differences and similarities between accreditation and certification

Accreditation	Certification
Third-party audit against defined criteria	Third-party audit against defined criteria
Common Laboratory Standard ISO/IEC 17025—for practically all laboratories (ISO 15189 for medical laboratories)	Common standard applicable to laboratory and nonlaboratory organizations—generally ISO 9001
ABs are MRA partners with ILAC and regional cooperative bodies like Asia Pacific Laboratory Accreditation Cooperation, European Cooperation for Accreditation, Inter-American Accreditation Cooperation, Southern African Development Community in Accreditation, and African Accreditation Cooperation	The certification bodies in India are approved by National Accreditation Board for Certification Bodies under Quality Council of India
NABL is an autonomous accreditation body under the DST in India	
Checks technical competence to perform tests/calibrations	Checks compliance to processes
Checks implementation of QMS and technical requirements	Checks implementation of QMS
In most countries there is a single AB, however, ILAC accepts many ABs in the same country	Each country has many certification bodies such as: TuV, UL, DNU, BSI< AENOR, CERMET, and IQNet
One step higher audit	One step lower audit
Test results from a laboratory accredited for ISO/IEC 17025 and/or ISO15189 accepted by MRA Partners	Test results from a laboratory certified for ISO 9001 is not being accepted, as it does not ensure technically valid results

Abbreviations: AENOR, The Spanish Association for Standardization and Certification; BSI, British Standards Institution; CERMET, Certificazione e ricerca per la qualita; DNV, Det Norske Veritas; IQNeT, The International Certification Network; QMS, Quality Management System; TUV, Technischer Überwachungs-Verein; UL, Underwriters Laboratories.
The terms accreditation and certification are used loosely and interchangeably by some.

Box 1

Accreditation bodies are MRA signatories to ILAC (www.ilac.org)

1. Organismo Argentino de Acreditacion (OAA), **Argentina**
2. National Association of Testing Authorities, Australia (NATA), **Australia**
3. Bundesministerium fur Wirtschaft, Familie und Jugend (BMWFJ), **Austria**
4. BELAC (Belgian Accreditation Body), **Belgium**
5. Coordenação Geral de Acreditação General Coordination for Accreditation (CGCRE), **Brazil**
6. Canadian Association for Laboratory Accreditation Inc (CALA), **Canada**
7. Standards Council of Canada (SCC), **Canada**
8. Instituto Nacional De Normalizacion (INN), **Chile**
9. Hong Kong Accreditation Service (HKAS), **Hong Kong, China**
10. China National Accreditation Service for Conformity Assessment (CNAS), **People's Republic of China**
11. Ente Costarricense de Acreditation (ECA), **Costa Rica**
12. Croatian Accreditation Agency (HAA), **Croatia**
13. National Accreditation Body of Republica de Cuba (ONARC), **Cuba**
14. Cyprus Organisation for the Promotion of Quality (CYS) - Accreditation Body (CYSAB), **Cyprus**
15. Czech Accreditation Institute (CAI), **Czech Republic**
16. Danish Accreditation (DANAK), **Denmark**
17. Egyptian Accreditation Council (EGAC), **Egypt** NLAB merged into EGAC as of 28 December 2009
18. Finnish Accreditation Service (FINAS), **Finland**
19. Comite Francais d'Accreditation (COFRAC), **France**
20. Deutsche Akkreditierungsstelle GmbH (DAkkS), **Germany** DAkkS was formed from a merger of DKD and DGA.
21. Hellenic Accreditation System S.A. (ESYD), **Greece**
22. Oficina Guatemalteca de Acreditacion (OGA), **Guatemala**
23. Hungarian Accreditation Board (NAT), **Hungary**
24. National Accreditation Board for Testing & Calibration Laboratories (NABL), **India**
25. National Accreditation Body of Indonesia (KAN), **Indonesia**
26. Irish National Accreditation Board (INAB), **Ireland**
27. Israel Laboratory Accreditation Authority (ISRAC), **Israel**
28. L'Ente Italiano di Accreditamento (ACCREDIA), **Italy**
29. International Accreditation Japan (IA Japan), **Japan**
30. Japan Accreditation Board for Conformity Assessment (JAB), **Japan**
31. Voluntary EMC Laboratory Accreditation Center INC (VLAC), **Japan**
32. National Centre of Accreditation (NCA), **Kazakhstan**
33. Korea Laboratory Accreditation Scheme (KOLAS), **Republic of Korea**
34. Office Luxembourgeois d'Accreditation et de Surveillance (OLAS), **Luxembourg**
35. Department of Standards Malaysia (STANDARDS MALAYSIA), **Malaysia**
36. entidad mexicana de acreditación, a.c. (ema), **Mexico**
37. Dutch Accreditation Council (RvA), **Netherlands**

38. International Accreditation New Zealand (IANZ), **New Zealand**

39. Norsk Akkreditering (NA), **Norway**

40. Pakistan National Accreditation Council (PNAC), **Pakistan**

41. Papua New Guinea Laboratory Accreditation Scheme (PNGLAS), **Papua New Guinea**

42. Philippine Accreditation Office (PAO), **Philippines**

43. Polish Centre for Accreditation (PCA), **Poland**

44. Instituto Portugues de Acreditacao (IPAC), **Portugal**

45. Romanian Accreditation Association (RENAR), **Romania**

46. Association of Analytical Centers "Analitica" (AAC Analitica), **Russian Federation**

47. Singapore Accreditation Council (SAC), **Singapore**

48. Slovak National Accreditation Service (SNAS), **Slovakia**

49. Slovenian Accreditation (SA), **Slovenia**

50. South African National Accreditation System (SANAS), **South Africa**

51. Entidad Nacional de Acreditacion (ENAC), **Spain**

52. Sri Lanka Accreditation Board for Conformity Assessment (SLAB), **Sri Lanka**

53. Swedish Board for Accreditation and Conformity Assessment (SWEDAC), **Sweden**

54. Swiss Accreditation Service (SAS), **Switzerland**

55. Taiwan Accreditation Foundation (TAF), **Chinese Taipei**

56. The Bureau of Laboratory Quality Standards, Department of Medical Sciences, Ministry of Public Health, Thailand (BLQS-DMSc), **Thailand**

57. National Standardization Council of Thailand—Office of the National Accreditation Council (NSC-ONAC).

Regional cooperation bodies

ILAC has peer reviewed these regional bodies and has signed MRAs with them **(Fig. 1)**. They include:

- Asia Pacific Laboratory Accreditation Cooperation, Secretariat—Australia
- European Cooperation for Accreditation, Secretariat—France
- Inter-American Accreditation Cooperation, Secretariat—Mexico
- Southern African Development Community in Accreditation, Secretariat—South Africa
- African Accreditation Cooperation (AFRAC), Secretariat—Republic of South Africa.

Regulation

Accreditation was predominantly a voluntary activity in the early part of the 20th century. The realization of the importance of providing reliable health care many countries has made accreditation a mandatory requirement before a laboratory can be licensed. In India, the National Accreditation Board for Testing and Calibration Laboratories (NABL) is the accreditation body for the testing and calibration laboratories.[16] It has signed an MRA with APLAC, the Regional Accreditation Cooperation, and with ILAC. Every 4 years, NABL undergoes peer evaluation by the APLAC team. NABL is an autonomous body under the Department of Science and Technology, Ministry of Science and Technology, Government of India. Initially, the accreditation was given only to industrial laboratories. In 1998, it added Medical/Clinical laboratories

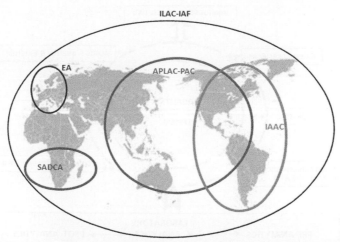

Fig. 1. Regional organizational structure showing system of cooperation amongst them. APLAC, Asia Pacific Laboratory Accreditation Cooperation; EA, European Cooperation for Accreditation; IAAC, Inter-American Accreditation Cooperation; IAF, International Accreditation Forum; ILAC, International Laboratory Accreditation Cooperation; PAC, Pacific Accreditation Cooperation; SADCA, Southern African Development Community in Accreditation.

in its scope of accreditation fields and prepared the Specific Guidelines for India. NABL extended its MRA for medical laboratories in 2008. Earlier, the accreditation was given per the requirements of ISO/IEC Guide 25 and later the standard ISO/IEC 17025. Since 2005, all clinical laboratory accreditations have been against the standard ISO 15189. NABL has accredited more than 350 clinical laboratories, and a large number of laboratories are in the pipeline. This is the rapidly expanding area and is overtaking all other accreditations. It is expected that by the end of the next 5 years, the figure may reach 5000. There are several reasons for this increase in number of laboratories seeking NABL accreditation. These include:

- Increase in awareness of general population
- Corporate houses referring their employees to NABL-accredited laboratories
- Companies supporting clinical trials accepting reports of NABL-accredited tests
- Government proposing to get all government laboratories accredited
- Most importantly, Government having higher test rates for accredited laboratories than for nonaccredited laboratories.

How

There is a common saying "What is not documented is not done." Accreditation requires extensive documentation and maintenance of records. This should become a habit. Most records can be maintained electronically. The second important requirement is acquiring competence at all levels, through appropriate training and education. The steps involved in getting accreditation against ISO 15189 are described below, taking example of the procedure in India:

- Contact the accreditation body and procure or download online (www.nabl-india.org), relevant accreditation documents eg, the application form and the country's specific guidelines, which in India is NABL document 112. (This

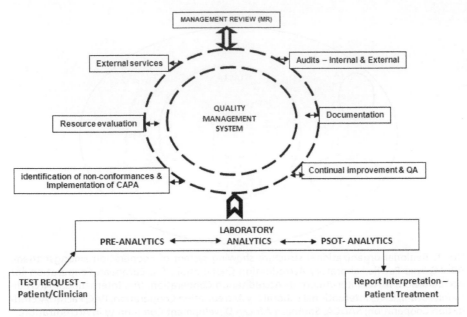

Fig. 2. Elements of Quality Management System (QMS) in a medical testing laboratory.

document gives clause-wise explanation of the requirements of ISO 15189 as applicable to India

- Obtain a copy of the standard ISO 15189, which is available from Bureau of Indian Standards or the government-approved booksellers
- Acquaint with all relevant documents and understand the assessment procedure and methodology of making an application
- Get at least 1 individual trained in QMS. Make him or her responsible to design the QMS (**Figs. 2** and **3**)
- Prepare an SOP for each investigation carried out in the laboratory; SOPs are required for other activities as well, for example, sample collection, equipment calibration, internal quality control, fire safety

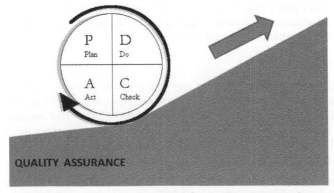

Fig. 3. Deming wheel of continual improvement for quality assurance in a medical testing laboratory.

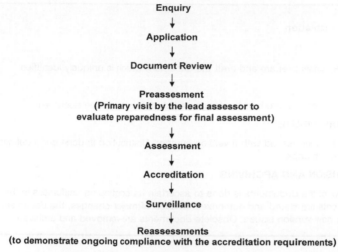

Fig. 4. Steps to accreditation.

- Ensure effective environmental conditions (ie, temperature, humidity, storage placement, etc)
- Get calibration of instruments/equipment, from accredited calibration laboratories
- Impart training on the key elements of documentation, such as document format, authorization of document, issue and withdrawal procedures, document review and change. Each document should have the identification number, name of controlling authority, and period of retention.
- Ascertain the status of the existing QMS and technical competence with regard to the accreditation authority recommendations and standards and address the question "Is the system documented and effective or does it need modification?"
- Implement all activities described in the Quality Manual and other documents
- Incorporate Internal Quality Control (IQC) practices. Record IQC data and determine uncertainty of measurements. Maintain Levy Jennings charts.
- Participate in External Quality Assessment (EQA) schemes
- Develop a system to detect nonconformities, take corrective and preventive actions as applicable, and monitor effectiveness of the actions
- Take corrective actions on IQC/EQA outliers.
- Conduct internal audit and management review
- Apply to accreditation authority along with appropriate fee (**Fig. 4**).

ELEMENTS OF A QMS ACCORDING TO ISO 15189

The primary step of introducing good quality management in the laboratory is the identification of the key elements of a QMS. Integration of these with the existing processes and organization, through documentation of SOPs and definition of objectives and policies in a quality manual form, is the foundation on which the other elements are laid. The important elements of QS are covered by the ISO 15189 accreditation standard in 2 distinct chapters: Management Requirements and Technical Requirements. Management aspects include document control; identification of nonconformances; implementing CAPAs and action plans to continuously improve; performance of internal audit and management review; resolution of complaints; and

---

Box 2
Steps in documentation

PREPARE

Competent personnel prepare and draft the document which is uniquely identified.

APPROVE

Once the document is authorized by designated staff, it is an active document.

ISSUE AND DISTRIBUTE

The document is then issued with a version number. Distribution is done per a defined list either electronically or on paper.

REVIEW REVISION AND ARCHIVING

Regular review of the documents is done to ascertain its continuing usefulness in the laboratory. Any amendments are dated and authorized. In case of major changes, the document should be revised and a new version issued. Obsolete documents are removed and archived.

---

evaluation of external services, suppliers, contracts, and referral laboratories (**Box 2**). Technical elements include personnel and training; accommodation; equipment; validation; and assuring quality of examination procedures by IQC, EQA, maintenance, and calibration. The same is depicted in the following flow chart (see **Fig. 2**).

The assurance of quality is a continuous process that needs regular checks, and the same can be depicted by the Deming wheel of continuous improvement (see **Fig. 3**).

CONCEPT OF QUALITY INDICATORS

The standard mentions that "Laboratory management shall implement quality indicators for systematically monitoring and evaluating the laboratory's contribution to patient care. When this program identifies opportunities for improvement, laboratory management shall address them regardless of where they occur (ISO 15189, 4.12.4)." **Box 3** enumerates some of the possible quality indicators that can provide a starting point for each laboratory.

Why

Laboratory accreditation ensures putting in place a QMS for achieving continuous improvement in laboratory. This is important for the acceptance of test results nationally and internationally. In turn, it helps in making decisions and formulating policies, which no longer remain regional but can be applied globally. Accreditation is immensely beneficial in supporting an achievable and efficient health-care system. Accreditation is used to attain needed confidence

- in the results obtained by a testing facility and in its operation
- in the certification system and the certificates
- in the results of any other accreditation body.

When

Seeking accreditation starts with planning. A laboratory needs to make a definite plan for obtaining accreditation and nominate a responsible person as quality manager (a

---

Box 3

Quality indicators that can provide a starting point for each laboratory

- Percentage of redos
- Repeat testing
- Turnaround times
- Number of contaminations
- Number of analytical failures
- Number of reporting mistakes
- EQA failure rate and comparison of EQA results with those of other laboratories
- IQC results
- Staff (health, vacancies)
- Number of complaints
- Customer feedback

---

person familiar with the laboratory's existing QMS) to coordinate all activities related to seeking accreditation.

Where

Given the importance of medical testing, it is essential to aim for the highest levels of quality assurance and continuous quality improvement. Accreditation formally and officially recognizes technical and scientific competence, facilitates exchange of services, provides a valuable management tool, and enhances confidence that the needs and requirements of all users (clinicians, patients, and families) are met.[17,18] Therefore, any organization, whether a standalone laboratory or a hospital-based laboratory, should opt for accreditation from the time of its inception. This will not only provide the benefits of accreditation mentioned before, but will also make quality a habit.

SUMMARY

Clear and tangible objectives should be spelled out for everyone to know and understand that laboratory accreditation is a system for developing laboratories to have a good QMS and maintain up-to-date competency. This will help provide an efficient health care system, thus saving the scarce resources of laboratories. Accreditation will provide a sustainable and good QMS for laboratories, as they will be assessed periodically. Accreditation is not a 1-time activity but a continuous process of improvement. Therefore, getting accreditation does not mean that a laboratory is perfect; it means that it is at an acceptable level according to the standard and requirements. The next assessment will aim for laboratories to improve performance. Accreditation should be taken as a positive tool for laboratory improvement.

ACKNOWLEDGMENTS

The authors are grateful to Anil Relia, Director NABL, Bipin Philip, Quality Officer, NABL, and Dr Punam Bajaj, Accreditation Officer, NABL for their valuable input and providing information on terminology.

REFERENCES

1. Lewis SM, Bradshaw A. Laboratory organization and management. In: Bain BJ, Bates I, Laffan MA, et al, editors. Dacie and Lewis practical haematology. 11th edition. London: Churchill Livingstone Elsevier; 2011. p. 564–84.
2. Burtis C, Ashwood A, Burns D. Tietz textbook of clinical chemistry and molecular diagnostics. 4th edition. Washington, DC: Saunders, 2005.
3. Williams LO, Cole EC. General recommendations for quality assurance programs for laboratory molecular genetic tests. Centers for Disease Control and Prevention Public Health Practice Program Office, Division of Laboratory Systems, Atlanta, Georgia. Available at: http://wwwn.cdc.gov/dls/pdf/genetics/dyncor.pdf. Accessed December 15, 2011.
4. Guidance for implementing a laboratory quality management system. Clinical Laboratory Evaluation Program. New York State Department of Health, Wadsworth Center, Clinical Laboratory Reference System, Version 1 August 2010. Available at: http://www.wadsworth.org/labcert/clep/ProgramGuide/NYS_QMS_Guidance_0810.pdf. Accessed December 15, 2011.
5. International Organization for Standardization: ISO/IEC 17025 general requirements for the competence of testing and calibration laboratories, 2005.
6. International Organization for Standardization: ISO 15189 medical laboratories—particular requirements for quality and competence, 2007.
7. Canadian Standards Association: The ISO 15189:2003 essentials—a practical handbook for implementing the ISO 15189:2003 standard for medical laboratories, 2004.
8. CPA Standards for the medical laboratory. PD-LAB-Standards, Version: 2.00 (September 2007). p. 1–57.
9. CAP 15189[SM] – Accreditation to the ISO 15189:2007 Standard. Why entrust the CAP with your organization's ISO 15189 accreditation? Available at: http://www.cap.org/cap15189. Accessed December 15, 2011.
10. International Organization for Standardization (ISO) Standard. ISO/IEC 17000:2004.
11. Kenny D. ISO and CEN documents on quality in medical laboratories. Clin Chim Acta 2001;309:121–5.
12. Burnett D. ISO 15189:2003—quality management, evaluation and continual improvement. Clin Chem Lab Med 2006;44:733–9.
13. Burnett D, Blair C. Standards for the medical laboratory—harmonization and subsidiarity. Clin Chim Acta 2001;309:137–45.
14. Burnett D, Blair C, Haeney MR, et al. Clinical pathology accreditation: standards for the medical laboratory. J Clin Pathol 2002;55:729–33.
15. Burnett D. A practical guide to accreditation in laboratory medicine London: ACB Venture Publications; 2002.
16. National Accreditation Board For Testing and Calibration Laboratories (NABL) introduction. Available at: http://www.nabl-india.org/nabl/html/about-intro.asp. Accessed December 15, 2011.
17. Silva P. Guidelines on establishment of accreditation of health laboratories. New Delhi, World Health Organization Regional Office for South-East Asia, 2007 (SEA-HLM-394).
18. Berwouts S, Morris MA, Dequeker E. Approaches to quality management and accreditation in a genetic testing laboratory. Eur J Hum Genet 2010;18:S1–19.

Blood Bank Regulations in India

Nabajyoti Choudhury, MBBS, PhD, MBA[a],*, Priti Desai, MBBS, MD, DCP[b]

KEYWORDS

- Blood bank regulation • Blood transfusion services • Blood bank license
- Drugs and Cosmetics Act • National Blood Policy • India

KEY POINTS

- Successful blood services depend on legally empowered regulatory services.
- Blood transfusion services are important constituents of national health services.
- Blood transfusion services in India are regulated by the Drugs and Cosmetics Act, 1940 and its subsequent amendments.
- The Drugs and Cosmetics Act, 1940 specifies about accommodation, manpower, equipment, supplies and reagents, good manufacturing practices, and process control to be followed in Indian blood transfusion services.
- Regulatory affairs in the Indian blood banking system are controlled by central and provincial Drug Control authority under Drug Controller General of India.
- National AIDS Control Organization (NACO) acts as a facilitator to Indian blood transfusion services on behalf of the Ministry of Health and Family Welfare, Government of India, especially to the government sector.
- The National Blood Policy was published by the Government of India in 2002 and it provides objectives to provide safe, adequate quantity of blood, blood components, and products.

A safe and adequate blood supply is essential in modern medicine. The Blood Transfusion Service (BTS) is an important part of the National Health Service, as there is no substitute for human blood and its components. A successful blood program depends on nationally coordinated blood services that operate under legally empowered regulatory authority.

The objective of safe blood transfusion requires a well-coordinated system of recruitment of safe donors; testing facilities for infectious disease markers and compatibility tests; and preparation and storage of blood components according to the defined quality standards and appropriate clinical use. To ensure quantity, quality, and safety, blood banks and transfusion services need to be coordinated and

[a] Transfusion Medicine, Tata Medical Centre, 14 MAR (EW), New Town, Rajarhat, Kolkata 700 156, India; [b] Department of Transfusion Medicine, Tata Memorial Hospital, Dr E. Borges Road, Parel, Mumbai 400012, Maharashtra, India
* Corresponding author.
E-mail address: nabajyoti_2000@yahoo.com

Clin Lab Med 32 (2012) 293–299
http://dx.doi.org/10.1016/j.cll.2012.04.002
0272-2712/12/$ – see front matter © 2012 Elsevier Inc. All rights reserved.

regulated. The ultimate responsibility for appropriate regulation and coordination is governmental (Health Authority).[1]

Appropriate blood transfusion legislation and adequate regulation is a public health priority to ensure the safety and availability of blood and blood products. Regulation of blood transfusion services is required to ensure compliance with all national legislation related to blood transfusion. A regulatory framework is necessary to establish and maintain an appropriate and effective system for the inspection, licensing, audit, and/or accreditation.[2]

The major difficulties associated with blood transfusion services include risk of transfusion of transmissible infections, inadequate supplies of safe blood and blood products, technical and clerical errors during processing and testing, and inappropriate use. There should be uniform standards to maintain the quality and safety of blood and blood products. The World Health Organization (WHO) Basic Requirements for Blood Transfusion Services provides guidance to countries in setting up the standards for quality, safety, adequacy, and accessibility of blood supply and the safety of the clinical transfusion process.[3]

To achieve the basic requirements for BTS and to bring uniformity across the country, it is necessary to establish a national blood program, which includes the involvement of the government or national health authority for the development of policy, plans, standards, and legislation. Proper organization, management, and effective regulation are important elements of a successful blood program. Regulation of the blood transfusion service indicates how the system is functioning for implementing the relevant policies, strategies, goals, and objectives. Strengthening of national and regional blood regulatory authorities has, therefore, been recognized as a fundamental need to assure availability of safe blood products.[4]

BLOOD BANK REGULATION IN OTHER COUNTRIES

In 2005, the WHO Expert Committee on Biological Standardization (ECBS), which is advisory to WHO, recognized the need for a global network of regulatory authorities in the blood field and recommended the cooperation of experienced regulatory authorities in risk assessment and information sharing through the establishment of a "peer regulators group." Subsequently, in 2006, WHO formed the Blood Regulators Network (BRN). The BRN provides a forum for the exchange of information and opinion among members on blood-related issues.[4]

In the United States, the Center for Biologics Evaluation and Research (CBER) is that part of the US Food and Drug Administration that regulates the collection of blood and blood components used for transfusion or for the manufacture of pharmaceuticals derived from blood and blood components, such as clotting factors, and establishes standards for the products themselves. CBER also regulates related products such as cell separation devices, blood collection containers, and human immunodeficiency virus (HIV) screening tests that are used to prepare blood products or to ensure the safety of the blood supply. CBER develops and enforces quality standards, inspects blood establishments, and monitors reports of errors, accidents, and adverse clinical events.[5]

In Europe, with the efforts made by regulatory authorities, there is now a comprehensive system of regulatory control, the basis of which is stringent legislation on both the European Community (EC) and member state (national) levels. Particularly, a dedicated "blood law," directive (2002/98/EC) and "daughter" directives provide a regulatory framework. Important technical standards are provided by the European Pharmacopoeia monographs and guidance documents issued by the Council of Europe and the European Medicines Agency.[2]

Within most of South East Asia, the regulation of blood does not fall under the sole purview of a single regulatory authority. Fresh blood and blood components are usually regulated through a combination of controls on practice, personnel, premises, and processes (eg, medical clinic and clinical laboratory licensing, professional registration of medical and nursing practitioners) enforced by the Ministry of Health. Plasma derivatives are separately regulated as medicinal products through medicine controls (eg, product evaluation, registration and licensing and postlicense monitoring) enforced by drug regulatory authorities.[2]

The blood services in South Africa are private, and they operate under license from the Ministry of Health. Current regulations governing Blood Transfusion in South Africa are found in Human Tissue Act. This legislation clearly outlines regulations pertaining to donor eligibility, blood collection, mandatory testing, and issuing. They also make provision for a Department of Health–appointed inspector to visit and audit blood services on a regular basis.[2]

LEGAL REQUIREMENT FOR BLOOD BANK IN INDIA

In India, human blood is covered under the definition of "Drug" under section 3(b) of the Drugs and Cosmetics Act, 1940[6,7] because blood and blood components are used as therapeutic agents to treat certain clinical conditions. As with drugs, adverse effects may occur after blood transfusion; therefore, it is imperative that Blood Banks be regulated under the Drugs and Cosmetics Act and rules, and the license is granted for operating a blood bank by the State Licensing and the Central Licensing Authority.

Drugs and Cosmetics Act, 1940 is the Indian regulation that governs the blood banking system in India. As mentioned in the name of the Act, it was enacted in 1940, but there were multiple amendments in between to cope with changes in the last 70 years. In India, the regulatory body is Central Drugs Standard Control Organization (CDSCO), which is headed by the Drugs Controller General (India) (DCGI). Every state government has state-level regulatory bodies for implementation of regulation inside regional boundaries. Indian regulators have many more areas to look after, and one of them is blood banks.[8] The DCGI is the Central License Approving Authority (CLAA), whereas the regulatory control remains under the dual authority of the State and the Central Government.

The requirements of a blood bank for collection, storage, processing, and distribution of whole human blood and blood components are given in Part X-B of the Drugs and Cosmetics Rules. The Rules from 122F to 122P explain the various procedures of making applications by a blood bank, fees to be paid for grant/renewal of license by the applicant, and conditions of license to be followed by the applicant after grant/renewal of license.[6]

In 1967, the government of India (Ministry of Health) enacted a separate provision in Schedule F Part XII B of Drugs and Cosmetics Rules. In this section, the requirement for the functioning and operation of a blood bank and/or for preparation of blood components is given. This includes various requirements such as accommodation, personnel, equipments, supplies and reagents, criteria for blood donation, blood donation camp, processing of blood components from whole human blood, plasmapheresis, plateletphersis, and leukapheresis.

The DCGI has issued a notification that the blood should not be collected from paid professional donors with effect from January 1998 to supply safe blood and blood components. The honorable Supreme Court of India delivered one verdict in response to a public interest litigation submitted in 1995. This judgment specified many legal provisions for the operation and management of Indian BTS. It even indicated a specified date to license all compliant blood banks and also to stop operation for those blood banks that do not comply.[9]

PREREQUISITE FOR GRANT OF LICENSE FOR BLOOD BANK

There should be adequate space, infrastructure, and equipment for any or all the operations of blood collection or blood processing and adequate storage of blood and blood components. Minimum total area should be 100 m² having appropriate lighting and ventilation with washable floors and shall consist of following rooms, namely:

1. Registration and medical examination room with adequate furniture and facilities for registration and selection of donors
2. Blood collection room (air conditioned)
3. Room for laboratory for blood group serology (air-conditioned)
4. Room for laboratory for transmissible diseases like hepatitis, syphilis, malaria, HIV antibodies etc (air conditioned)
5. Sterilization and washing room
6. Refreshment room
7. Store and records room.

The operation of the Blood Bank or processing of whole human blood for components or manufacture of blood products should be carried out under the personal supervision of competent technical staff. A blood bank medical officer is required at a minimum to be a graduate in medicine of a recognized university preferably having work experience in a blood bank for at least 1 year with adequate knowledge and experience in blood group serology, blood group methodology, and medical principles involved in the procurement of blood.

- The manufacturing of blood components requires additional space of 50 m² area, which should be fully air conditioned
- Adequate and qualified technical staff is required to carry out routine blood bank activities
- Appropriate equipment, required consumables and reagents, and forms and labels should be available.

LICENSING PROCEDURE

License from Food and Drugs Control Administration (FDCA) is a must for operating a blood bank. Under the legal provisions laid down in of Drugs and Cosmetics Act, 1940 a blood bank cannot be run without a valid license. Application for grant (first time) or renewal of license for operation of a blood bank should be submitted to the Licensing Authority in Form 27-C, accompanied by license fee of and inspection fee in the case of renewal of license.

For the purpose of obtaining a fresh license, certain necessary formalities are to be followed. The management of the proposed blood bank should submit the floor plan of the blood bank to the provincial (state) FDCA and a copy to the CDSCO office at zonal level. Once FDCA approves the floor plan, the interested management should submit the application in Form 27-C along with requisite fees. The application form should accompany multiple documents like legal status of the organization, no objection certificate (NOC) from local municipally, clinical license (in case of hospital-based blood bank), list of competent personnel, list of equipment, standard operating procedures for all major technical and nontechnical areas, and samples of all stationeries to be used in the blood banks.

Once the application is in order, a joint inspection is conducted by the provincial FDCA and CDSCO officials. During onsite inspection, the inspectors examine all sections of the premises, infrastructure, and equipment and also inspect the process of manufacture proposed to be used or being used along as well as testing facilities, personnel, standard operating procedures, and calibration of equipment. After completion of joint inspection and favorable recommendation by the team of inspecting officers, the state licensing authority examines the suitability and eligibility of the applicant with respect to the facilities provided. If the applicant is able to fulfill the conditions of license, rules, regulations, and provisions of the act, recommendation to grant the license is forwarded to the CLAA, New Delhi for approval. The power of CLAA has been designated to DCGI, New Delhi. Once the license has been duly approved and signed by CLAA, it is handed over to the applicant to allow blood bank activities. Every blood bank license is valid for a period of 5 years. After approval of license, the state licensing authority may carry out surprise inspections any time in addition to regular yearly surveillance. During this visit, if any noncompliance is observed, the blood bank has to correct the deficiency to continue to have the license for operations.

ROLE OF FACILITATORS IN BLOOD BANK OPERATIONS AND REGULATIONS IN INDIA

Consequent to a public litigation case, the honorable Supreme Court of India has directed the government of India. In this judgment, the Supreme Court has given a number of directions, the most important of which is the ban on professional blood donation.[7,9] Under the direction of the Supreme Court, a National Blood Transfusion Council (NBTC) was formed under the ministry of Health and Family Welfare at Delhi. The NBTC was started with the objective to strengthen the blood bank system in country and to cover the entire blood bank services including voluntary blood donor motivation program, proper storage and utilization of blood, quality control program, education training, and research.

NBTC is a registered society headquartered in New Delhi. It has representatives from the Directorate General of Health Services of the Government of India, the Drug Controller of India, Ministry of Finance, Indian Red Cross Society, private blood banks, major medical institutes of the country, and nongovernment organizations active in voluntary blood donations. The council is headed by Additional Secretary in Ministry of Health who is also in charge of the National AIDS Control Organization (NACO). The NBTC has a similar society in every state and union territory (SBTC) with same representative body. The NBTC and SBTCs aim at ensuring safe and quality blood for transfusion services, promoting voluntary and nonremunerated blood donors, following up with quality control/assurance programs in blood-banks, and conduct training programs. NBTC has the major advisory role in the formulation of policy on safe blood transfusion services in the country. NACO is responsible for collection of safe blood and also the provision of financial assistance to blood banks, mainly in government sectors. NACO was established under the blood safety program in 1987.[10]

While the Drug Controller General is the licensing authority, the NACO and State AIDS Control Societies (SACSs) aims to prevent the transmission of HIV and ensure 100% screening of all collected blood units and provide training and financial assistance to blood banks for technical modernization for ensuring the quality of blood banks.

Currently, the blood safety section of NACO centrally procures consumables and nonconsumable items and also provides manpower to blood banks. It takes the help of outside procurement agencies by tender as per-government rules. It procures infectious disease marker kits, blood bags, and other relevant consumables as well. NACO also procures almost all required equipment for blood banks at different stages. It even procures vehicles centrally at all India level for blood donation and distribution. This program is supported by various international organizations and internal resource mobilization by the government of India.

NATIONAL BLOOD POLICY

The National Blood Policy was published by the Government of India in 2002. The objective of the policy is to provide safe, adequate quantity of blood, blood components, and products. There are 8 main objectives coving all spectrums of BTS. The main issue of the blood banking system in the country is fragmented management. The standards vary from state to state, city to city, and centre to centre in the same city. In spite of a hospital-based system, many large hospitals and nursing homes do not have their own blood banks, and this has led to stand-alone private blood banks.

The availability and utilization of blood components is limited. There is shortage of trained health care professionals in the field of transfusion medicine. There is a need to develop well-equipped blood centers with trained man power to achieve quality, safety, and efficacy of blood and blood products. It is essential to have good manufacturing practices and implementation of a quality system to achieve total quality and safety. The need for modification and change in the blood transfusion service has necessitated formulation of a National Blood Policy and development of a National Blood Programme, which will also ensure implementation of the directives of Supreme Court of India–1996. The main aim of the policy is to procure blood from nonremunerated regular blood donors by the blood banks to ensure blood safety. The policy also addresses various issues with regard to technical personnel, research and development, and the elimination of profiteering by the blood banks by selling blood. The policy also envisages that fresh licenses to stand-alone blood banks in the private sector shall not be granted, and renewal of such blood banks shall be subject to thorough scrutiny.

The policy aims to ensure easily accessible and adequate supply of safe and quality blood and blood components collected/procured from a voluntary nonremunerated regular blood donor in well-equipped premises, which is free from transfusion-transmitted infections and is stored and transported under optimum conditions. Transfusion under supervision of trained personnel for all who need it irrespective of their economic or social status through comprehensive, efficient, and a total quality management approach will be ensured under the policy.[11]

AMENDMENTS IN THE DRUGS AND COSMETICS ACT

The Drugs and Cosmetics Act, 1940 are amended from time to time to meet the latest standards. The DCGI issued a notification following an order from the Supreme Court in January 1998 that blood should not be collected form paid professional donors. The Government of India issued a notification under the Drugs and Cosmetics Act and Rules and made the test for HIV mandatory in 1989. The Drugs and Cosmetics Act (Part X B and Part XII B of schedule F) were again amended in 1992-93; the DCGI and CLAA must approve the license of notified drugs (ie, blood and blood products, intravenous fluids, vaccines, and sera).

In accordance with the Supreme Court order, blood bank legislation has been extensively revised in April 1999 to include good manufacturing practices, standard operating procedure, and validation of equipment. The rules thereafter were amended thrice until 2003. Under these rules, no blood bank can function without having license from the CLAA of the Ministry of Health and Family Welfare, and the license has to be renewed on expiry of validity. The outdoor blood donation camp can be held only by a licensed Government Blood Bank, Indian Red Cross Society, and a licensed Regional Blood Transfusion Centre approved by State Blood Transfusion Council.

Per an announcement made on the Website of the Central Drugs Standard Control Organization (CDSCO)[12] there are about 2517 blood banks in India. The Website was last updated in June 2011. Per the Website, there are about 973 (38.6%) blood banks managed by the central or state government; 1544 (61.3%) blood banks are designated as private charitable type. All these blood banks are governed by the Drugs and Cosmetics Act, 1940, which needs revision because of advancement in transfusion science and new practices coming into the routine blood bank management. This was a recent attempt by the CDSCO in this direction and the draft was discussed among many experts at different state levels. Recommendations are also sent to the DCGI (I) by multiple groups. Per the available document from expert groups, proposed amendments need more discussions at the time of this writing. This document should serve as a model regulatory document for all Asian countries, as there are many similarities in standards in this region. Hopefully, there will be a new Drugs and Cosmetics Act in the near future.

REFERENCES

1. Sibinga CT. Transfusion medicine in developing countries. Transfus Med Rev 2000; 14(3):269–74.
2. Epstein J, Seitz R, Dhingra N, et al. Role of regulatory agencies. Biologicals 2009;37: 94–102.
3. World Health Organization. Blood Transfusion Safety. Available at: www.who.int/ bloodsafety. Accessed December 20, 2011.
4. Epstein J. Best practices in regulation of blood and blood products. Biologicals 2012;40(3):200–4.
5. US Food and Drug Administration. Blood and Blood Products. Available at: www.fda. gov/blood & blood product. Accessed December 20, 2011.
6. Drugs and Cosmetics Act and Rules. Government of India, Ministry of Health & Family Welfare, 1940.
7. Transfusion Medicine Technical Manual. 2nd edition. Directorate General of Health Services, Ministry of Health & Family Welfare; 2003. p. 384.
8. Choudhury N. Need to change present regulatory framework for blood banks in India. Asian J Transfus Sci 2011;5(1):1–2.
9. Sarin ML, Giani HS, editors. The Blood Bankers' Legal Handbook. Chandigarh: Sarin Memorial Legal Aid Foundation; 2003.
10. Ramani KV, Mavlankar DV, Govil D. Study of Blood-transfusion Services in Maharashtra and Gujarat States, India. J Health Popul Nutr 2009;27(2): 259–70.
11. National AIDS Control Organization, Department of AIDS Control, Ministry Health & Family Welfare, Government of India. National Blood Policy. Available at: www.nacoonline.org/upload/publication. Accessed December 21, 2011.
12. Central Drugs Standard Control Organization, Directorate General of Health Services, Ministry of Health & Family Welfare, Government of India. Number of Licensed Blood Banks in the country up to July 2011. Available at: www.cdsco. nic.in. Accessed December 21, 2011.

Distant Testing in Laboratory Hematology and Flow Cytometry— The Indian Experience

Amar Das Gupta, MD, PhD[a,b,*]

KEYWORDS

- Distant testing • Laboratory hematology • Preanalytic variables
- Transportation-associated changes

KEY POINTS

- Outsourcing or sending out of patients' samples to other laboratories for hematologic investigations is a common practice these days.
- Preanalytic variables that alter cellular parameters and levels of analytes in transit and on storage can significantly and adversely affect interpretation of test results in hematology.
- Awareness of these changes is necessary to avoid misinterpretation of results that in turn could influence medical management decisions.

WHY DO WE NEED DISTANT TESTING?

All health care providers, for example hospitals, nursing homes, clinics, laboratories, and so forth, outsource or send out tests to laboratories outside their premises. Important considerations that prompt sending out of samples to an outside laboratory are listed as follows. One or more of these factors apply to a given situation:

- Nonavailability of specialized tests locally or at a nearby location.
- Geographic vastness of the region; good laboratories are sparsely distributed.
- Limited capability of in-house or nearby laboratories in performing specialized assays. The outside laboratory has greater testing capability and offers a different and/or wider test menu.

The author has nothing to declare.
[a] Hematology Services, Super Religare Laboratories, S.V. Road, Goregaon (West), Mumbai, Maharashtra, India; [b] International Operations, Super Religare Laboratories, S.V. Road, Goregaon (West), Mumbai, Maharashtra, India
* Super Religare Laboratories, Prime Square Building, Gaiwadi Industrial Estate, S.V. Road, Goregaon (West), Mumbai 400062, Maharashtra, India.
E-mail address: adasgupta@srl.in

Clin Lab Med 32 (2012) 301–314
http://dx.doi.org/10.1016/j.cll.2012.04.004
0272-2712/12/$ – see front matter © 2012 Elsevier Inc. All rights reserved.

labmed.theclinics.com

- Setting up of complex tests requires major investment in equipment, space, and manpower. Smaller laboratories have limited capability and affordability in this respect.
- Small number of complex tests requires batching of assays for cost-effectiveness. This requirement in turn leads to delay in report. Reference laboratories can address this issue.
- For central testing of clinical trial samples.

Therefore, availability of distant testing facilities offers several advantages to the patients and the medical community:

- Focus on and availability of esoteric testing.
- Technologies and resources pooled, greater feasibility and viability.
- Complex tests made cost-effective.
- Wider range of tests.
- Availability of tests to a larger population directly or through network laboratories and collection centers.
- This arrangement creates logistic and information technology (IT) infrastructure that is not available otherwise.

Operational success of reference laboratories that aim to offer the previously mentioned services would obviously depend on successful implementation of effective logistic and IT supports that ensure quality of systems and processes at every step in the testing chain.

COMPLETE BLOOD COUNT

Complete blood count (CBC) is one of the most commonly prescribed investigations. This fact coupled with the ready availability of facilities for performing CBC preclude the need to transport samples for this investigation to a distant laboratory in day-to-day medical practice. Hence, awareness and knowledge of changes in cellular parameters brought about by storage and transport of blood samples over long periods of time are not commonplace. However, this issue can assume importance in the context of clinical trials, which require samples from various trial sites located in different parts of the country to be sent to a central clinical laboratory. Reference laboratories too receive samples for CBC as a part of a test panel containing tests that are not available at the local laboratories, for example, a hemoglobinopathy screening panel consisting of a CBC, hemoglobin (Hb) electrophoresis, and high-performance liquid chromatography (HPLC) for Hb.

A variety of hematology analyzers are available that follow impedance or flow cytometry principles for performing CBC. Blood samples for CBC are collected in evacuated tubes containing di- or tripotassium ethylenediamine tetra-acetic acid (K_2 or K_3EDTA). These samples are normally transported at ambient temperature. Each of the cellular constituents of blood shows changes in its number and volume with passage of time at this temperature. According to some studies, K_2 EDTA has been shown to maintain the stability of cellular parameters for a longer period of time than K_3 EDTA, especially when the ratio of blood to the anticoagulant is incorrect,[1] although others have not confirmed this finding.[2]

Aging-related changes start appearing early in these cells and manifest as increased volume due to swelling of the cells and progressive reduction in their number. Initially though, these changes are mild, progress slowly, and do not alter the cellular parameters significantly for a considerable period of time. Different types of cells are affected differently, for example, platelets and white blood cells (WBCs) are more vulnerable to these changes than red cells. Also, analyzers differ in their ability to capture these changes depending on the measuring principles used. An earlier study using a particular brand of hematology analyzer has shown that normal and high WBC and platelet counts are stable for up to 7 days at ambient temperature whereas low counts tend to decline faster, and significantly lower counts are observed after 3 to 4 days' storage.[3] The mechanism for reduction in the WBC and platelet counts in stored samples seems multifactorial and extends from cell death and disintegration to trapping of these cells in microclots that are generated over time in blood samples, especially when the latter are transported. Excessive shaking of the tubes and high ambient temperature in transit in tropical climates (if samples are not transported on cool packs) could also contribute to this process. The automated differential white cell counts were found to be very unstable in the study cited above with relative increase in the percentage of neutrophils, lymphocytes, and eosinophils as early as day 2 on storage at room temperature. Monocyte percentage declined during this period. Other studies have made similar observations.

Red blood cell (RBC) parameters that are independent of the red cell volume, for example, Hb, RBC count, and mean corpuscular hemoglobin (MCH) are the most stable parameters. They are stable beyond 7 days.[3] However, RBC volume, similar to the volume of the other blood cells, is sensitive to changes introduced in the milieu in vitro on storage at ambient temperature beyond 8 hours and tends to cross the normal upper limit within 2 days of storage under these conditions. Potassium efflux and entry of sodium and water inside the red cells as a result of progressive depletion of intracellular adenosine triphosphate (ATP) and consequent failure of the energy-dependent (sodium and potassium ATPase) membrane pumps[4,5] result in cellular swelling. This change has a significant impact on other important red cell parameters that are dependent on RBC volume such as hematocrit, mean corpuscular volume (MCV), and mean corpuscular hemoglobin concentration (MCHC).

One aspect of this issue that has not received the attention of the medical community it deserves is the influence of the measuring principles used by different analyzers on the cellular parameters in aging blood samples. The measurement technologies used by different types of analyzers are impedance, laser-based, flow cytometry, and so forth. Some analyzers pretreat the RBC with chemical reagents, for example detergent, to reduce the influence of poikilocytosis on the measurement of red cell indices (isovolumetric sphering). The red cell reagent causes sphering and partial fixation of the cells.[6] Such procedures compromise the integrity of the red cell membrane and the effects of aging, for example spherocytosis, are magnified[7,8] leading to increase in MCV as early as 8 hours from collection of the sample. In contrast, instruments that analyze RBC in their native state and without any pretreatment show stable results in much older samples.[3]

To determine the magnitude and extent of the problem the author and colleagues conducted a time-scale study to compare the changes in cellular parameters of blood on storage as measured by automated hematology analyzers using different technologies.[9] They sequentially measured red cell parameters of 7 anticoagulated (K$_2$ EDTA) blood samples, preserved continuously at ambient (20–24°C) temperature, at the time of collection and at 12, 24, 36, and 48 hours after collection on three different types of analyzers (one each from Messers Beckman Coulter, Messers Sysmex Corporation, and Messers Bayer Healthcare). The technologies used by the analyzers for cellular analysis are impedance measurement, hydrodynamic focusing, and differential count detection and laser light scattering, respectively. In Bayer analyzer, the red cells are specially treated to render them spherical to reduce the influence of poikilocytosis. Increase in MCV was significantly higher with passage of time in both

Bayer (coefficient of variance [CV] 6.1–7.7) and Sysmex (CV 8.1–10.3) analyzers as compared with Beckman Coulter analyzer (1.8–3.3). Correspondingly, changes in hematocrit and MCHC were more marked in the former two analyzers. Changes in Hb, red cell count, and MCH were not significantly different among the three analyzers. As mentioned, these three parameters are independent of volume changes and therefore also are more stable over time.

Because MCV is an important parameter for determining the red cell size and therefore the type of anemia, instruments that more accurately reflect the actual changes in the red cell parameters on storage should be preferred for analyzing these parameters in blood samples older than 8 hours. This concern assumes greater significance in the diagnosis of the type of anemia in stored blood samples at least in two specific situations, namely, beta-thalassemia trait wherein a mildly low MCV could be masked by swelling of the red cells and a misdiagnosis of latent vitamin B_{12} deficiency (normal Hb but macrocytic red cell indices) could be made in otherwise normal individuals due to an artificial increase in MCV on storage. The artificial treatment of the red cells by the Bayer analyzer to render them spherical seems to enhance the increase in MCV that normally occurs in stored blood with passage of time. Both the conditions are quite prevalent in several communities in the Indian subcontinent. Therefore, the chances of missing a diagnosis of beta-thalassemia trait and of overdiagnosis of latent vitamin B_{12} deficiency will be higher under these circumstances.

The author's data confirmed that analyzers that enhance aging-related changes in the RBC are unsuitable for red cell analysis in older blood samples. This unsuitability has a direct bearing on the type of laboratory where such equipment can be placed—they are not suitable for laboratories that test samples older than 8 hours, for example reference laboratories and clinical trial laboratories, whereas they would be perfectly all right for a hospital laboratory. Therefore, the suitability and the choice of a hematology analyzer should be determined by the type of samples to be processed by the laboratory, and laboratories need to find out this fact by conducting appropriate in-house studies.

COAGULATION ASSAYS

Most coagulation proteins are inherently labile at ambient temperature. Hence if there is a possibility of delay beyond 4 hours prior to testing, the samples need to be frozen down to ultra cold temperature for storage and/or transport. Freezing to −20°C preserves these proteins for a few weeks.[10] For longer storage, the plasma samples need to be kept at or below −40°C, preferably below −80°C.[11] Frozen plasma maintained at or below −20°C can be safely transported from the site of collection to a testing laboratory located far away if all steps in preparation of platelet-poor plasma (PPP) are strictly adhered to. Freezing of plasma samples is also necessary for improving cost-effectiveness of tests, especially while performing specialized coagulation assays because it allows batching of samples and improves efficiency of the laboratory.

Thawing of frozen plasma can lead to precipitation of cryoproteins including factor VIII, von Willebrand factor, and fibrinogen. Inadequate mixing of thawed plasma samples can lead to erroneous results because of unequal distribution of the precipitated proteins in the aliquots dispensed for the actual assays. Centrifugation of thawed plasma is also contraindicated for this reason.

A major yet less appreciated factor that influences results of coagulation assays in transported samples is the time taken for the samples to be frozen down after collection of blood and separation of plasma. Hence in a distant testing scenario, the plasma sample might reach the testing laboratory in a frozen state if transported on dry ice, yet the coagulation factors might have already deteriorated in the sample prior to freezing because of a long time gap between separation of plasma and freezing. This situation not only leads to erroneous results but also wastage of precious time, energy, and money. Obviously, variables that influence results of coagulation tests in near testing conditions are also applicable to distant testing. Therefore, it is important that sample collection and processing centers should minimize the time gap between blood collection and freezing and record this information in the request form for the benefit of the testing laboratory. Only samples processed strictly within the allowable time limit should be accepted by the laboratory to avoid the issues mentioned previously. Of course, strict maintenance of the cold chain is of paramount importance to ensure reliable results.

It has been recommended by some that the sample collection center in a distant testing scenario should include a "pilot" plasma sample from a normal individual in all consignments containing patients' samples for coagulation assays. This approach is based on the premise that abnormal results in the pilot plasma sample would suggest deterioration of the coagulation factors being tested in the patients' samples as well. However, a practical problem in following this recommendation is the potential wastage of the reagent kit anyway if the results of tests in the pilot sample suggest evidence of its deterioration and therefore the laboratory decides not to proceed with the testing of the patients' samples. This necessity is because of the short open-vial stability of most of the reagents for coagulation assays. So once the reagents have been used for testing of the normal sample they are unsuitable for another batch of assay at a later date.

SCREENING COAGULATION ASSAYS

Whereas on one hand freezing of PPP preserves the coagulation proteins, on the other hand some coagulation factors, for example, factor VII, reportedly get activated in cold.[12] Therefore, it has been recommended that samples destined to be tested for prothrombin time (PT) should not be kept in refrigerator or be frozen. This action would impose a serious restriction on the performance of factor VII–dependent assays in plasma samples transported to a central laboratory. Because PT is widely used for monitoring oral anticoagulation therapy, the author and colleagues conducted a study to examine the magnitude of this issue. They froze multiple aliquots of PPP samples from normal adults at −25°C for variable periods of time and estimated PT in these samples sequentially at different time points. As shown in **Table 1**, the author did not observe any significant shortening of PT of either normal PPP on freezing for up to 72 hours. The interassay CV for all the 10 samples tested in this manner was less than 2%. Therefore, contrary to popular belief, freezing of PPP samples does not seem to shorten PT. This finding is of great practical value for it allows performance of PT and PT-based assays on frozen plasma days after collection of the blood sample. This result has a practical bearing especially in the context of central testing of clinical trial samples.

Activated partial thromboplastin time (APTT) is a temperature- and time-sensitive assay. Extremely high APTT (eg, >300 seconds) in a plasma sample that was received from another location (even in a frozen state) should arouse the suspicion of sample deterioration prior to freezing and should be processed further only after verification of sample integrity. This approach would save precious reagents and technologists' time. It is advisable for central laboratories to identify sample collection and processing centers that are chronic offenders in this respect and take appropriate corrective measures.

Table 1 PT of 10 plasma samples							
Sample No.	0 h	24 h	CV (%) 0 vs 24 h	48 h	CV (%) 0 vs 48 h	72 h	CV (%) 0 vs 72 h
1	13.2	13.4	1.44	13.8	3.14	13.3	0.53
2	12.9	12.8	0.55	12.9	0.00	13.1	1.09
3	12.5	12.8	1.68	13.5	5.44	13.0	2.77
4	13.4	14.4	5.09	13.0	2.14	12.7	3.79
5	12.6	12.5	0.56	13.1	2.75	12.5	0.56
6	12.4	12.7	1.69	12.7	1.69	13.1	3.88
7	12.7	12.9	1.10	12.9	1.10	12.3	2.26
8	12.5	12.7	1.12	12.6	0.56	13.0	2.77
9	14.1	13.9	1. 05	13.9	1.01	14.2	0.50
10	13.8	13.7	1.01	13.9	0.51	14.0	1.02
Mean	13.0	13.0	1.44	13.2	1.84	13.0	1.92

Samples were tested fresh (0 hours) and subsequently in parallel aliquots frozen at −25°C for 24, 48, and 72 hours. No shortening of PT is seen in these samples on freezing.

The influence of platelet contamination in shortening the results of all types of APTT-based assays, especially those for detection of lupus anticoagulant, is also well-known.[13] Inadequate removal of platelets because of suboptimal centrifugation of the blood sample results in platelet contamination of plasma (platelet count $>10 \times 10^9$/l). Freezing, thawing, and vortexing of such samples prior to testing lead to breakdown of platelets and generation of membrane fragments rich in phospholipids. These fragments provide more than the required quantity of phospholipid for APTT-based assays thereby shortening the time taken for the clot to form and masking coagulation abnormalities that cause prolongation of APTT. Results of a host of important coagulation assays are adversely affected by this factor.

NATURAL INHIBITORS OF COAGULATION

Inherited deficiencies of protein C (PC), protein S (PS) and antithrombin (AT) are responsible for approximately 3%, 2%, and 1% of cases of venous thrombosis (VT), respectively, in Western populations.[14] The incidence of deficiencies of these three anticoagulants has been reported to be higher in Indians and other South Asian patients with VT.[15,16] Although the difference in the two sets of data could reflect a genuine difference in the incidence of deficiencies of these anticoagulants in the two populations, the role of reduced levels of these proteins following prolonged storage of plasma samples even at an ultra cold temperature needs to be considered. This possibility assumes significance in view of the fact that most laboratories carry out assays for these proteins on batches of plasma samples frozen at or below −20°C for variable lengths of time to reduce the cost of tests. The same logic also holds true for plasma samples transported to reference laboratories in frozen conditions. Furthermore, in the absence of locally established normal ranges for these proteins on account of the high cost of such an exercise, most laboratories in this subcontinent report results of these tests using reference ranges provided by the manufacturers of reagents established in freshly drawn plasma specimens from whites. These facts could be responsible for a falsely higher incidence of deficiencies in PC, PS, and AT in the populations examined by these laboratories as referred to previously. Therefore, the author and colleagues examined the levels of PC, free protein S (FPS), and AT at different time points in plasma samples from normal adults frozen at −25°C to assess the effect of freezing of normal plasma samples on PC, FPS, and AT levels and to determine its potential impact on the interpretation of results of similarly frozen patients' samples.[17]

PC, FPS, and AT levels were measured by clotting-based test, by sandwich enzyme-linked immunosorbent assay and by chromogenic assay respectively in 50 normal plasma samples prior to freezing, and 2 and 4 weeks later in parallel aliquots frozen at −25°C. The mean levels of the three proteins dropped significantly after a fortnight's freezing, PC: 130.7% to 122.8% (P<.0246); FPS: 105.9% to 94.1% (P<.0016); AT: 103.2% to 95.8% (P<.0001). The corresponding interassay CVs of the two sets of results were 8.9%, 6.6%, and 9.3%. Thereafter, only FPS declined significantly (84.3%) (P<.0001) (**Table 2**). In 2 of 48 and 5 of 48 cases at the end of 2 and 4 weeks, respectively, the levels of FPS values went below the lower limit of the normal range established from the 50 plasma samples. Freezing of plasma at −25°C for 24 hours per se did not alter the levels of PC and AT and caused only a negligible change in FPS levels (**Table 3**). Because 6%, 4%, and 14% of normal plasma samples would have been labelled as AT-, PC-, and PS-deficient, respectively, had the tests been performed after 4 weeks of freezing, the author recommends that for correct interpretation of the results, laboratories should establish their reference ranges on normal samples frozen for the same period of time as the patients' samples. Alternatively, all samples awaiting assays for these proteins should immediately be frozen down to or below −40°C prior to testing.

HEMOGLOBINOPATHY TESTING

An accurate diagnosis of thalassemia and structural Hb variants is of great clinical and epidemiologic importance in this subcontinent. HPLC-based technologies have been found very useful in the diagnosis of hemoglobinopathies, in terms of automation, accuracy, capability of handling large number of samples, and speed. However, limited availability of this technology in laboratories in this country dictates that samples for hemoglobinopathy diagnosis would have to be transported to distant laboratories.

In a study extending over a year, a total of 12,866 samples received from various parts of the country were examined by the author and colleagues for hemoglobinopathy diagnosis.[18] Seventy-six (.59%) of these samples were labeled as "problem samples," the reasons being clotted samples: 30, hemolyzed samples: 14, aged samples (> 5 days old): 10, and improper samples: 22. All samples were analyzed on Hb Variant II HPLC system (M/s Biorad, USA) using the "beta-thalassemia short" program. The retention time, the relative percentage of hemoglobin fractions, and the chromatograms were studied in all cases with normal and abnormal Hb.

In addition to a wide variety of beta and some alpha globin chain structural variants and cases of beta and alpha thalassemia, the author observed abnormal Hb peaks in P3 window in 108 cases (.84%). These results were in addition to the Hb variants eluting in P3 window. That these peaks indeed represented an aging-related change was proven by progressive increase in the peaks on further incubation of the sample at ambient temperature (**Fig. 1**). The quantity of these peaks in all the cases was less than 10%. If present in a significant percentage (15%–25%), they need to be distinguished from abnormal Hb variants that elute with retention time (RT) of 1.40 to 1.90 minutes (P3 window), for example Hb J-Norfolk (RT 1.47 minutes), Hb Camden (RT 1.48 minutes), Hb N-Baltimore (RT 1.58 minutes), Hb Grady (RT 1.60 minutes), Hb

Table 2
Levels of natural anticoagulants at different time points on continuous freezing at −25°C

Anticoagulant (Number of Samples)[a]	Day 0 (D0)	Week 2 (W2) Significance (D0/W2)	% Mean CV (D0/W2)	Week 4 (W4) Significance (D0/W4)	% Mean CV (D0/W4)	Significance (W2/W4)	% Mean CV (W2/W4)
Antithrombin activity (%) (50)	103.2 (80–125)[b]	95.8 (70–122)[b] $P<.0001$ (significant)	8.9	95.0 (60–122)[b] $P<.0001$ (significant)	7.9	$P<.5885$ (not significant)	7.8
Protein C activity (%) (40)	130.7 (80–200)[b]	122.9 (67–195)[b] $P<.0246$ (significant)	6.6	116.8 (70–200)[b] $P<.0008$ (significant)	10.6	$P<.1431$ (not significant)	7.9
Free protein S level (%) (48)	106.0 (70–153)[b]	94.1 (70–151)[b] $P<.0016$ (significant)	9.3	84.3 (40–110)[b] $P<.0001$ (significant)	20.5	$P<.0001$ (significant)	12.9

Statistical significance of the changes in the levels of the three anticoagulants at week 2 and week 4 compared with day 0 and the mean interassay CV of the paired results of each sample for each anticoagulant at these time points are also indicated.

[a] PC and FPS were estimated in 40 and 48 samples, respectively.

[b] Values in parenthesis are ranges.

Table 3
Levels of AT, PC, and FPS in 20 plasma samples before and after freezing at −25°C for 24 hours

Anticoagulant	Day 0	After 24 Hours of Freezing	% Interassay CV (Mean)
Antithrombin activity (%)	111.0 (96–126)[a]	112.0 (99–125)[a]	1.5
Protein C activity (%)	134.0 (103–184)[a]	136.0 (105–177)[a]	3.8
Free protein S level (%)	96.0 (66–110)[a]	92.0 (62–114)[a]	4.5

Mean CV derived from assay results in paired aliquots of each sample before and after freezing for 24 hours is also indicated for each anticoagulant.

[a] Values in parenthesis are ranges.

Fannin Lubbock (RT 1.68 minutes), Hb J-Baltimore (RT 1.72 minutes), Hb J Meerut (RT 1.88 minutes) and Hb J-Bangkok (RT 1.90 minutes). This issue can be settled by the fact that (a) the quantity of structurally abnormal Hb eluting in P3 window is usually more than 25%, and (b) in the case of acquired P3 peak further incubation of the sample leads to increase in the level of the peak as described previously (**Fig. 1**). Finally, electrophoresis of the sample at the right pH and medium would clinch the diagnosis in most cases.

FLOW CYTOMETRIC IMMUNOPHENOTYPING

The high cost and complexity of the technology involved in flow cytometric immuno-phenotyping of hematolymphoid cells demand that facilities for performing these tests be centralized. Therefore, the number of laboratories performing these tests is very small in resource-poor countries. This limitation also implies that samples from remote locations need to be transported to central laboratories for testing with the associated risk of cellular changes in transit that could affect the final result. Awareness of these changes mandates that the testing laboratories should establish criteria for accepting and processing of transported samples. This consideration is true for both lymphocyte subset enumeration and immunophe-notyping of hematolymphoid neoplasms. Guidelines for collection and transport of samples for flow cytometry–based assays that could reduce artificial changes in cells on account of storage and transport are available.[19]

CD4 LYMPHOCYTE SUBSET ENUMERATION

There are several strategies for measuring lymphocyte subsets. Single-platform technologies use multicolor (2–4) reagent panels and a predefined number of fluorescent beads to measure the absolute CD4 lymphocyte counts, whereas dual platform techniques use the percentage CD4 lymphocyte count from the flow cytometer and absolute lymphocyte count from the hematology analyzer to derive the absolute CD4 count.[20] Whichever strategy is used, the most essential requirement for accuracy of lymphocyte subset counts is the ability of the flow cytometer to separate the various subpopulations of leucocytes in the primary scatter plots used for this purpose, for example CD45/side scatter channel (SSC) or forward scatter channel/SSC. With aging of blood samples distinction among these subpopulations becomes increasingly blurred because of a number of cellular changes that include downregulation of CD4 and other leucocyte-associated antigens and changes in cell size and granularity. They in turn result in

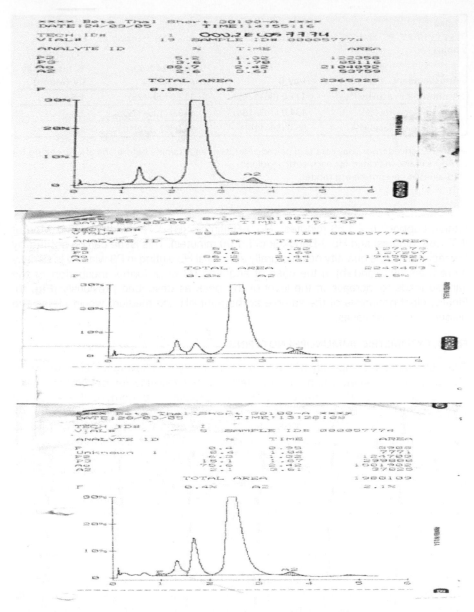

Fig. 1. Progressive increase in P3 peak from 1.70 % on day 2 to 5.6% on day 3 and 6.3% on day 4 in the same sample on storage at room temperature for 4 days.

inaccuracies in the counts. The matter is further complicated by progressive cell death as the sample becomes older. Downregulation of CD4 receptors on lymphocytes and cell death also occurs in human immunodeficiency virus (HIV) infection. Although published data and guidelines for acceptability of older blood samples for lymphocyte subset enumeration are available, the actual experience may vary from laboratory to laboratory depending on the ground realities.

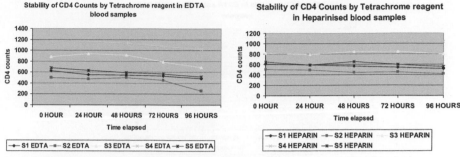

Fig. 2. CD4 lymphocyte counts in the same five samples as shown in Fig. 3A but processed using PLG CD4 reagents. Contrary to expectations, the counts were found to be more unstable than those obtained by the 4-color antibody panel. Counts in EDTA anticoagulated samples were again more unstable than those in heparinized samples.

Therefore, it is recommended that laboratories involved in lymphocyte subset enumeration in transported and aged samples should establish their acceptability criteria through appropriately conducted in-house studies. The author's own experience, as described later, strongly supports this approach.

Some equipment and reagent manufacturers have marketed reagents and software that circumvent the issues referred to above. PanLeucogating (PLG) CD4 reagent (M/s Beckman Coulter, USA) is one such reagent that is reported to have yielded more accurate CD4 counts in older blood samples compared with other similar reagent combinations by virtue of a clear separation between CD4 lymphocytes and monocytes.[21] This two-color (CD45-fluorescein isothiocyanate/CD4-phycoerythrin) single-platform reagent was field tested in South Africa to determine CD4 lymphocyte counts in samples transported to a central laboratory and was found to yield stable counts in up to 5-day old samples.[22–24] The author and colleagues reevaluated the actual performance of this method and compared the results with those of another established, more expensive single-platform technology. EDTA and heparinized blood samples from 127 healthy adult men and 128 women were tested by two-color PLG CD4 reagents (CD45/SSC/CD4 sequential gating), and 20 of these were tested in parallel by a four-color tetrachrome reagent from the same vendor (CD45/SSC/CD3/CD4/CD8 gating). Stability of the counts was checked by both the methods at timed intervals in samples retained up to 5 days at room temperature.

There was a high degree of correlation between the CD4 counts obtained by PLG and by tetrachrome reagents ($r^2 = .97$). Results from EDTA anticoagulated samples tested by PLG CD4 reagents showed a better stability (up to 48 hours) compared with those from heparinized samples (up to 24 hours). However, the stability of the counts in heparinized samples by PLG was significantly inferior to that by tetrachrome (72 hours) (**Figs. 2** and **3**).

CD4 enumeration by PLG CD4 reagents is cheaper and is comparable in accuracy and reproducibility to more expensive reagent panels. However, this technology seems less suitable for samples more than 48 hours old, especially if collected in EDTA. This time frame is contrary to the claim made by the manufacturer of the reagents and some published studies referred to previously. It is noteworthy in this context that the time scale study conducted by the author and colleagues was in controlled temperature of the laboratory (22–25°C) whereas in reality samples are

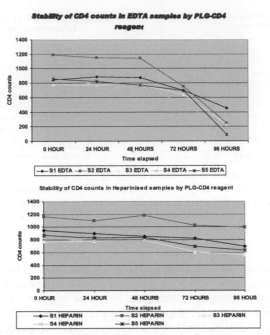

Fig. 3. CD4 lymphocyte counts at different time points in five samples collected in parallel in EDTA and in heparin using a 4-color reagent panel. Counts are more stable in EDTA anticoagulated samples than those in heparin.

transported in ambient temperature that can reach very high levels in tropical countries. This factor could further lower the already low CD4 lymphocyte counts in HIV-infected patients.

IMMUNOPHENOTYPING OF HEMATOLYMPHOID NEOPLASMS

By virtue of their abnormal metabolic pathways secondary to the disease-associated molecular lesions, neoplastic cells in some hematolymphoid malignancies are more prone to cell death compared with the normal cells or even other types of neoplastic cells. Burkitt lymphoma cells and T-cell malignancies are examples of such diseases. Therefore, preferential loss of cells of interest could pose a major problem in transported samples in these conditions. The problem gets further compounded if the number of such cells in the sample is low to start with. However, in view of the precious nature of the cells, the laboratory should try to interpret the results and give a diagnosis as far as is practical under the circumstances.

REFERENCES

1. Goossens W, Van Duppen V, Verwilghen RL. K_2- or K_3-EDTA: the anticoagulant of choice in routine haematology? Clin Lab Haematol 1991;13:291–5.
2. Hess R, Greenwalt TG. Storage of red blood cells: new approaches. Transfus Med Rev 2002;16:283–95.
3. Gulati GL, Hyland LJ, Kocher W, et al. Changes in automated complete blood count and differential count results induced by storage of blood at room temperature. Arch Pathol Lab Med 2002;12:336–42.

4. Dern RJ, Brewer GJ, Wiorkowski JJ. Studies on the preservation of human blood. II. The relationship of erythrocyte adenosine triphosphate levels and other in vitro measures to red cell storageability. J Lab Clin Med 1967;69:968–78.

5. Wolfe LC. The membrane and the lesions of storage in preserved red cells. Transfusion 1985;25:185–203.

6. Lippi G, Salvagno GL, Solero GP, et al. Stability of blood cell counts, hematologic parameters and reticulocyte indexes on the Advia A120 hematology analyzer. J Lab Clin Med 2005;146:333–40.

7. Raat NJ, Verhoeven AJ, Mik EG, et al. The effect of storage time of human red cells on intestinal microcirculatory oxygenation in a rat isovolemic exchange model. Crit Care Med 2005;33:39–45.

8. Moser K, Seelenbinder F, McFadden S, et al. Selecting a new analyzer for the hematology laboratory; the experience at Ohio Health Hospitals. Laboratory Hematology 2001;7:245–54.

9. Das Gupta A, Jeswani K, Khadapkar R, et al. Changes in red cell indices in stored blood are instrument and method dependent. Laboratory Hematology 2006;12(Suppl 1):181–2.

10. Arkin CF. Collection, transport and processing of blood specimens for coagulation testing plasma-based coagulation assays: approved guideline. 4th edition. Wayne (PA): National Committee for Clinical Laboratory Standards; 2003.

11. Woodham B, Girardol O, Blanco MJ, et al. Stability of coagulation proteins in frozen plasma. Blood Coagul Fibrinolysis 2001;12:229–36.

12. James H, Morrissey B, Macik G, et al. Quantitation of activated factor VII level in plasma using a tissue factor mutant selectively deficient in promoting factor VII activation. Blood 1993;81:734–44.

13. Tripodi A. Laboratory testing for lupus anticoagulants: a review of issues affecting results. Clin Chem 2007;53:1629–35.

14. Rosendaal FR. Venous thrombosis: a multicausal disease. Lancet 1999;353:1167–73.

15. Angchaisuksiri P, Atichartakarn V, Aryurachai K, et al. Risk factors of venous thromboembolism in Thai patients. Int J Hematol 2007;86:397–402.

16. Ghosh K, Shetty S, Madkaikar M, et al. Venous thromboembolism in young patients from western India: a study. Clin Appl Thromb Hemost 2001;7:158–65.

17. Das Gupta A, Sharma A. Impact of reduced levels of protein C, free protein S and antithrombin in normal frozen plasma on the interpretation of patients' results. Blood Coagul Fibrinolysis 2012;23:51–5.

18. Das Gupta A, Ghosh S, Syed K, et al. Spectrum of hemoglobinopathies encountered on HPLC analysis at a central reference laboratory. Int J Lab Hematol 2008;30(Suppl 1):129–30.

19. Stetler-Strevenson M. Clinical flow cytometric analysis of neoplastic hematolymphoid cells-approved guidelines. 2nd edition. Wayne (PA): Clinical and Laboratory Standards Institute; 2007.

20. Das Gupta A, Ochani Z. Single platform enumeration of lymphocyte subsets in healthy Indians aged between 18 and 49 years. Cytometry B Clin Cytom 2006;70B:361–2.

21. Glencross D, Scott L, Jani I, et al. CD45-assisted PanLeucogating for accurate, cost-effective dual-platform CD4+ T-cell enumeration. Cytometry 2002;50:69–77.

22. Glencross DK, Stevens W, Mendelow BV. Laboratory monitoring of HIV/AIDS in a resource poor setting. S Afr Med J 2003;93:262–3.

23. Glencross DK, Janossy G, Coetzee LM, et al. Large-scale affordable PanLeucogated CD4+ testing with proactive internal and external quality assessment: in support of the South African national comprehensive care, treatment and management programme for HIV and AIDS. Cytometry B Clin Cytom 2008;74B(Suppl 1):S40–51.

24. Mandy FF, Nicholson JK, McDougal JS. Guidelines for performing single-platform absolute CD4 T-cell determinations with CD45 gating for persons infected with human immunodeficiency virus. CDC and prevention. MMWR Recomm Rep 2003; 52:1–13.

Clinical Trials and Contract Research Organizations in India

Shoibal Mukherjee, MD, DM

KEYWORDS

- Clinical trials • Research • India • CRO • Research quality • Compliance

KEY POINTS

- Economics and demography are driving drug development to the developing world. India needs this opportunity to build research skills required to combat its enormous disease burden.
- A variety of global and local contract research organizations (CROs) that specialize in the execution of research to develop health care products operate in India today.
- CROs assure quality and compliance to regulations while coordinating with tertiary providers such as a site management organization and the central laboratory.
- Back room operations to manage, analyze, and report data form a bulk of the employment generated by clinical research, absorbing programmers, data managers, biostatisticians, and medical writers.
- Despite rapid growth and strong potential, India remains a minor contributor to global pharmaceutical research because of policy stagnation, regulatory gaps, and misinformed controversies in the media.

Clinical trials are integral to the development of new medicines, diagnostics, and medical devices. Because there is no other way to demonstrate the effectiveness and safety of new therapeutic modalities for human use or their equivalence or superiority over existing therapy, regulatory authorities require a series of clinical trials to be conducted and their results analyzed before a new treatment can be introduced for general consumption. Every claim that is made in the package insert of a pharmaceutical product must be backed up with evidence from clinical trials. Consequently, clinical trials account for almost 60% of the time and resources required to bring a new drug to market.[1] Yet most of this investment is wasted, because over 80% of new products tested in clinical trials fail to live up to the promise of improvement over existing therapy, and therefore have to be abandoned.

Indeed, the explosive growth of life science technologies juxtaposed with the growing complexity of the science behind discovery and development of new

Quintiles Research Private Limited, 8th Floor, DLF Square, Jacaranda Marg, DLF City Phase II, Gurgaon, Haryana 122002, India
E-mail address: shoibal.mukherjee@quintiles.com

Clin Lab Med 32 (2012) 315–320
http://dx.doi.org/10.1016/j.cll.2012.04.008
0272-2712/12/$ – see front matter © 2012 Elsevier Inc. All rights reserved.

medicines have led to a situation where, despite the plethora of new leads, the conventional research pathway in the developed world has become too expensive and increasingly unaffordable, even for the largest corporate entities.[2] The lower cost of research talent in developing countries, the larger size of study populations in countries like China and India, and the fact that the pharmaceutical markets in these countries is now approaching the size of historically large markets of Europe and North America, are driving pharmaceutical research to developing countries. In India this trend is further accentuated by public health investments being made by nonprofit organizations and investments in drug development research by the local industry. Indeed, given the fact that India is home to the world's highest disease burden in absolute terms,[3] it is imperative that the country take steps to combat that burden through prowess in the development of breakthrough health care products.

CONTRACT RESEARCH ORGANIZATIONS

The early part of the last decade saw substantial growth of clinical research capability. Many local and multinational companies set up clinical development units in the country,[4] as did several nonprofit entities and publicly funded research bodies under the Department of Biotechnology and the Indian Council of Medical Research. These units were supplemented by contract research organizations (CROs)—companies with specific specialization in the execution of research for the development of health care products. Today there are a variety of CROs operating in India—from those involved in discovery research to those specializing in the various aspects of preclinical and clinical research. The clinical CROs are the most numerous because entry barriers are relatively low.

Clinical CROs undertake execution of clinical projects on behalf of a sponsor. This practice is good for sponsors because the skills necessary to execute a clinical trial are very specific and divorced from the basic research, manufacturing, and marketing competencies that sponsors may have. For smaller sponsors who have a single or small number of products to develop, this partnership ensures that they do not have to hire an army of staff to execute a single project and then lay them off once the project is over. So, once an entrepreneur has translated an original scientific idea into a molecule that can combat disease and has put it through the animal tests required to prove that it can be given to patients without unacceptable safety risks, a CRO can be hired to conduct the clinical trials that will be required to collect the data necessary to define the use of the product by patients. CROs are generally capable of doing the rest, which includes preparing a clinical development plan, writing the clinical protocols, obtaining regulatory approvals to conduct clinical trials, contacting health care practitioners to recruit patients into the study using informed consent procedures approved by an ethics committee, ensuring meticulous documentation of the effects of the drug when administered according to the protocol, collecting and analyzing the data, and writing a final report for regulatory submission.

To accomplish these tasks a CRO usually has several departments of qualified and trained individuals: a regulatory department trained in the rules and regulations governing clinical trials; a site identification and start-up unit that maintains contact with health care professionals and institutions that may serve as investigators and sites for the study and ensures that these sites have the necessary infrastructure and staffing to undertake trials; a clinical operations group that works with the investigators at the site to train the team on the study protocol and ensure that the study is conducted in line with complex Good Clinical Practice[5] guidelines; a quality assurance department that conducts periodic audits of study to point out deficiencies if any and ensure that these are corrected and preventive measures put in place; a medical

Table 1	
Parties to a clinical trial: the role of various bodies involved in the clinical trial process	
Sponsor	Discovers, funds, and develops new therapies from bench to bedside. Has commercial incentives to ensure appropriate funding and progress of each project. Has high stakes in the accuracy and validity of data. Bears high reputational risk and financial penalties for misconduct.
Regulator	Reviews protocols and data to ensure compliance to regulations and ethical guidelines for each trial at the national level. Conducts inspections to monitor compliance.
Contract research organization	Coordinates the conduct of clinical trials across sites, countries, and regions. Reviews data to ensure accuracy and eliminate fraud. Organizes and analyses data for reporting and submission to regulators.
Investigator	Supervises the informed consent and patient recruitment process, is responsible for care and well-being of patients and compliance to protocol, regulations, documentation.
Ethics committee	Reviews protocols and safety data to safeguard the rights and well-being of patients locally at the site level.
Data safety monitoring board	Periodically reviews data to determine whether it is safe and meaningful to continue with a trial. Recommends changes to the protocol to safeguard patient safety.
Site management organization	Coordinates clinical trial activities at the site level. Ensures appropriate documentation of all trial-related activities.
Central laboratory	Used to ensure standardization for key laboratory tests, including pathology, imaging, and electrophysiological studies across multiple sites worldwide.

department to review medical aspects of the protocol and product safety; a data management group that is responsible for designing and commissioning electronic databases for the patient data that would emerge from the study; a biostatistics department that would analyze the data using scientific techniques; and a medical writing group that would prepare the final report in line with regulatory guidances (**Table 1**).

ASSURING QUALITY AND COMPLIANCE

An important aspect of the CRO's role is to assure compliance to the myriad rules and regulations governing clinical trials. CROs do this by employing trained monitors (also called clinical research associates or CRAs) who frequently visit the sites and review the documentation at the sites to preclude fraud, ensure that informed consent procedures are followed, ensure that the data captured by the investigators are accurate and verifiable, and ensure that the study drugs are being stored and used in line with the protocol. Site staff often need to be trained on Good Clinical Practice guidelines and other aspects of managing trial activities at the site. In the past CROs have organized such training programs. More recently, public-private partnership initiatives have been put in place with active involvement of federal government agencies toward this end in order to build capacity in clinical development with particular focus on public health interventions.[6]

CROs often need to work with other third party providers. One such is the site management organization, which provides trained staffing resources to guarantee quality of documentation at sites. For busy investigators this function can be the difference between research excellence and a critical audit observation. Many large hospitals set up their own site management department that keeps track of all clinical research activities being undertaken in the hospital and, for a fee, helps sponsors coordinate with investigators, the ethics committee, pathology and imaging departments, and the pharmacy—all within the hospital.

The central laboratory is another such provider. Use of a central laboratory for key laboratory tests, especially when such tests are part of the primary or secondary end-points being studied, ensures that the conduct of these tests is standardized across sites and patients and that accreditation and audit requirements can be applied to a single laboratory rather than a multiplicity of laboratories across sites.

Laboratories that participate as a central laboratory in clinical trials must consistently live up to expectations that go beyond what is usually required in the course of routine clinical care. Central laboratories can expect to receive samples for testing from diverse locations within the country and overseas. They therefore need to collaborate with a courier facility for smooth pick-up and dispatch of samples, with minimal sample miscarriage so that need for resampling is minimized, if not eliminated. This function requires thorough training of site teams on sample collection and storage. Reagents and sampling equipment must be shipped to sites before the start of the study and replenished in a timely manner. The central laboratory must have quicker testing turnaround time, when possible, to make up for time lost in sample transportation because clinicians are loath to have to wait longer for test results. The results themselves must be communicated back to the clinician by swift electronic means. Record-keeping and long-term record traceability are essential. Special foolproof systems are required to avoid sample mixups, and the laboratory must be open to audits and possible inspection by regulatory authorities. Participation in external quality control programs and advanced accreditations are now basic requirements. In India, certification by the National Accreditation Board for Testing and Calibration Laboratories is considered mandatory, and accreditation by the College of American Pathologists is highly desirable.

THE LARGE BACK ROOM

The back end activities of a CRO can be quite extensive. Electronic data capture systems must be programmed to receive data from the sites, a process of data triage and cleaning is necessary to ensure that the data entered into the database are internally consistent and complete. Data sets are then passed on to the biostatisticians who supervise programming of the statistical software and run the programs on the dataset received from the data managers. The tables, lists, and figures thus generated are passed on to the medical writers for preparation of the final report in the exhaustive ICH E3[7] format that is accepted across most of the world. The nonclinical work involved may account for as much as 40% (and sometimes more) of the effort involved in a clinical trial. India has now grown to become an important location for off-shoring such back end work in clinical data management, biostatistics, pharmacovigilance, and medical writing, employing more people than in the core clinical domain.

A FUTURE WITH POTENTIAL AND UNCERTAINTY

Clinical research in India grew at a fast pace between 1995 and 2008, and by 2008–2009 there were several hundred projects ongoing across the country. The global financial crisis of 2009 led to a slowing down of that pace, and in 2010 the

Table 2
Current issues surrounding clinical trials in India

Informed consent	Sporadic reports of patients signing informed consent without adequate comprehension of the information in the consent form points to the need for closer scrutiny of the process. Video recording of the informed consent discussion between the investigator and patient has been suggested as a means of ensuring that investigators spend time with patients to explain the risks and benefits of participating in a clinical trial.
Compensation for trial-related injury	Inadequate process detail and lack of fair balance in the determination of causality and compensation payouts has led to uncertainties that have resulted in sponsors hesitating to include India in their global drug development plans.
Deaths reported from clinical trials	Misinterpretation of figures by the media has led to the impression that clinical trials are to blame for deaths of patients participating in clinical trials. Closer analysis should reveal the potential for clinical trials to reduce mortality not only because commercial incentives drive sponsors toward more effective and safer drugs, but also because in resource-starved situations, clinical trials assure better access to health care.
Financial irregularities at sites	Alleged cases of investigators working in public institutions diverting clinical trial funding into personal accounts has led sponsors to insist on tripartite arrangements with institutional administrators in order to ensure transparency of funding and of the utilization of funds.
Fraud and data manipulation	Occasional cases of fraud by investigator or site staff have been identified by CRO monitors. Cases of fraudulent ethics committees have also come to light. These instances highlight the need for proscriptive regulatory provisions against fraud and a system of approval and accreditation of ethics committees.

number of projects submitted for regulatory approval in India shrunk by about 25%. Although the demand has picked up again thereafter, India remains a very small player in the global clinical development effort, with no more than 2% to 3% of the world's trials including India as a location.[8]

Despite great potential, regulatory delays and controversies surrounding clinical trials in India (**Table 2**) threaten to further stagnate the country's transition toward becoming a global hub for drug discovery and development. Misconceptions about clinical trials in India generally stem from ignorance of the processes and safeguards inbuilt into the system. In addition there are gaps in regulatory oversight and enforcement that keep regulators from being able to ensure and certify compliance to guidelines at the site level across a multiplicity of sites. Technicalities involved in the analysis and interpretation of outcomes have often led to misrepresentation of facts. It is hoped that these uncertainties will resolve over time. Much will depend on the development of science-based regulatory reforms and the success of indigenous entrepreneurship.

REFERENCES

1. DiMasi JA, Hansen RW, Grabowski HG. The price of innovation: new estimates of drug development costs. J Health Econ 2003;22:151–85.

2. Grabowski H. Are the economics of pharmaceutical research and development changing? Productivity, patents, and political pressures. Pharmacoeconomics 2004;22(Suppl 2):15–24.
3. World Health Organization. The global burden of disease: 2004 update. Geneva (Switzerland): WHO; 2008. Available at: http://www.who.int/evidence/bod. Accessed December 21, 2011.
4. Mukherjee S. Pharmaceutical research development in India – looking up? Business briefing: Future Drug Discovery 2006:73–7. Available at: http://www.touchhealthsciences.com/authors/dr-shoibal-mukherjee. Accessed December 21, 2011.
5. Guideline for Good Clinical Practice E6(R1). International Conference on Harmonisation of Technical Requirements for Registration of Pharmaceuticals for Human Use. Available at: http://www.ich.org/fileadmin/Public_Web_Site/ICH_Products/Guidelines/Efficacy/E6_R1/Step4/E6_R1_Guideline.pdf. Accessed December 21, 2011.
6. Clinical Development Services Agency. Progress Report for the period September 2010 to August 2011. Available at: http://cdsaindia.in/Progress_Report_CDSA_Sep_2010_to_ Aug_2011.pdf. Accessed December 21, 2011.
7. Structure and Content of Clinical Study Reports E3. International Conference on Harmonisation of Technical Requirements for Registration of Pharmaceuticals for Human Use. Available at: http://www.ich.org/fileadmin/Public_Web_Site/ICH_Products/Guidelines/Efficacy/E3/Step4/E3_Guideline.pdf. Accessed May 3, 2012.
8. ClinicalTrials.gov. Location-wise map of open studies. Available at: http://clinicaltrials.gov/ct2/results/map?recr=Open. Accessed December 21, 2011.

Medical Tourism in India

Vijay Gupta, PGDBM[a],*, Poonam Das, MD[b]

KEYWORDS

- Medical tourism • India • Health care • Nonresident patients

KEY POINTS

- The term *medical tourism* is under debate because health care is a serious business and rarely do patients combine the two.
- India is uniquely placed by virtue of its skilled manpower, common language, diverse medical conditions that doctors deal with, the volume of patients, and a large nonresident Indian population overseas.
- Medical tourism requires dedicated services to alleviate the anxiety of foreign patients. These include translation, currency conversion, travel, visa, posttreatment care system, and accommodation of patient relatives during and after treatment.

Medical tourism is an activity wherein people travel to another country for medical, surgical, or dental care that is either not available or not affordable in their own country. The term *tourism* also suggests combining health care with leisure travel.[1] The term *medical tourism* is debatable. A number of alternate terminologies like *medical value travel* and so forth are being used. The industry can be divided into three groups:

- Outbound: patients traveling to other countries for medical care
- Inbound: foreign patients traveling into the developed countries for medical care
- Intrabound: patients of any country traveling within their own country for medical care.

Health care in India has emerged as one of the largest service sectors in India. It is expected to contribute 8% of gross domestic product and employ about 9 million people this year.

A Price Water House Report titled "Healthcare in India", indicates that Indian Healthcare sector will reach $40bn by 2012. It is estimated to be growing at 13–15% CAGR.

The ratio of doctors to patients—at 60 per 100,000 people—is also relatively high, although the quality of medical training varies.

The authors have nothing to declare.

[a] P.D. Hinduja National Hospital and Medical Research Centre, Veer Savarkar Marg, Mahim, Mumbai 400016, Maharashtra, India; [b] Laboratory and Transfusion Services, Max Healthcare, 2, Press Enclave Road, Saket, New Delhi 11017, India
* Corresponding author.
E-mail address: vijay.gupta@hindujahospital.com

Clin Lab Med 32 (2012) 321–325
http://dx.doi.org/10.1016/j.cll.2012.04.007
0272-2712/12/$ – see front matter © 2012 Published by Elsevier Inc.

labmed.theclinics.com

Medical tourism is a fast-growing industry in many developing nations. India boasts of internationally accredited multi- and superspecialty hospitals having some of the world's most talented doctors combined with advanced facilities. Multispecialty hospitals in metropolitan areas offer excellent standards of quality with a sterile environment and tailored care.

According to a Wharton School article published in IndiaKnowledge@Wharton in June 2011, India's share in the global medical tourism industry will reach around 3% by end of 2013. The December 2010 report titled, "Booming Medical Tourism in India," says that the industry should generate revenues of around US $3 billion by 2013.

Today, India offers the most advanced equipment and procedures, for example robotic surgery and cutting-edge radiosurgery cancer treatment for tumors under nonstationary therapy. The success rates are very high with mortality rates comparable to or better than anywhere in the world. These results in some cases even surpass those of the developed world. The multispecialty hospitals are designed to cater to the international patients.

MARKET SIZE AND TRENDS

World Medical Tourism market is estimated to be close to $100bn currently. It is estimated that 1.3 million medical tourists go to Asia each year. South Korea, Singapore, Hong Kong, Malaysia, and Thailand are emerging as important medical tourism destinations in Asia (**Table 1**).

Table 1
Comparison of major Asian destinations for medical tourism

Major Destination	Medical Tourists, Millions	JCI-Accredited Hospitals	Range of Costs (% of US cost)	Popular Treatment Options
India	0.45 (in 2007)[2]	19	6%–21%	Alternative medicine, bone marrow transplant, cardiac bypass, eye surgery, and hip replacement
Thailand	1.54 (in 2007)[3]	34	6%–28%	Alternative medicine, cosmetic surgery, dental care, gender realignment, heart surgery, obesity surgery, oncology, and orthopedics
Singapore	0.41 (in 2006)[4]	22	8%–33%	Organ transplants, stem cell transplants, and other high-end procedures
Malaysia	0.29 (in 2006)[5]	9	6%–23%	Cardiovascular surgery, cosmetic surgery, dental care, eye surgery, general surgery, orthopedic surgery, and transplant surgery

Abbreviation: JCI, Joint Commission International.
Joint Commission International website . Available at: http://www.jointcommissioninternational.org/JCI-Accredited-Organizations/. Accessed April, 2012; Deloitte Center for Health Solutions. Medical tourism: consumers in search of value. 2 Joint Commission International Web site; 2008. p. 1–30. Available at: http://www.deloitte.com/view/en_HR/hr/industries/lifescienceshealthcare/964710a8b410e110VgnVCM100000ba42f00aRCRD.htm. Accessed April 20, 2012; and Grail Research (A division of Integreon). Preview document. Available at: http://www.grailresearch.com/Solutions/ViewSolution.aspx?id=62. Accessed April 20, 2012.

The medical tourism market in India is fast-growing and is expected to touch US $2 billion in 2012 according to Forbes Magazine. India's medical tourism industry is projected to grow at an annual rate of 20% to 30 % by 2015. A study conducted by the Confederation of Indian Industry says that in 2005 around 150,000 foreigners visited India for medical treatment, and the number is rising by 15% every year. By 2015, 3.2 million medical tourists are estimated to arrive in India. States of Andhra Pradesh, Karnataka, Tamil Nadu, Maharashtra, West Bengal, and New Delhi have been acknowledged as the foremost destinations for medical tourists when visiting the country. These states have excellent quality medical infrastructure for complex medical operations.

The patient inflow distribution data show that about 22% of medical tourism to India comes from the nonresident Indians residing abroad, 18% comes from Africa, 16% to 17% comes from the Middle East and Bangladesh, Sri Lanka, and Nepal. Around 8% to 9% comes from Afghanistan and Iraq, and 4% to 6% comes from Europe and the United States.

India offers high – cardiac, Obesity, pediatric, dental, cosmetic and orthopedic surgical services as well as traditional healing systems. It is also recognized as the cradle for test – tube babies and is popular for surrogacy services.[6] The medical tourism does not cater to emergency services. The services provided are largely knee joint replacement, hip replacement (mostly orthopedic), bone marrow transplant, bypass surgery, cosmetic surgery, and so forth. Hospitals also advertise for preventive health checkups for family members accompanying the patients in addition to alternative medicine services.

Some of the major advantages to medical tourists include:

1. **Virtually no waiting time** even for advanced treatments.
2. **Availability of latest medical technology, skills, knowledge, and resources.**
3. Highly qualified surgeons of hospitals with **international accreditations**, complying with high quality standards. India has 19 Joint Commission International–accredited hospitals in major metropolitan areas. Similarly, National Accreditation Board for Hospitals and Healthcare Providers, the Indian quality standard, is becoming rigorous and widely acceptable. The same goes for other types of quality accreditation in health care including International Organization for Standardization, and so forth.
4. **No language barrier in most cases.** The travel industry is well-understood, and in most cases the providers are in a position to set seamless processes to alleviate patient anxiety. Medical tourism–focused hospitals usually have an International Patients' Department that interacts with the consultant after receiving a query and even arranges for a telephone meeting if required. Interested patients are issued a visa facilitation letter for the embassy. If needed, the department also facilitates stay, travel, and currency exchange facilities besides a translator.
5. **Traditional Indian alternate medicine and wellness systems.** With Ayurveda gaining popularity worldwide, this ancient Indian therapy can be used as a nonsurgical treatment for various ailments along with meditation and yoga.[7]
6. **Diverse availability of tourist destinations.** Leisure tourism is in great demand in India because of the country's rich diverse cultural and scenic beauty. India offers a diverse choice of leisure destinations, ranging from high mountains, vast deserts, scenic beaches, historical monuments and religious places.
7. **Comparative cost of treatment.** Health care assumes a very high cost in the developed world compared with India. The treatment costs in the United States can be as high as10 times those in India. Currently in the United States, there are

Table 2 Cost of various surgeries (amount in US $)				
	United States	India	Thailand	Mexico
Heart bypass	130,000	7000	11,000	20,000
Angioplasty with one stent	57,000	7000	13,000	15,000
Knee replacement	48,000	8000	14,000	11,000
Hip replacement	43,000	8000	12,000	14,000
Bariatric surgery	65,000	9000	14,000	9000

These costs are indicative, and actual expenses would vary based on the specific treatment package of the patient.
Peacock L. Medical tourism in India. Smart Travel Asia; 2009. Zenith International Journal of Multi Disciplinary Research 2011;2. Available at: http://www.zenithresearch.org.in. Accessed April 20, 2012.

approximately 47 million people without health insurance and 120 million without dental coverage. When an emergency strikes the common man, especially the uninsured, they find it hard to meet estimated expenses. This is a major reason for travel. **Table 2** gives a comparison of costs for major surgeries in the United States and other countries.[7,8]

India is in a strategically advantageous position to further tap global prospects in the medical tourism sector. The role of government as a facilitator is important even though the private sector along with trade bodies have taken lead in developing this segment. Convenient visa processing mechanism along with tracking of such travel besides better infrastructure for patient transport will help India realize it's true potential. Today the healthcare services in India are concentrated in large metros, which are endowed with better infrastructure and treat almost all such medical tourists.

International market is changing with more and more countries entering into the fray, to the benefit of the international patients who now have wider choice. This is beginning to show its impact on the Indian healthcare sector, as well, with many Indian providers are expanding their network overseas through development, acquisitions or affiliations tapping into the advantage of various geographic locations and making their brand more familiar.

These recent developments have also facilitated the return of many doctors who had gone overseas to study, as they can now practice in an environment they are familiar with. Besides the skills these doctors bring with them international associations. For international patients this has meant familiar practices and continuity in treatment, once they return to their home countries.

Cultural, racial and geographic diversity, coupled with large population also means a wide range of conditions to treat in large numbers. This results in better experience for Indian doctors to treat a wider range of conditions compared to many other countries. For an international patient medical travel overseas is worthwhile only for high-end procedures. Going forward India will have to develop strong position, for itself or specific regions within, for specific treatments to make choice easier. This means clear communication and showcasing specific strengths rather than all.

The insurance companies also need to develop new products that allow for coverage in distant locations through international partnerships. Already the new cross-border health care legislation allows European Union citizens to travel and receive medical treatment in any European Union country. This legislation could be a model that can be perfected at a regional level. Travel agents and the hotel industry also have a part to play.

The general image of a destination as a hygienic and tourism-friendly country goes a long way in developing medical tourism. Of course publicity, particularly negative, needs to be managed carefully to ensure a fair share of medical tourism.

REFERENCES

1. Medical Tourism: Consumers in Search of Value (Deloitte). Available at: http://www.deloitte.com/view/en_HR/hr/industries/lifescienceshealthcare/964710a8b410e110VgnVCM100000ba42f00aRCRD.htm. Accessed April 20, 2012.
2. Deloitte Center for Health Solutions. Medical tourism: consumers in search of value. 2 Joint Commission International Web site; 2008. p. 1–30. Available at: http://www.deloitte.com/view/en_HR/hr/industries/lifescienceshealthcare/964710a8b410e110VgnVCM100000ba42f00aRCRD.htm. Accessed April 20, 2012.
3. Grail Research (A division of Integreon). Preview document. Available at: http://www.grailresearch.com/Solutions/ViewSolution.aspx?id=62. Accessed April 20, 2012.
4. Top 5 medical tourism destinations. Nuwire Investor. March 2008.
5. Numbers of note. Business Today. December 2008.
6. Imrana Q, John ME. The business and ethics of surrogacy. Economic and Political Weekly 2009;44(2):10–2.
7. Dawn SK, Pal S. Medical tourism in India: issues, opportunities and designing strategies for growth and development. International Journal of Multidisciplinary Research 2011;1(3):7,10.
8. Peacock L. Medical tourism in India. Smart Travel Asia; 2009. Zenith International Journal of Multi Disciplinary Research 2011;2. Available at: http://www.zenithresearch.org.in. Accessed April 20, 2012.

International Reference Laboratories

Palat K. Menon, MD, PhD

KEYWORDS

- Overview • International reference laboratories in India
- Quality Management Systems • Laboratory Information Management system
- Accreditations

KEY POINTS

- International reference laboratories hold many benefits for India. They invest in innovation technology and large-scale operations and try to attain cost-efficient testing.
- These laboratories set up good quality management systems with good laboratory practices and excellent laboratory information management systems.
- Continuous improvement in operations is driven by Lean and Six Sigma.
- These laboratories are globally harmonized using similar testing platforms, kits, reagents, and controls.
- International reference laboratories help to enhance the quality of diagnostic testing as well as provide globally harmonized testing for clinical trials.

INTRODUCTION

Laboratories working across international boundaries can generate information that cannot be achieved by any one institution working in isolation. New world-class clinical laboratory networks are expanding in developing countries such as India, facilitated through transfers and exchanges of methods, data and information, people with expertise, and biological materials. Constraints to this process include limited funding, protection of intellectual property rights, communication barriers, and legal and regulatory controls. Formal Networks of Excellence, established and funded by the European Union, and global initiatives inspired by international organizations such as the Food Agriculture Organization and World Health Organization have established standardized public laboratories in different parts of the world.[1,2] Enhancing public and private laboratory capabilities and capacity is essential for generating reliable and

DISCLOSE ANY RELATIONSHIP: The author works as the Senior Medical Director for Quest Diagnostics Laboratory at Gurgaon in India.
Quest Diagnostics India Pvt. Ltd, A17, Info City, Gurgaon, Haryana, India 122001
E-mail address: pkmenon@airtelmail.in; pkrish@vsnl.com

Clin Lab Med 32 (2012) 327–340
http://dx.doi.org/10.1016/j.cll.2012.04.013
0272-2712/12/$ – see front matter © 2012 Elsevier Inc. All rights reserved.

accurate data from clinical research and providing laboratory testing, especially in resource-constrained settings.

In this article the author describes many of the multinational private clinical laboratory chains and discusses the unique information and technical support they provide in establishing new world-class clinical laboratory operations, thus expanding capabilities and capacity. The specific focus is on the opportunities for multinational clinical laboratories in India.

Establishing clinical laboratory networks involves more than acquiring new equipment and reagents; it also requires a long-term commitment to staff training and development, quality control, and biosafety. Four key areas are of importance in such laboratory chains.

1. Understanding the testing menu appropriate at each level of a tiered, integrated clinical laboratory network and how this evolves over time.
2. Standardization of laboratory equipment and supplies at each level of the tiered network; ready availability of reagents, calibrators, controls, and facility for ready maintenance and servicing of equipment.
3. Selection and provision of consistently high-quality training and development for laboratory scientists and personnel are vital. All personnel must actively participate in continuing education programs and technical assessments to ensure ongoing standardized quality across the globe.
4. A comprehensive quality system and safety program are essential in ensuring consistency of reliable laboratory results and the safety of personnel and patients served.

India is an economically emerging nation, with a population that is young (median age of 25 years vs 36 years in China and 45 years in Japan), growing, earning more, and simultaneously becoming more aware of its human rights and environmental and international obligations. In general, industry and government are struggling with the transition from traditional mediocrity on one side to its more recent quest for excellence on the other. Customer awareness of quality is increasing, and quality services are being increasingly sought after. Health care is no exception to these dynamics.

Currently, outside of the government, nearly all health care expenses are paid out of pocket. Recently, the population covered by health insurance has been increasing, driven in part by the influx of international companies that provide medical insurance coverage in their home countries. Accordingly, health insurance is emerging as one of the primary sources of funding individual and family health care. The need for high-quality clinical laboratory testing is a cornerstone for evidence-based medicine with laboratory results involved in more than 70% of health care decisions. Good health care decisions will rely on the emergence of only those laboratories following good laboratory practice (GLP) and with accreditation from reputable international organizations such as the College of American Pathologists (CAP) and with International Organization for Standardization (ISO) certification. Sophisticated testing requirements, especially in the areas of personalized medicine and companion diagnostics, are coming of age as specific less toxic therapies emerge for targeted therapy. International reference laboratories play an important part to fulfill these requirements. International reference clinical laboratories, by virtue of their scale and scope of operations, are able to invest in innovation, make the significant initial and ongoing investments in latest technology, transfer innovations and expand licenses, provide for cost efficacies, and weather the time investment in new operations. Over time, the new clinical laboratories may provide specialized testing and evolve as centers of excellence as their turnovers increase. International reference laboratories form the nidus from which will emerge scientists and technicians with exposure to GLP, good quality management systems (QMSs), laboratory operations, standardizations, validations, and advanced technology, thus providing the seeds for further expansion of local capabilities and capacity.

Many reference laboratories have set foot tentatively into India. This article examines the various factors that are driving this move and its significance.

WHY DO BUSINESS IN INDIA

Multinational companies seeking long-term growth that may be limited in the United States and Europe are focusing their attention on fast growing economies of India and China with a combined population of 2.4 billion. India and China will be the global economic center of gravity by 2050. Accordingly, most multinational companies have either entered India and China or are in the process of establishing themselves in this region. The barriers to invest and conduct business in India are falling. Among the top reasons[3] making India an attractive industrial destination are

1. In terms of population, by 2025, India will likely be the most populous country in the world. With continually extended life expectancies since its independence, by 2025 the number of people 60 years and older is estimated to be 189 million, creating a large demand for chronic disease care.
2. India's gross domestic product is increasing every quarter at more than 7%, making it the 11th largest economy in the world. India is increasingly turning into an industrialized economy and is ranked 12th in the world in terms of nominal factory output.
3. India's gross national income (GNI) per capita is growing, and in less than 10 years the GNI per capita doubled (from $1560 in 2000 to $3250 in 2009). The middle and upper classes are growing rapidly.
4. India is a democratic country with a system of laws based on the English system. Historically imposing bureaucratic barriers and corruption are being addressed.
5. There are nearly 800 million mobile phone subscribers in India, and it is also the second largest telecommunication network in the world in terms of number of wireless connections (after China). Wireless Internet is going to massively enhance the access of millions of Indians across the subcontinent.

Regarding the health care industry, English is the primary language in medicine, making language less of an issue than in other countries. Medical practice is a combination of traditional medicine (Ayurvedic medicine, Unani, and acupuncture), especially in rural areas, and modern (Western) allopathic medicine, especially in urban areas. Medical infrastructure is being built throughout the country with approximately 70% of hospitals being privately funded and operated.

As with other industries that have planted roots in India, private multinational clinical laboratories are establishing themselves in India too. The immediate need perceived in setting up of networks of harmonized laboratories worldwide is to cater to the need of multinational clinical trials (CTs) for the pharmaceutical industry. Pharmaceutical companies are attracted to India because of the ease in recruiting investigators and study participants who have not been previously exposed to many treatments, the high compliance rate among study investigators and participants, and the lower operational costs compared with the United States, Europe, and Japan.

GLOBAL PRESENCE OF INTERNATIONAL REFERENCE LABORATORIES

Ten major multinational laboratory networks are outlined in **Table 1**. There are no global laboratory networks that operate in countries serving most of the world's population. In addition to the companies listed, there is a new wave of investors in clinical laboratories including General Electric and Nestlé, companies with extensive international experience and deep financial resources.

INTERNATIONAL REFERENCE LABORATORIES
Eurofins

Eurofins operates central laboratories through its six facilities in the United States, Netherlands, France, India, Singapore, and China.[4] The predecessor of Eurofins Global Central Laboratory was founded in 1973 as SML/BCO, an independent spinoff from the Saint Ignatius hospital in Breda, Netherlands. In 1992, Sandoz set up Medinet as a joint venture with BCO, a network of routine testing laboratories in Breda; Paris; Cologne, Germany; Copenhagen, Denmark; and London. In the 1990s, this European network was replaced to meet the need to accommodate globalization of clinical trials and the joint venture Clinical Reference Laboratory Medinet was established. Medinet was acquired by Analytico in 1999. In 2001 Analytico itself was acquired by Eurofins. Since 2006, Eurofins Medinet added wholly owned laboratories in the United States, France, Singapore, China, and most recently India, to replace the partner laboratory network. The global infrastructure has included fully standardized partners in Argentina, South Africa, and Japan. The laboratory testing portfolio is broad and offers the synergy of integrated safety assessment, biomarkers, bioanalysis, therapeutic drug monitoring, pharmacokinetics of biopharmaceuticals, immunogenicity testing, genomic testing, and a full range of services to support drug development. Certified and licensed laboratories perform a comprehensive menu of routine and customized safety and efficacy tests, including biochemistry, hematology, urinalysis, flow cytometry, and many more to support clinical research programs of any size and complexity.

Eurofins in India

Eurofins Global Central Laboratory in Bangalore, India, is part of the chain of laboratories set up by Eurofins across globe to cater to local needs of global studies. The Bangalore laboratory complements the Eurofins Global Central Laboratory's current global footprint of wholly owned laboratory facilities in the United States, Europe, Singapore, and China. Eurofins Global Central Laboratory, Bangalore, has put in place a similar quality management system as in its either Europe or United States laboratories, which confirms to ISO 15189 and/or CAP requirements. Eurofins uses globally identical platforms, calibrators, and controls at their facilities, thus giving the vendors a result that is harmonized. The QMS of Eurofins Global Central Laboratory is designed to encompass both the international and country-specific quality standards. A high level of standardization enables collecting and integrating laboratory data from multiple laboratories. Utilization of global standard operating procedures, uniform instruments, reagents, and analytical methods for safety testing enables the use of global reference ranges, generating laboratory data that are globally harmonized. Eurofins Global Central Laboratory has a dedicated global standardization team responsible for executing internal and external proficiency programs including CAP, Bio-Rad, and National Glycohemoglobin Standardization Program (NGSP) level 1 testing programs. Between the Eurofins facilities, the same lot numbers of quality control materials are used, and quality control results are monitored on a continuous basis (Karanth R, MD, Bangalore, Karnataka, India, personal communication, December 2011).

Table 1
Major multinational laboratory networks

Company	North America	Europe	India	China	Other–Asia Pacific	Known Affiliate Laboratories
ACM Global	Rochester, NY	New York, United Kingdom	Mumbai			Beijing, China; Melbourne, Australia
Clearstone	Ontario, Canada	France; Germany		Beijing	Singapore	
Covance	Indianapolis, IN	Geneva, Switzerland		Shanghai	Singapore	Japan
Eurofins	Washington, DC	Netherlands; France	Bangalore	Shanghai	Singapore	
Icon	Farmingdale, NY	Dublin, Ireland	Bangalore	Beijing	Singapore	
LabCorp	Burlington, NC with United States national operations	Belgium				Australia; India; Israel; Singapore; South Africa
PPD	Highland Heights, KY	Belgium		Beijing	Singapore	
Quest Diagnostics	Valencia, CA; Madison, NJ with United States national operations	Heston, United Kingdom; Ireland	Gurgaon			Brazil; Argentina; Shanghai; Singapore
Quintiles	Durham, NC	Edinburgh, Scotland	Mumbai	Beijing	Singapore	
Sonic Healthcare	Operates in multiple states	Belgium; Germany; Ireland; Switzerland; United Kingdom			Australia; New Zealand	

ICON Central Laboratories

ICON Central Laboratories (ICL), Inc, is headquartered in Farmingdale, New York.[5] ICON provides global central laboratory services from core facilities in New York; Dublin, Ireland; Singapore; India; and China. Since 2000, ICON has successfully managed the laboratory and associated investigator and logistical support requirements for hundreds of clients in virtually every phase and therapeutic area of clinical development. Its laboratories are accredited by the CAP and also have the ISO 17025 quality certification. Its parent company, ICON plc, is a global provider of outsourced development services to the pharmaceutical, biotechnology, and medical device industries. The company specializes in the strategic development, management, and analysis of programs that support clinical development—from compound selection to phase I to IV clinical studies. ICON teams have successfully conducted over 5500 development projects and consultancy engagements across all major therapeutic areas. ICON currently has over 6500 employees, operating from 72 locations in 38 countries. ICON is dedicated exclusively to central laboratory testing and the associated services for clinical trials. ICL's global network of facilities in the United States, Ireland, Singapore, India, and China operate with identical analytical platforms, standard operating procedures (SOPs), quality control materials, and reagents to support large global studies.

ICON in India

Since their inception in Bangalore, India, in the year 2008, ICON has successfully managed the laboratory and associated investigator and logistical support requirements for thousands of clients in virtually every phase and therapeutic area of clinical development. Clinical research and development is a global endeavor, and every aspect of ICL's central laboratory service revolves around that requirement. From the time of study setup to data lock, every department at ICL works to blend the global consistency in operating procedures and database management with the unique local needs of investigator sites to offer a comprehensive service package (Rajput A, MD, Bangalore, Karnataka, India, personal communication, December 2011).

LabCorp

Laboratory Corporation of America Holdings,[6] with approximately 26,000 employees, is an independent clinical laboratory company headquartered in Burlington, North Carolina. LabCorp has approximately 1500 patient service centers along with a national network of laboratories and rapid response laboratories. Through its national network of laboratories, the company offers a wide range of clinical laboratory tests that are used by the medical profession in routine and specialized testing, LabCorp tests on more than 440,000 patient specimens daily and provides clinical laboratory testing services to clients throughout the United States, Puerto Rico, Belgium, and three provinces in Canada. Its clients include physicians, hospitals, managed care organizations, governmental agencies, employers, pharmaceutical companies, and other independent clinical laboratories. LabCorp also offers paternity testing, often used by the courts. LabCorp earned $5.0 billion in revenue and $1.22 billion in earnings before interest, taxes, depreciation, and amortization (EBITDA) in 2010.

In December 2010, Genzyme Corporation sold its genetic testing business to the LabCorp Esoterix Genetic Laboratories, LLC (Genzyme Genetics), a provider of complex reproductive and oncology testing services and the preferred provider for such services to maternal fetal medicine specialists and obstetrician/gynecologists in the United States. In December 2011, the company completed the acquisition of Orchid Cellmark, Inc. LabCorp has many specialty facilities that include the Center for

Molecular Biology and Pathology (molecular pathology); National Genetics Institute, Inc (Genetics); Viro-Med Laboratories (virology), and others.

LabCorp in India
LabCorp is setting up operations in India.

Quest Diagnostics

Originally founded in 1967, Quest Diagnostics was spun off from Corning, which owned the company from 1982 through 1996. Quest Diagnostics, with 42,000 employees, is the leading provider of diagnostic testing, information, and services. Quest Diagnostics offers a broad test menu in the industry with more than 3000 tests covering all medical specialties including dentistry.[7] It provides harmonized testing operations globally by standardized equipment, kits, controls and calibrators, and constant peer group review of its data. SOPs are constantly revised to ensure best practices. Its clients include physicians, hospitals, managed care organizations, governmental agencies, employers, pharmaceutical companies, and other independent clinical laboratories. The company is focused primarily in the United States, with US sales accounting for greater than 90% of overall sales. Quest Diagnostics also operates in Puerto Rico, Mexico, South America, Europe, and Asia. An interesting innovation is Care360, used by over 165,000 physicians in the United States to order laboratory tests, deliver timely test results, share clinical information quickly and securely, and prescribe drugs. Quest Diagnostics earned $7.4 billion in revenue in 2010. Quest Diagnostics provides testing services for clinical trials, risk assessment services for the life insurance industry, preemployment drug testing, and employer-sponsored wellness programs. In addition, Quest Diagnostics manufactures and markets diagnostic tests for sale to other laboratories and directly to physicians.

Some of the specialty facilities include Nichols Institutes (esoteric testing), Focus Diagnostics (infectious disease), Oral DNA Labs, AmeriPath (histopathology), HemoCue (point-of-care testing), Celera (genome sequencing), ExamOne (insurance testing), and so forth.

Quest Diagnostics in India
In India Quest Diagnostics[8] has set up a 65,000 square foot laboratory with all pathology subspecialties including safety testing, microbiology, molecular diagnostics, biomarkers, anatomic pathology, and cytogenetics in 2007. Its aim in India is to bring a quantum change in the availability, accuracy, reproducibility, and reporting of diagnostic testing and therapeutic monitoring services. The quality standards followed are as prescribed by National Accreditation Board Laboratories (NABL) (under ISO 15189) and the CAP. The laboratory in India is NABL and CAP accredited. It has also acquired NGSP level I certification.

Quintiles

Quintiles Transnational is a pharmaceutical services company offering clinical, commercial, consulting, and capital services. It was founded in 1982.[9] The network consists of more than 20,000 employees in 60 countries. It manages clinical trials on behalf of pharmaceutical customers and provides the following services:

- Management of clinical trials, data, projects, and laboratory services
- Providing customers with sales force, product, and brand solutions
- Providing data-driven recommendations to help customers achieve success
- Creating strategic partnerships through financing and operational solutions.

It has helped develop or commercialize a majority of the best selling drugs. It operates a network of wholly owned, CAP-accredited central laboratories that offer therapeutically-focused solutions to meet the clinical trials safety and esoteric testing and services needs of the biopharmaceutical industry.

Quintiles in India

The Quintiles Central Laboratory in Mumbai, which opened in 2007, has provided investigators with all of the quality, flexibility, and speed needed to run efficient clinical trials. There are uniform instrumentation and SOPs similar to all laboratories in Quintiles, so that results from Mumbai are directly comparable with those from a similar laboratory anywhere else in the world. The Mumbai laboratory operates in an area of 8300 square feet, employs a staff of 48 professionals, and offers project management, protocol planning and management, sample management, archival services, investigator support services, quality assurance, preanalytical services, kit building services, and logistics support services (S. Menon, Director, Lab Operations, Quintiles, Mumbai, Maharashtra, India, personal communication, December 2011).

Sonic Healthcare

Based in Sydney, Australia, Sonic Healthcare, with more than 23,000 employees, is a multinational medical diagnostics company offering extensive laboratory medicine, pathology, and radiology services to the medical community. Sonic Healthcare's revenues are nearly US $3.4 billion, with EBITDA of US $618 million. Approximately 30% of its overall business is laboratory testing based in Australia, 23% in United States, and 18% in Germany. The company seeks fragmented markets and then bolsters operations by its economies of scale and by identifying synergies with ongoing operations.

Sonic Healthcare has no operations in India.

MENU

The majority of international laboratory networks in India have established themselves as a means of supporting international clinical trials from a laboratory perspective. Specimen viability, turnaround time, and logistics costs are the primary factors to establish these laboratories. The clientele dictate the testing menu of these laboratories and are predominantly into safety testing.

Laboratory networks like Quest Diagnostics have invested in infrastructure to cater not only to CT but also to the diagnostic marketplace. They have been instrumental in bringing new technology and new tests into the Indian market. They provide laboratory investigations for various diseases ranging from the most routine to the most advanced molecular genetic disorders based on clinical chemistry, hematology and coagulation, microbiology, enzyme immunoassays, anatomic pathology and cytology, flow cytometry, and conventional and molecular cytogenetics. There are few small niche laboratories in India that focus only on one or a select specialty or technology.

ACCREDITATIONS

Accreditations help ensure central laboratory testing standards are maintained and that results are accurate, reliable, and comparable wherever they are produced. Through education and promotion of best practice, accreditation helps ensure that the results of investigations are reliable and harmonized wherever they are produced. The accreditations acquired by International laboratories include

- The College of American Pathologists, United States.
- The NABL, Department of Science and Technology, Government of India, with reciprocal accreditations to International Laboratory Accreditation Council and the Asia Pacific Laboratory Accreditation Council. The standards laid down by NABL are in accordance with ISO 15189:2003.
- ISO 9001 certification (global).
- ISO 27001 for information technology (code federal regulations [CFR] part 11 audit and compliance) for information technology systems.
- Northwest Lipids Certificate of Traceability (global).
- NGSP certification.

All international reference laboratories performing diagnostic testing in India have obtained CAP certification. Additionally, laboratories in India have obtained certification for local regulatory purposes from NABL under the ISO 15189. CAP has interestingly started to provide accreditation under ISO 15189 in the United States. Another certification commonly acquired by international reference laboratories in India is the NGSP, for hemoglobin A1c testing.

EXTERNAL QUALITY ASSURANCE SERVICE PROVIDERS

Participation in high-quality interlaboratory programs is important for laboratories to ensure the reliability and precision of their testing systems. It is a powerful and effective mechanism for providing information and improving laboratory analytical performance and harmonization between interlaboratory groups, which are critical to significant peer comparisons. These external quality assurance services (EQAS) programs help the laboratory recognize analytical process improvement opportunities and increase confidence in proficiency survey outcomes.

National EQAS Programs (India)

National EQASs are basic programs and do not segregate data obtained from participating laboratories based on type of instrumentation/kits used.

- The Department of Hematology at the All India Institute of Medical Sciences runs a cost-efficient hematology EQAS program.
- The Department of Biochemistry at the Christian Medical College Vellore runs a cost-efficient biochemistry EQAS program.
- The Microbiology Department at the Shankar Nethralaya Eye Institute runs a microbiology EQAS program.

International EQAS Programs

International EQAS programs segregate data obtained from participating laboratories based on type of instrumentation/kits used. The commonly subscribed EQAS programs include

- CAP
- UK National EQAS
- Bio-Rad.

STAFFING AND TRAINING

Despite having English language–based training, recruitment of good well-trained staff and staff retention are issues. Most laboratory staff require retraining in fundamentals of GLP, computer skills, electronic document management, record keeping, archival of documents and specimens, and the QMS. There is an extreme shortage of well-trained technologists, cytotechnologists, molecular biology technologists, diagnostic technologists, cytogenetics technologists and genetic counsellors for cytogenetics. There is a lack of opportunity for training in the local laboratories, and reference laboratories need to invest a lot of time and effort to ensure optimal training of staff to meet regulatory requirements. Once trained in GLP, they become extremely valuable and are actively recruited by competing laboratories.

LABORATORY OPERATIONS

The necessity and importance of harmonizing laboratory operations to ensure that the laboratory results generated in facilities around the world can be easily combined cannot be overemphasized. Utilization of global SOPs, uniform instruments, reagents, and analytical methods for safety testing enable the use of global reference ranges, resulting in global laboratory data that are truly combinable. A global footprint ensures specimen integrity, optimal turnaround time of results, and manageability of the logistic process and associated costs. It also helps optimize profits by assessing workflow and updating methodologies to reflect technical opportunities and clinical needs. It is important to be aware of the global changing regulatory requirements that impact upon a laboratory's compliance and ability to do business. It is important to optimize operations by increasing laboratory utilization and enhancing the clinical and financial value of laboratory services.

LABORATORY INFORMATION MANAGEMENT SYSTEMS

As the needs of the modern laboratory vary widely from laboratory to laboratory, similarly, expected deliverables from a laboratory information management system (LIMS) also shifts.[10] LIMS is a software-based system that offers a set of key features that support a modern laboratory's operations. Those key features include workflow, sample management, assay data management, data mining, data analysis, risk calculations, algorithms, data reporting, billing, and other support functions. Ideally these functions should be accomplished completely within a single software solution. This goal may not be possible and may require other software in the database to provide a complete solution. LIMS needs a flexible architecture, standardized databases, and smart data exchange interfaces with equipment that fully supports its use in regulated environments.

From the initial LIMS in the 1970s that were developed by a few individual laboratories, LIMS have evolved over time to use of automated reporting tools, use of relational databases, use of client/server architecture, advanced data processing capabilities, web-enabled LIMS, the adoption of XML standards, and the development of Internet ordering and reporting.

The core function of LIMS has traditionally been the seamless management of samples to result delivery. This function typically is initiated when a sample is registered in the LIMS. This registration process may involve preaccessioning a sample at the collection point, accessioning the sample on receipt in the laboratory, and producing barcodes to enable the analytical equipment to recognize the sample tube and carry out the relevant tests. Various other parameters such as clinical or phenotypic information corresponding with the sample are also often recorded. Reports are generated with age- and sex-appropriate normal ranges. The LIMS then tracks chain of custody as well as sample location often down to the granular level of shelf, rack, box, row, and column. The successful transfer of data files in Microsoft Excel and other formats, as well as the import and export of data to Oracle, SQL, and Microsoft Access databases are pivotal aspects of a the modern LIMS.

Regulatory Requirements

LIMS users may also have regulatory concerns to comply with such as Clinical Laboratory Improvement Amendments, Health Insurance Portability and Accountability Act, GLP, and Food and Drug Administration specifications (CFR part 11 compliance). One key to compliance with many of these standards is an audit trail of all changes to LIMS data, and in some cases a fully electronic signature system is required for rigorous tracking of field-level changes to LIMS data.

The exponentially growing volume of data created in laboratories coupled with increasing business expectations and focus on profitability have pushed LIMS to enhance ability for large volume electronic data processing and exchanges. 3G (and futuristic 4G and 5G) personal digital assistants and tablets will integrate with the LIMS. Standardized database management systems such as Oracle and SQL play an important role in how data is managed and exchanged in laboratories.

LIMS systems are commercially available off the shelf, for example, NeTLIMS and STARLIMS. Many laboratories use legacy system LIMS that have evolved with their growth over time. LIMS in the United States provide bidirectional communication with physician and hospital practices. Laboratory tests requests are electronically received, and test reports are electronically delivered. Test results are incorporated into patients' electronic health records that encompass pharmacy, radiology, consults, and the breadth of medical services.

ELECTRONIC DOCUMENT CONTROL AND TRAINING MANAGEMENT SYSTEMS

Conventionally, SOPs are created using Microsoft Word, printed out, and stored in binders. The binders are physically sent from one approver to the next. Once approved, the contents of the binder are photocopied so every affected department will have one binder handy. A manual system poses many challenges, including inefficiency, poor communication, lack of training, ineffective documentation, poor revision control, poor collaboration, and lack of visibility. Development of effective SOPs and proper implementation require continued management commitment and oversight. Implementation of appropriate software solutions to facilitate and improve SOP management is important and decreases document control challenges seen in a paper-based SOP system. An efficient and effective electronic SOP management system is a foundation for an organization's sustainable compliance and long-term success in the market. Most reference laboratories rely on electronic document control (EDC) and training management systems (TMSs)–based SOPs.[11] An EDC system addresses the challenges by automating routing, delivery, and storage of SOPs with a secure, centralized electronic repository that makes search and retrieval easy. The system will continue to send notifications until the person acts on an SOP. It incorporates escalation, so if the person is unavailable for a period of time, the SOP will move to the next person authorized to approve it.

By integrating training control with SOP management and other quality processes, all employees affected by new or revised SOPs are automatically sent training tasks. Implementation of a progressive training program by sequencing training courses becomes possible. The system thus provides a time-stamped audit trail that captures the identity of anyone who creates, views, or changes an electronic record; when the action occurred; and the changes made. Along with the stamp, users are asked to enter a reason for every change. Only approved documents are released and made available to the users. Obsolete SOPs do not resurface. Setting an expiration date makes an SOP obsolete on that date, and it will automatically be archived. Automatic revision control ensures that when an SOP is revised it is available for checkout until approval of the revision.

SITE SELECTION FOR A REFERENCE LABORATORY

Site selection for a central laboratory in India is a challenge. It cannot be located in residential areas primarily because of its size and nature of business. Recently the Government of India passed a gazette notification deeming laboratories to be small-to medium-scale enterprises. Following this notification it is possible to locate central laboratories in business parks as small medium enterprises. This regulation has advantages in terms of power supply, licensing, labor, and logistics approach. Also, the local supply of skilled technologists and scientists may influence site location.

INDIAN LABORATORY NETWORKS DEVELOPING A GLOBAL FOOTPRINT

The Indian laboratory market is consolidating and spreading its wings to neighboring countries. The laboratories with branches outside India are Dr Lal Pathlabs (laboratories/collection centers: Saudi Arabia, Sri Lanka, Kuwait, Nepal, and Bangladesh), Super Religare Laboratories (which through its network of reference laboratories within and outside India, network laboratories, and collection centers provides routine and specialized testing services to customers outside India, including leading hospital chains in the United Arab Emirates, Oman, Qatar, Kuwait, Bahrain, Sri Lanka, Bangladesh, Nepal, the Maldives, Tanzania, and Zambia), and Metropolis Labs (Africa, Sri Lanka, and United Arab Emirates).

LOGISTICS

Logistics is a necessary competency for an international reference laboratory. It is vital to develop a courier and shipping system infrastructure that transports fragile biological specimens from doctor's offices and hospitals from around the world to international central laboratory facilities for rapid and accurate processing.[12] The ability to prepare, organize, and manage the delivery of prevalidated sample collection kits with unique bar-coded patient identification labels and to ensure that sufficient supplies are on hand with the client is the first part of the process. In addition, SOPs and training are provided to each client during an on-boarding process to ensure complete and proper handling, packaging, and delivery of the specimens. Biological research materials shipped domestically and internationally (import and export) are subject to a number of local, state, federal, and international regulations. All infectious and noninfectious human biological-based materials are packaged and handled by International Air Transport Association trained and certified individuals using project-specific packaging, labeling, marking, and documentation that comply with United Nations regulation 6.2 for transport of dangerous goods. Most countries have regulatory differences, and knowledge of country-specific regulations for transportation of samples to and from a country is an important aspect of intercountry logistics of patient samples.

LONG-TERM SPECIMEN STORAGE AND ACCESSIONING FACILITIES

Where required, international reference laboratories provide long-term storage with continuous monitoring of storage temperature with the ability to access and accurately pull in and pull out samples. This ability is an especially important service for CTs. Storage conditions may vary from ambient (20°C to 25°C), to refrigerated (2°C to 8°C), to frozen (−20°C to −80°C) to cryopreservation (−196°C). Calibrated temperature monitoring devices with capabilities of around-the-clock monitoring and the ability to sound alarms and send a text message to the process owner in case of temperature outliers are essential and play a vital role in the monitoring of specimens stored in these systems.

CHALLENGES SPECIFIC TO REFERENCE LABORATORIES IN INDIA
Power Supply

Constant good quality power supply in India is a scarce resource. For high-end laboratories it becomes vital to have an online uninterrupted power supply–based system backed up by diesel generators to ensure trouble-free operations.

Water Supply

Water supply is often augmented by ground water sources, and it becomes imperative to control the pH and mineral content of water input for laboratory work. Water from the primary source needs an initial water filtration step followed downstream by a reverse osmosis water plant for general use. For specific cases this process is followed downstream by a deionizer system to provide deionized water. Millipore-based systems form the final layer of equipment ensuring high-quality water is supplied to the analysers.

Equipment and Support

Liaison with vendors and adequate engineering support become vital when new instruments and technologies are imported into the country. The long lead time required for procuring yearly licenses for import of reagents necessitates adequate inventory levels of reagents.

Export and Import of Time-Sensitive Clinical Samples

Export and import of time-sensitive clinical samples is an important factor that will determine future growth of this industry. Emergence of centers of excellence in this field will require regulatory support enabling smooth movement of time-sensitive, temperature-controlled international shipments to and from the country. This attainment will ensure control of preanalytical variables and output of reliable reports.

Other Challenges

Other Challenges include sustainable funding, competition from emerging foreign destinations in southeast Asia, good quality and cost-effective physical infrastructure, development of technical and operational capabilities, forging alliances to enable a sustainable sample flow, the financial strength to sustain early operations, and the ability to innovate and adapt to local market conditions.

ADVANTAGES FOR INDIA
Laboratory Process Outsourcing

Several Indian laboratories are now stepping out gingerly into the international arena. As an English speaking country with availability of high numbers of educated young people, laboratory capability and capacity, and good laboratory practices, establishment of international reference laboratories with a view to get large quantities of specimens into India for high volume low cost testing with high revenue yield can be an interesting business proposition. Indian Council of Medical Research has recently outlined a methodology for the same; however, it requires more input from the industry to make it more industry-friendly.

Continuous Improvement, Lean and Six Sigma

Lean and Six Sigma are the new tools available for developing efficient laboratories. The partnership of Six Sigma and best practices will help develop an alignment driving corporate-wide standardization and world-class performance. Combining the expertise of technical knowledge with a process-focused mindset puts in place effective teams to drive change and excellence in the business.

SUMMARY

International reference laboratories are here in India. They offer best of class in terms of QMS, GLP, LIMS, EDC, TMS, and Lean and Six Sigma–driven operations. They are a part of global clinical laboratory networks that aim to provide harmonized testing services across the globe primarily for the pharmaceutical industry. This network results in the best of global practices and standards being implemented and will enhance the quality of health care in India. Esoteric testing, personalized medicine, and companion diagnostics offered by international reference laboratories in India will enhance health care, and when locally set up will become cost-effective and will provide competitive centers for testing of samples sourced from around the globe. Laboratory business process outsourcing as a business wave may become possible and have high synergy with medical tourism once regulatory barriers are removed and other synergistic processes combine to enable free flow of samples and data across continents.

REFERENCES

1. Kirk CJ, Shult PA. Developing laboratory networks: a practical guide and application. Public Health Rep 2010;125(Suppl 2):102–9.
2. Edwards S. International reference laboratory networks: challenges and benefits. Dev Biol (Basel) 2007;128:97–102.
3. 10 reasons why one should do business in India. Rediff Business. Available at: http://www.rediff.com/business/slide-show/slide-show-1-10-reasons-why-one-should-do-business-in-india/20110909.htm. Accessed December, 2011.
4. Eureofins. Available at: http://www.eurofins.com/pharma-services/pharma-services/pharma-central-laboratory/about-us/company-history.aspx. Accessed May 25, 2012.
5. Global central laboratories. ICON. Available at: http://www.iconplc.com/__uuid/dcb31c1e-916b-4164-8e4b-02558370b857/. Accessed December, 2011.
6. LabCorp. Wikipedia. Available at: http://en.wikipedia.org/wiki/Laboratory_Corporation_of_America_Holdings. Accessed December, 2011.
7. Quest Diagnostics. Available at: http://questdiagnostics.com/home/about/brands.html. Accessed December, 2011.
8. About us. Quest Diagnostics. Available at: http://www.questdiagnostics.in/about-quest-diagnostics.aspx. Accessed December, 2011.
9. Quintiles. Wikipedia. Available at: http://en.wikipedia.org/wiki/Quintiles. Accessed December, 2011.
10. Laboratory information management system. Wikipedia. Available at: http://en.wikipedia.org/wiki/Laboratory_information_management_system. Accessed December, 2011.
11. White paper: SOP Management as a Compliance Tool in FDA and ISO Environments. At: Document control software systems. Master Control Compliance Accelerated. Available at: http://www.mastercontrol.com/document-control-software/. Accessed April 23, 2012.
12. Eudaric A. Managing clinical logistics for clinical trials. Parexel. Available at: www.parexel.com/index.php/download_file/view/69/. Accessed December, 2011.

Index

Note: Page numbers of article titles are in **boldface** type.

Clin Lab Med 32 (2012) 341–352
http://dx.doi.org/10.1016/S0272-2712(12)00067-4
0272-2712/12/$ – see front matter © 2012 Elsevier Inc. All rights reserved.

labmed.theclinics.com

Moving?

Make sure your subscription moves with you!

To notify us of your new address, find your **Clinics Account Number** (located on your mailing label above your name), and contact customer service at:

Email: journalscustomerservice-usa@elsevier.com

800-654-2452 (subscribers in the U.S. & Canada)
314-447-8871 (subscribers outside of the U.S. & Canada)

Fax number: 314-447-8029

Elsevier Health Sciences Division
Subscription Customer Service
3251 Riverport Lane
Maryland Heights, MO 63043

*To ensure uninterrupted delivery of your subscription, please notify us at least 4 weeks in advance of move.

Printed and bound by CPI Group (UK) Ltd, Croydon, CR0 4YY

03/10/2024

01040461-0020